SIXTH EDITION

Law, Liability, & Ethics

for Medical Office Professionals

SIXTH EDITION

Law, Liability, & Ethics

for Medical Office Professionals

Myrtle Flight
J.D., M.Ed., CMA (AAMA)

Wendy Mia Pardew, Esq.

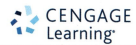

CENGAGE
Learning®

Australia • Brazil • Mexico • Singapore • United Kingdom • United States

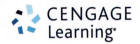
CENGAGE
Learning®

Law, Liability, and Ethics for Medical Office Professionals, **Sixth Edition**
Myrtle Flight, Wendy Mia Pardew

SVP, GM Skills & Global Product Management:
Jonathan Lau

Product Director: Matthew Seeley

Product Team Manager: Stephen Smith

Senior Director, Development:
Marah Bellegarde

Senior Product Development Manager:
Juliet Steiner

Content Developer: Kaitlin Schlicht

Product Assistant: Mark Turner

Vice President, Marketing Services:
Jennifer Ann Baker

Marketing Manager: Jonathan Sheehan

Senior Content Project Manager: Thomas
Heffernan

Art Director: Angela Sheehan

Cover image: iStock.com/Thomas_EyeDesign

For product information and technology assistance, contact us at
Cengage Learning Customer & Sales Support, 1-800-354-9706

For permission to use material from this text or product,
submit all requests online at **www.cengage.com/permissions.**
Further permissions questions can be e-mailed to
permissionrequest@cengage.com

Library of Congress Control Number: 2017935644

ISBN: 978-1-305-97272-8

Cengage Learning
20 Channel Center Street
Boston, MA 02210
USA

Cengage Learning is a leading provider of customized learning solutions
with employees residing in nearly 40 different countries and sales in more
than 125 countries around the world. Find your local representative at
www.cengage.com.

Cengage Learning products are represented in Canada by
Nelson Education, Ltd.

To learn more about Cengage Learning, visit **www.cengage.com**

Purchase any of our products at your local college store or at our preferred
online store **www.cengagebrain.com**

Notice to the Reader

Printed in the United States of America
Print Number: 01   Print Year: 2017

Dedication

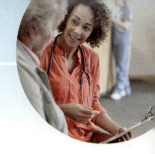

I dedicate the sixth edition of *Law, Liability, and Ethics for Medical Office Professionals* to Myrtle Flight, who conceived of and authored the first five editions of this gem of a text. Her vision was light years ahead of the pack, and the medical profession is better because of her. Ms. Flight's path to authoring this book is inspiring.

Wendy Mia Pardew

HISTORY OF THIS TEXT

Approximately thirty years ago, the seed for this book was planted by Sister Winifred Kelley at Aquinas Junior College in Milton, Massachusetts. I was struggling to teach medical assistants office procedures with a limited text, while Sister Winifred was struggling to teach medical assistants law and ethics without text. She was adamant that the students learn about the interaction of law and medicine. With the exception of a few articles in **Medical Economics** and a couple of drug companies' pamphlets on upcoming medical malpractice crises, there was little material available geared to the medical office assistant.

At the time, Dr. Jules Ribin of Canton, Massachusetts, provided us with his medical periodicals, which we clipped and cut in our search to develop a resource file of relevant case material. A few years later, on a trip to New York, I purchased the book **Medical Malpractice Law**, by Angela Roddy Holder, from a secondhand bookstore; this provided at least one factual pattern for each legal point. At this stage, the complexities of substantive law, coupled with ignorance of procedural matters, yielded nothing but confusion.

The experience of being involved in a labor lawsuit (sex discrimination in promotion) further developed my interest in law, and the professionalism of Alan McDonald, the attorney who successfully represented me in the case, challenged my stereo-type of lawyers. I applied and was accepted in 1979 to the New England School of Law evening program, graduated in 1983, passed the Massachusetts Bar in 1984, and have been a sole practitioner since November 5, 1985. While I was in law school, Professor Jonathan Brant, now Judge Brant, allowed me to independently research the materials fundamental to the chapters on law. My interest in ethics developed at a later date.

Myrtle R. Flight

Contents

Preface xiii
Acknowledgments xix

1 The Big Business of Health Care and You 1

2 Laws and Regulations You Will Encounter 23

3   From the Constitution to the Courtroom   51

4   Criminal Acts and Intentional Torts   73

5   What Makes a Contract   111

6 Medical Malpractice and Other Lawsuits   131

7 The Health Record   169

8 Introduction to Ethics   193

12 Death and Dying   275

Preface

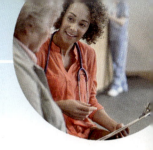

As part of the frontline of health care, medical office professionals have a critical need to understand medical law and ethics. This text is designed specifically with them in mind, to help them excel in an environment rife with legal and ethical issues, and to educate in a way that helps minimize the risk of lawsuits by discussing the concepts of standard of care, scope of employment, criminal and civil acts, contracts, negligence, health care ethics, and more. This text has been updated to reflect new health care regulations and technology, and it will prepare future medical office professionals for the changing health care environment. The sixth edition also features a contemporary voice that will resonate with students. The spectrum and depth of topics contained in this text makes it valuable as a resource that would be wise to keep handy long after graduation.

The issues discussed in this text occur in the real world. As a result, actual legal decisions and real-life anecdotes illustrate concepts and enhance understanding. The underlying concept coupled with the cases and anecdotes ensure readers can understand, digest, and apply the material, while also sparking interest and engagement.

This sixth edition reflects the numerous changes in health care regulations. Patients' health care needs will continue to expand. And just as methods of treatment will change, methods of health care delivery and compensation will also change. The law strives to keep pace with the new issues raised due to new maladies, treatments, technology, and regulations. This text serves as an invaluable resource for medical office professionals working in the center of this exciting and often challenging time of change.

Organization of the Text

The sixth edition is designed to cover the most common legal and ethical issues. Chapters start by exploring the business of health care and the legal system in general (Chapters 1–4) and then move through legal topics students need to know, such as standard of care, employment laws, criminal and tortious acts, contractual issues, negligence, medical malpractice, and more (Chapters 5–7). The conversation then turns to ethics, presenting the basics of health care ethics, and moving on to discussions of the allocation of scarce resources, medical research, reproductive issues, and end-of-life issues (Chapters 8–12). Each chapter is designed in a similar fashion: first providing student focus through Objectives and Key Terms; then presenting concepts coupled with relevant legal cases and news stories; and ending with a summary and activities for students to apply what they have learned:

Features

The key features in this text are designed to support learning and show real-world context of chapter concepts. The following is a brief description of each feature:

- **Quotes:** Relevant and thought-provoking quotes appear at the start of each chapter and throughout the text.
- **Objectives:** Each chapter begins with a list of objectives to focus student attention on what they need to learn.
- **Key Terms:** A list of key terms appears at the start of each chapter, and each key term is presented in boldface and defined in the margin of the text where the term first appears in the chapter.
- **News Stories:** Timely examples of legal and ethical health care dilemmas in the news illustrate chapter concepts and promote engaging discussions.
- **Legal Case Studies:** Summaries of actual legal cases highlight the legal issues and actions most prevalent in health care today.
- **Summary:** A bulleted list of key concepts serves as an at-a-glance study tool.
- **Suggested Activities:** Students can complete a list of additional activities to further engage with the chapter material through research, role play, field trips, and other exercises.
- **Study Questions:** These questions quiz students on their ability to understand and apply key chapter concepts.
- **Case for Discussion:** Real and fictional court cases allow students to practice applying what they have learned.

New to This Edition

The sixth edition seeks to make health care law and ethics accessible, interesting, and relevant for students. As such, chapters have been reorganized to build on content from preceding chapters to deliver a clearer, deeper picture of legal realities in modern health care, and updated content has been added. New content reflects recent legislation, including the Affordable Care Act (ACA), telemedicine, and euthanasia, among other critical topics. In addition, new legal cases and news stories have been added throughout the text to address some of the most recent dilemmas in medical offices and hospitals throughout the United States. To assist with comprehension, summaries at the end of each chapter have been revised and are now presented as a bulleted list to help readers understand core chapter content at-a-glance. And throughout the sixth edition there is a new, contemporary voice that is sure to resonate with students.

In addition to the changes outlined above, a chapter-by-chapter summary of major content updates is included below:

Chapter 1—The Big Business of Health Care and You

- New content on locum tenens
- New content on the patient bill of rights and how it relates to a patient's choice of, consent for, and refusal of treatment
- New and updated explanations of health care delivery and compensation systems, including MCO, HMO, PPO, and ACO
- New and updated information about telemedicine describing its applications and a real-life "doctor on demand" anecdote

Chapter 2—Laws and Regulations You Will Encounter

- New information on the Health Information Technology for Economic and Clinical Health Act (HITECH)
- New information on Genetic Information Nondiscrimination Act (GINA)
- New and updated explanation of the Lilly Ledbetter Fair Pay Act of 2009

Chapter 3—From the Constitution to the Courtroom

- New information on the U.S. Constitution, the supremacy clause, enumerated powers, and the interstate commerce clause
- New information on the executive, congressional, and judiciary branches of government
- New information on Federalism and its intersection with health care's regulation

Chapter 4—Criminal Acts and Intentional Torts

- Additional information about child abuse, elder abuse, domestic violence, and sexual assault
- New information on reporting illegal activity in the health care setting following proper protocol
- New information on completing an incident report related to an error in patient care

Chapter 5—What Makes a Contract

- Additional information about the elements of a contract

Chapter 6—Medical Malpractice and Other Lawsuits
- Additional information about statute of limitations

Chapter 7—The Health Record
- New information on electronic health records
- New information on HITECH and the "meaningful use" of electronic health records
- Additional information on HIPAA and a HIPAA-related activity

Chapter 8—Introduction to Ethics
- Minor content updates and reorganization include an updated news story illustrating the interplay of medical technology and ethics

Chapter 9—Laws and Ethics of Patient Confidentiality
- Additional information on HIPAA and protected health information (PHI)
- New information about the high-profile patient

Chapter 10—Professional Ethics and the Living
- New information about AAMA's Medical Assisting Code of Ethics and AMT's Standards of Practice and related activity
- New information on medical tourism
- Additional information about the Tuskegee Study

Chapter 11—Birth and the Beginning of Life
- New information about ethical issues associated with in vitro fertilization, embryos, and embryonic stem cells

Chapter 12—Death and Dying
- New information about the Uniform Determination of Death Act (UDDA)
- Additional information about the Patient Self-Determination Act (PSDA)
- Additional information about advance directives
- New information about terminally ill patients and euthanasia

Learning Package for the Student

MindTap
(Printed Access Code, 2 Semesters, ISBN 978-1-337-09011-7)

(Instant Access Code, 2 Semesters, ISBN 978-1-305-97278-0)

(Printed Access Code, 4 Semesters, ISBN 978-1-337-09008-7)

(Instant Access Code, 4 Semesters, ISBN 978-1-337-09007-0)

MindTap is a fully online, interactive learning experience built upon authoritative Cengage Learning content. By combining readings, multimedia, activities, and assessments into a singular learning path, MindTap elevates learning by providing real-world application to better engage students. Instructors customize the learning path by selecting Cengage Learning resources and adding their own content via apps that integrate into the MindTap framework seamlessly with many learning management systems.

This MindTap includes the following:

- An interactive eBook with highlighting, note-taking, and more
- Polling
- Video case studies
- Computer-graded activities and exercises
- Easy submission tools for instructor-graded exercises
- Flashcards for practicing chapter terms

To learn more, visit www.cengage.com/mindtap.

Teaching Package for the Instructor

Instructor Companion Web Site

(ISBN 978-1-305-97274-2)

Spend less time planning and more time teaching with Cengage's Instructor Companion Web site to accompany *Law, Liability, and Ethics for Medical Office Professionals, sixth edition.* As an instructor, you will have access to all of your resources online, anywhere and at any time. All instructor resources can be accessed by going to www.cengage.com/login to create a unique user login. The password-protected instructor resources include the following:

- An electronic Instructor's Manual that is packed with everything an instructor needs to be effective and efficient in the classroom. The Instructor's Manual includes answer keys to the Study Questions and Cases for Discussion from the text, as well as a sample syllabus.
- Customizable PowerPoints® for each chapter
- Cengage Learning Testing Powered by Cognero, which is a flexible, online system that allows you to:
  - Author, edit, and manage test bank content from multiple Cengage Learning solutions
  - Create multiple test versions in an instant
  - Deliver tests from your LMS, your classroom or wherever you want

Acknowledgments

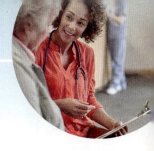

Several people deserve acknowledgment, praise, and thanks: Stephen Smith, for inviting me to take on this rewarding project and for his boundless professionalism; Kaitlin Schlicht, for patiently, precisely, and perfectly guiding me through the process; Wendy Berninger, for being the quintessential wordsmithing mentor for almost three decades; Albany Law School's Professor Dale Moore for igniting my interest in health care and tort law more than two decades ago; and many others for their support and for enduring the many times I had to say, "I can't, I am writing."

I am also indebted to the sixth edition reviewers listed below whose experience and willingness to contribute helped make this edition one we can all be proud of.

Wendy Mia Pardew

REVIEWERS

Chantelle Blakesley-Boddie, BS, CMA (AAMA)
Lake Washington Institute of Technology
Kirkland, WA

Estelle Coffino, MPA, RRT, CPFT, CCMA
Program Director, Chairperson and Associate Professor, Allied Health
College of Westchester
White Plain, NY

Jennifer Helfrich, HFA, MSM, RMA (AMT), AHI
Online College Instructor
Grantham University
Evansville, IN

Kathy Locke
Instructor
Spartanburg Community College
Spartanburg, SC

Michelle R. McClatchey, BS, CMRS
Program Chair
Westwood College—CHR
Calumet City, IL

Sandra Metcalf
Professor
Grayson College
Denison, TX

Cheryl A. Miller, MBA/HCM
Program Director / Assistant Professor
Westmoreland County Community College
Youngwood, PA

Pamela Sanborn, CMA (AAMA), M.Ed
Medical Assisting Program Director
Cabrillo College
Aptos, CA

Lara Skaggs, MA
State Program Manager / Health Careers Education
Oklahoma Department of Career and Technology Education
Stillwater, OK

Carol Turner, HIPAA Compliance Officer, NCICS, Certified Medicaid Representative, CCDI
Program Director / Faculty of Medical Office Technology
Lamar State College—Orange
Orange, TX

Marilyn M. Turner, RN, CMA (AAMA)
Medical Assisting Program Director
Ogeechee Technical College
Statesboro, GA

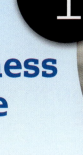

1

The Big Business of Health Care and You

 Wherever the art of medicine is loved, there is also a love of humanity.

Hippocrates

OBJECTIVES

After reading this chapter, you should be able to:

1. Recognize the importance of the business aspect of the health care industry.
2. Recognize the importance of your role on the frontlines of the health care industry.
3. Identify the different types of legal entities.
4. Identify the many types of managed care delivery systems.
5. Explain the benefits of telemedicine.

BUILDING YOUR LEGAL VOCABULARY

Agent	Investment
Bylaws	Joint venture
Capitation	Legal entity
Certification	Negligence
Conglomerate	Negotiated fee schedules
Directors	Notice
Dividends	Officers
Fee-for-service	Per capita payment

(continues)

Reasonable person

Registration

Respondeat superior

Shares

Stockholders

Utilization review

Vicariously liable

INTRODUCTION TO THE BUSINESS OF HEALTH CARE

Today's health care industry looks nothing like it did when you were born. Law that requires all Americans to have health insurance, technological advances, medical malpractice lawsuits, and changes to health care delivery and compensation systems, among others, have all contributed to the health care industry becoming big business. In 2015, the health care industry accounted for almost 18 percent of all goods and services produced in the United States.

As a medical office professional, you will be on the frontlines of this multi-trillion-dollar industry. How you perform on the frontline matters. You will be entrusted with tasks and information that, in the most extreme situation, could mean the difference between life and death. The number of medical malpractice lawsuits continues to rise, and the business of health care continues to become increasingly complex. Now more than ever, frontline health care professionals need to be familiar with risks that can result in a lawsuit or other unwanted action.

The health care industry has many competing interests as the various parties work to achieve their objectives. Physicians, nurses, hospital employees, and others employed in the field look to balance maximum personal financial gain through the health care services they provide while providing quality health care and complying with laws, regulations, and health insurance company protocols. The health insurance companies seek to reduce costs and maximize profits. Employers want to reduce the cost of the health insurance they provide to their employees. The government wants to protect its citizens and manage health care costs. And, patients want the best possible care at the lowest possible price. These competing interests form the framework of the big business of the health care industry.

The industry relies upon competition and regulation to control health care costs. Competition in business has led employers, governments, and health insurance companies to seek control of escalating costs through regulation. Health insurance companies, eager to gain market share, develop new products intended to help manage ever-increasing health care costs. This competitive approach has given rise to managed care organizations (MCOs), which are health care delivery and compensation systems that are different from the traditional pay-for-fee service.

A solid and well-rounded understanding of the health care business will ensure you are the best professional possible while on the frontlines. The framework of the health care business includes business structures and how health care is delivered and compensated.

THE FRONTLINE IS YOU

A patient's first interaction at a health care facility is usually with a frontline professional such as you. It is the frontline professionals who communicate most frequently with patients. What you know and how you conduct yourself can influence a patient's experience. The health care industry is a complex maze of laws, regulations, protocols, and interactions that you will want to understand. To be the best professional you can be, a well-rounded understanding of the health care industry is a must. For your patients, "the best professional" means providing the most professional, efficient, and effective service for them that you can. For your employer, it means representing your employer in a professional manner, as well as ensuring you do all that you can to prevent complaints, lawsuits, regulatory violations, mistakes, and any other act that creates risk for you, your patient, or your employer.

THE IMPORTANCE OF LEGAL KNOWLEDGE

Medical malpractice, licensing and regulations, employment law, and corporate mergers are just some of the legal issues that arise in the health care industry. When you understand the nature and scope of these issues and how they arise and affect a business, you are in a much better place to avoid lawsuits and other risks for yourself and for your employer. That is the purpose of this text: to provide you with the basics of law so that you will recognize situations that may lead to an unwanted legal action and know what to do when you see such situations.

Medical office professionals participate in many aspects of the delivery of health care. They are held to a higher standard of care than laypersons who do not have your special knowledge and training. Other professionals, such as physicians and nurses, are held to the standard of care established by state law, their state licensing organizations, and **registration** boards at the national or state level. **Certification** means that the individual has attained the levels of education and training necessary to meet minimum qualifications required by the certifying agency.

Part of being a medical office professional includes knowing the scope within which you can practice. Most medical office employees are not licensed to practice medicine and must carry out their responsibilities without making medical decisions or acting outside their area of expertise.

registration fulfilling administrative qualifications for a licensed profession; may require special testing or training or other vetting

certification a record of being qualified to perform certain acts after passing an examination given by an accredited professional organization

Personal Protection

By understanding basic principles of the law, you can protect yourself from needless litigation and loss of reputation, personal wealth, or earning power. This text should help you develop thought patterns that can help you avoid legal pitfalls. For example:

A young woman, nineteen years of age, who had just completed an accredited medical assisting course, found her first job with a specialist in internal medicine. Seventy-five to one hundred individuals walked daily by her desk to meet with the physician. Approximately twenty-five were scheduled in her appointment manual.

One afternoon the police came, and she was arrested along with the physician. The physician was indicted on several counts of illegal narcotic distribution, and she was indicted as a conspirator. Her salary stopped. The profession for which she had trained was no longer a potential source of employment, and she was faced with the reality of having to defend herself in a court of law.

The case took three years to go through the legal system. The physician was convicted of twenty counts of illegal distribution of narcotics; the charges against her were dismissed without trial. She was never proven innocent or guilty.

Now she is twenty-two years of age, tainted by her employment record, and unable to find a job in a physician's office or any other health care facility in the area. Potential employers will not hire her for fear that she might have been involved in illegal narcotics distribution and that their offices might, therefore, become suspect of the same by her presence.

Author Myrtle Flight's Experience

As a medical office professional, you will want to be aware of the nature of your employment. In addition, you must remember that you work in a field that is highly regulated by federal and state legislation. Ignorance of a law or a regulation does not excuse a medical office professional's violation. You are a professional and expected to know the laws and regulations that govern your profession.

Although the professional status of medical assistants has increased during the past few years, many state laws and regulations, including medical practice acts and nursing practice acts, either do not acknowledge the existence of the medical assisting profession or do not authorize the delegation of administrative and clinical duties to medical assistants.

As members of society, we are all expected to conduct ourselves in a responsible manner that will not cause harm. This is known legally as holding an individual to a **reasonable person** standard of care. Physicians, nurses, and other health care professionals are held to a higher standard of care than what is demanded under the reasonable person standard of care. Violations of this professional standard of care are the basis of medical malpractice lawsuits, certificate or license revocations, and, in extreme cases, criminal charges.

Locum tenens is used to describe physicians, nurses, and physician assistants who are temporarily performing the duties of another. Physicians who are practicing "locum tenens," which is Latin for "to hold the place of," are held to the same standard of care as other physicians.

> " "
>
> Currently, more than 60 percent of medical assistants work in physicians' offices, 15 percent work in hospitals, 10 percent work in other healthcare offices and 7 percent work at outpatient care offices. In 2016, there were more than 600,000 medical assistants in the United States. That number is projected to grow by almost 25 percent by 2020. The average growth rate for all occupations is 7 percent.
>
> Bureau of Labor Statistics, U.S. Department of Labor. (2015). *Occupational outlook handbook, 2016–17 edition. Medical assistants.* Retrieved from http://www.bls.gov/ooh/healthcare/medical-assistants.htm

For medical assistants, the required standard of care is difficult to predict. For physicians and nurses, professional guidelines for accepted practices are more clearly defined. When a physician allows a medical assistant to perform certain functions, that is, to act as the physician's agent, the delegation of responsibility is based on the premise that the assistant can perform the functions as well as the physician, or as well as the nurse if the procedure is usually performed by a nurse. It also follows that, in those situations, the assistant may be held to the same standard of care as the physician or nurse.

In a 1986 case, *Riff v. Morgan Pharmacy*, it was held that each member of the health care team "has a duty to be, to a limited extent, his brother's keeper." The plaintiff was given a prescription for Cafergot suppositories with instructions for using the medication (one every four hours), but neither the prescribing physician nor the dispensing pharmacist added the admonition that no more than two should be used per headache and that no more than five should be used per week. The warning was included in the product's package literature and was well known to health care professionals. The plaintiff, who did not read the product's literature, used the medication as directed and suffered toxic effects.

reasonable person a prudent person whose behavior would be considered appropriate under the circumstances

Fallibility is a condition of human existence. Physicians, like other mortals, will, from time to time, err through ignorance or inadvertence. An error in the practice of medicine can be fatal, and so it is reasonable that the medical community—including physicians, pharmacists, anesthesiologists, nurses, and support staff—have established professional standards that require vigilance not only with respect to primary functions, but also regarding the acts and omissions of the other professionals and support personnel in the health care team.

Riff v. Morgan Pharmacy, 508 A.2d 1247 (Pa. 1986)

As medical office procedures became more sophisticated and complex, the modern health care office staff came into being. In most situations, nurses, licensed technicians, and medical office receptionists share office responsibilities. In other practices, a "hybrid" health care professional known as a medical assistant serves as a combination nurse-receptionist-technician. The scope of knowledge required and the amount of responsibility carried by this employee is extensive.

Medical office professionals are the link between the patient and the physician when arranging office visits, laboratory tests, therapeutic appointments, and hospital admissions. They are crucial in the development of good relations between the patient and the physician. It is important that medical office professionals understand the legal issues involved with providing health care and the importance of good patient relations. Positive patient interactions minimize the nonmedical and nonlegal variables involved in malpractice and may prevent a legitimate complaint from developing into a full-blown lawsuit.

Patient Protection

Patients trust that they are being treated by qualified health care professionals. State licensure laws protect patients by defining the education and experience required to perform certain procedures. A license indicates that the holder has the basic minimum qualifications required by the state for that occupation. License requirements also control employers by setting standards for hiring that ultimately protect patients. Licenses are granted by licensing boards, which also have the power to revoke the licenses. Although the grounds for revocation may vary slightly from state to state, they always include unprofessional conduct, substance abuse, fraud in connection with examination or application for a license, alcoholism, conviction of a felony, and mental incapacity.

Often medical office professionals are closer to the patients and more sensitive to their needs than are physicians. The requirements of privacy and respect for the confidential relationship between patient and physician must be met: Privacy and confidentiality have ethical and legal bases. Permission to touch and the right to perform certain procedures are interwoven with state medical practice acts.

The Health Insurance Portability and Accountability Act (HIPAA), which is further discussed in Chapter 2, is a federal law requiring every health plan and provider to maintain "reasonable and appropriate" safeguards to ensure the confidentiality of patient health information.

Many patients refer to everyone who works in a physician's office as a nurse, regardless of whether the individual is a registered nurse, licensed practical nurse, nurse's aide, medical technician, certified medical assistant, or receptionist. Today, many unlicensed personnel are assuming and performing tasks formerly done by an office nurse. These unlicensed employees may have been trained through a variety of disciplines.

In addition to protecting the patient, the law also operates to protect the public as a whole. Certain health matters must be reported by physicians in every state, including births and deaths, venereal and other communicable diseases, injuries resulting from violence such as stab and gunshot wounds, child and elder abuse, blindness, immunological proceedings, requests for plastic surgery to change a person's fingerprints, and cases of industrial poisoning, among others.

Patient Bill of Rights Health care facilities and providers have creeds entitled "Patient Bill of Rights," which establish standards, including ethical standards, for patient care. A Patient Bill of Rights is not always required by law, so each health care facility or provider has a version that best suits its needs. There may be as many versions of a Patient Bill of Rights as there are health care facilities and providers. A Patient Bill of Rights conveys patients' legal and ethical rights and includes acknowledgment of a patient's right to choose treatment, to consent to treatment, and to refuse treatment, among others. The following is a list of rights that may be included in the Patient Bill of Rights:

- To be treated with courtesy and respect in an environment free from discrimination.
- To be treated confidentially, with access to your records limited to those involved in your care or otherwise authorized by you.
- To be informed by your health care provider about your diagnosis, scheduled course of treatment, alternative treatment, risks, and prognosis.
- To use your own financial resources to pay for the care of your choice.
- To refuse medical treatment, even if your physician recommends it.
- To create Advance Directives and have your physician(s) or hospital staff provide care that is consistent with these directives.

- To be informed about the outcomes of care, treatment, and services that have been provided, including unanticipated outcomes.
- To be provided an estimate of charges for medical care, a reasonably clear itemized bill, and, if needed, an explanation of the charges.
- To receive prompt and reasonable responses to questions and requests.
- To know what patient services are available, including whether an interpreter is available if you do not speak English.
- To be informed if medical treatment is for experimental research and to give your consent or refusal to participate.

Physician Protection

vicariously liable legally obligated for the acts of others

respondeat superior legal theory that requires an employer be responsible (vicariously liable) for the behavior of an employee working within the scope of employment

Physicians and corporate employers are liable for their own conduct, as well as being **vicariously liable** for their employees' conduct while working within the scope of their employment. In the employment setting, this is known as **respondeat superior**, which is Latin for "let the master answer." It is sometimes difficult to determine whether an employee is acting within the scope of employment. The test is whether the employee's behavior serves the interest of the employer or furthers the employer's business. For example, a physician tells a medical assistant to give a patient an injection of penicillin and asks the nurse to prepare the syringe. The physician leaves the examining room. The nurse, without being directed to do so, gives the patient the injection but neglects to tell the patient what is being injected or ask if the patient is allergic to penicillin. The patient suffers a severe allergic reaction. The physician is vicariously liable under the doctrine of respondeat superior for the **negligence** of the nurse if the patient is injured and sues. This is because the nurse has acted as the physician's **agent** and the nurse was subject to control and direction of the physician. Basically, when one person acts on another's behalf, the person for whom the action was taken—even if it was the wrong thing to do—is responsible for the acts of that person.

negligence failure to act with reasonable and prudent care given the circumstances

agent one who has authority to act on behalf of another

THE BUSINESS STRUCTURE: LEGAL ENTITIES

conglomerate a corporation diversifying operations by acquiring varied enterprises

legal entity an individual or organization that has legal capacity to contract, incur and pay debts, and sue and be sued

A medical practice can be a solo practitioner operating from a single office, or it may be a group of physicians who have agreed to share the costs and sometimes the liability of a group practice with several office locations. It may be a corporation, or a **conglomerate** controlling hospitals or other health care facilities. Each medical practice has an underlying **legal entity** that governs matters such as ownership, profit distribution, liability, taxes, and control, among others. State, county, or city law governs the structure and requirements. Legal entities include sole proprietorships, partnerships, limited liability companies, professional associations, limited liability partnerships (LLPs), and corporations.

Any legal entity can choose to operate and hold itself out to the public under a name that is different than its registered name. The alternate name is referred to as a DBA, short for "doing business as." Companies that operate as a DBA (sometimes referred to as a trade name, a fictitious name, or an assumed name) usually have to file state or local registrations that identify the people or legal entity that is responsible for the DBA. The main purpose for these filings is to let others know with whom they are doing business.

Sole Proprietorship

A sole proprietorship is a legal entity that requires no state filing to create it. A sole proprietorship is simply one person operating a business for profit. That person has unlimited personal liability for the business. A sole proprietor can have employees, including other physicians. The person who chooses this business structure does so for two main reasons. First, individual ownership is the simplest and most basic business structure and appeals to a person who wants to be independent and free from the laws that govern other legal entities. Second, any financial rewards from the practice are for the owner and do not have to be shared with anyone else. However, any losses are also the owner's.

A sole proprietorship should not be confused with a solo practice, which is a type of medical practice where the practice includes just one physician. A solo practice can be one of the many legal entities discussed in this chapter. Most solo practitioners choose legal entities other than a sole proprietorship for liability and tax reasons. In fact, all medical practice types, such as solo practices, group practices, and employed physician practices may choose their legal entity type.

Partnership

A partnership, sometimes called a "general partnership" (GP), is two or more people who combine their work, money, and talents to achieve a common goal. It is a more complicated form of legal entity than a sole proprietorship. A partnership is formed when two or more parties agree—in compliance with state and local law—to certain business aspects such as ownership, profit distribution, liability, taxes, and control. Many states require a document or registration that serves as **notice** to the public that the partnership members are doing business together. Unless the terms of the partnership provide otherwise, each partner has a right to participate in managing the business and making decisions.

A high degree of mutual trust and confidence must exist between partners. For example, if one partner's personal debts become so large

notice an announcement of pertinent information to those interested

they cannot be satisfied by his or her private assets, creditors may go after that partner's share of the business property, thereby threatening the partnership.

In conducting the affairs of a partnership, all partners are bound by the acts of the others. This affects them as individuals. If, for example, one partner places an order for equipment beyond the financial means of the partnership, the other partners are required to share payment of the bill, possibly by using their personal funds. A notable exception is an LLP. In such cases, personal assets can be protected. The partners can agree that liability extends no further than the partnership.

Limited Liability Companies

A limited liability company (LLC) is a legal entity, created by one or more individuals or other legal entities, to further a common goal and to create ground rules for matters such as ownership, profit distribution, liability, taxes, and control. Individuals who have an interest in an LLC are usually referred to as "members." Most states have laws that govern LLCs.

Business owners have increasingly used LLCs because they provide protection from being held personally liable and can be advantageous from a tax perspective. The word *limited* in the name suggests that some wrongful acts of the members or employees may not provide the protection from personal liability. LLCs also require less legal and accounting work to get started. In addition, members can decide among themselves who has authority to perform acts such as hiring or firing employees, contributing capital, and earning profits, among others.

Some states allow for certain professionals, such as physicians, lawyers, architects, and accountants, to form professional limited liability companies (PLLCs). A PLLC is very similar to a LLC, but the governing statutes dictate that the limits of liability may only be applied to certain aspects of the business, such as creditors. A PLLC limits the liability protection that certain professionals can expect. In a health care scenario, PLLCs do not allow physicians to limit their liability for patient wrongs, such as malpractice.

Corporations

A corporation is a legal entity created by one or more individuals to further a common goal and to make use of corporate tax and legal advantages. A corporation is formed in accordance with the state laws in which it is registered. State law usually requires that a corporation's name includes a corporate designation such as "Corporation," "Co.," "Corp.," or "Inc."

Much thought is often given to the corporate name. The corporation may use any name, provided it has not been taken by some other legal entity in the state or does not too closely resemble the name of an existing legal entity. Health care providers usually try to choose a name that will instantly indicate to the public the services they provide.

The life of a corporation does not end upon the death of its **officers**, **directors**, or **stockholders**. Even if all died in a common disaster, **shares** of the corporation would generally be passed on to the officers', directors', or stockholders' heirs. The corporation will not cease to exist until it is dissolved by the requisite legal process. This is true even in a corporation where only one individual holds all of the stock.

One of the most desirable features of a corporation is the protection given to investors. For example, if the corporation loses money and the debts become greater than the assets, the creditors may not collect from the individual owners, known as stockholders. Only the capital of the corporation is available for the payment of debts. It is important to remember that judgments resulting from lawsuits are indeed debts. The most an individual investor may lose is the amount of the original **investment**.

Management responsibility is in the hands of the corporation's board of directors. The number of directors is usually set in the **bylaws** of the corporation, which are drawn up and adopted at the first stockholders' meeting. Directors answer to the stockholders, who elect and can terminate them. A member of the board of directors is expected to be loyal to the corporation and its shareholders. It is improper for a director to have an interest in any business that competes with the corporation. Officers of a corporation include the president, vice president, treasurer, secretary, and any other officers the board of directors appoints. They are employees of the company and need not be stockholders. Profits of a corporation are distributed to stockholders as **dividends**.

Not-for-profit organizations may also be corporations; there are no shareholders and no dividends. Revenue in excess of expenses is reinvested in the organization. Members of the board are chosen by the board, usually after screening by a committee.

Similar to a PLLC, a professional corporation (PC) or a professional association (PA) are legal entities that are designed for business endeavors of professionals such as physicians, attorneys, architects, and accountants. They are both governed by state law.

HEALTH CARE DELIVERY AND COMPENSATION SYSTEMS

As cost management in health care rose to crisis levels, alternative delivery and compensation systems have largely replaced traditional health care business practices. In the past, a patient who felt unwell would decide when and whom to visit for health care. The patient would then pay a fee for the physician's service either directly or through an insurance company. The traditional **fee-for-service** payment system has shown that it

officers persons holding formal positions of trust in an organization, especially those involved in high levels of management

directors those elected and terminated by stockholders to manage a corporation

stockholders those who hold an interest (stock) in a corporation

shares units of stock giving the possessor part ownership in a corporation

investment expenditure of resources (money, effort, etc.) to secure income or profit

bylaws regulations adopted by a corporation or association to govern its internal affairs

dividends distributed profits of a corporation

fee-for-service basis of professional billing, either so much per hour or per identified procedure encourages increased costs and reduces the quality of care patients receive as compared to other health care delivery systems. Consequently, those with a stake in the matter (health insurance companies, government, employers, patients, and physicians) have developed alternative delivery systems that reward cost management, quality care, and efficiency.

Managed care organizations seeking to manage health care costs and improve health care contract with physicians and health care facilities to provide health care services for the MCOs' insured in accordance with certain requirements. The two longstanding forms of alternative delivery systems are health maintenance organizations (HMOs) and preferred provider organizations (PPOs). The Affordable Care Act of 2010 has resulted in the promotion of another primary MCO, the accountable care organization (ACO), as well as variations of all three. In addition, Medicare and Medicaid have experienced similar changes as the government seeks to contain costs and improve the quality of health care.

The Affordable Care Act

The Patient Protection and Affordable Care Act (PPACA), more commonly referred to as the Affordable Care Act (ACA), is relatively new. The ACA was signed into law on March 23, 2010, but many of its provisions did not take effect immediately. As a result, the government, employers, health care industry, and patients had time to prepare for the changes that the ACA requires. The ACA is expansive, and it touches on many subjects including:

- use of electronic medical records,
- prohibition of coverage denials based upon preexisting conditions,
- requirement that insurance companies offer all applicants of the same age and locality the same premium without consideration of most preexisting conditions or age,
- imposition of minimum standards for health insurance companies,
- requirement that, with very narrow exceptions, all Americans have some form of health insurance,
- provision of government subsidies for insurance premiums based upon financial considerations,
- introduction of state run health insurance exchanges that allow comparison shopping for health insurance policies,
- revisions to Medicaid eligibility,
- requirement that dependents can remain on their parents' health insurance until their 26th birthday,
- prohibition on canceling policies when policyholders become ill, and
- requirement that new health insurance plans must fully cover certain preventive treatment and medical tests, without charging co-payments or deductibles.

The ultimate goal of the ACA is to encourage health care that increases the quality and affordability of health insurance, lowers the uninsured rate by expanding public and private insurance coverage, and reduces the costs of health care. The ACA seeks to ensure that all have health care, and since its passage, the number of uninsured Americans has decreased significantly.

In the first quarter of 2016, the uninsured rate among all U.S. adults was 11.0%, down from 11.9% in the fourth quarter of 2015. This marks a record low since Gallup and Healthways began tracking the uninsured rate in 2008. The uninsured rate has declined 6.1 percentage points since the fourth quarter of 2013, which was right before the individual mandate provision of the Affordable Care Act took effect in early 2014 that required Americans to carry health insurance.

Marken, S. (2016). *U.S. uninsured rate at 11.0%, lowest in eight-year trend.* Retrieved from http://www.gallup.com/poll/190484/uninsured-rate-lowest-eight-year-trend.aspx

Managed Care Organizations

Managed care is a term used to describe a method of delivering and compensating health care with a pointed focus on lowering costs and improving quality. An MCO is simply an organization that provides managed health care. Managed care typically includes a wide spectrum of health care services, including preventative care, diagnosis and treatment of illness, prescriptions, and mental health care. Managed care contracts with doctors, hospitals, clinics, and other health care providers to create provider networks. An in-network physician or health care facility is part of a MCO's network if there is a preexisting agreement between the MCO and the health care provider. The agreement dictates the protocols for patient care and the compensation system. An out-of-network provider is a physician or health care facility that does not have an agreement with the MCO. To discourage the use of out-of-network providers, a patient's reimbursement for services provided by an out-of-network provider is not compensated at the same level as an in-network provider. Managed care focuses on various aspects of health care and can include characteristics such as:

- networks of health care providers or facilities, who have agreed to predetermined protocols and compensation,
- primary care physicians (PCPs), who coordinate all of a patient's health care,
- preauthorization for specific treatments,

- limited reimbursement for out-of-network providers,
- claim filing assigned to the provider rather than the patient, and
- tiered coverage of prescription drugs.

There are many different ways that MCO's members contribute to the cost of their health care. A member will typically pay a monthly premium, some or all of which may be paid by a third party, such as an employer or the government. In addition, members may be responsible for satisfying an annual deductible before certain coverages are effective. With a few exceptions, each office or emergency room visit or prescription requires that members contribute in the form of a co-payment. MCOs manage prescription-drug costs by charging members a lower co-payment for drugs that cost the MCO less. See Table 1-1 for an MCO matrix that includes the characteristics of HMOs, POSs, EPOs, and PPOs.

MCOs use PCPs as gatekeepers to control the cost-effectiveness of services offered to members. Gatekeepers control access to specialists. In addition, many MCOs have adopted authorization requirements, meaning that the MCO must approve some procedures before the PCP orders them. The payers are controlling access to health care by denying approval for certain procedures and allowing payment for others. They make decisions that reduce the number of hospital admissions, shorten the time until discharge, control the number of expensive diagnostic procedures, and, in the mental health field, substitute medication for therapeutic counseling treatment. When gatekeepers have an incentive to deny referrals to specialists, limit diagnostic treatments, and shorten hospital stays, the integrity of the patient–physician relationship is

Table 1-1 MCO Characteristics Matrix

	Requires PCP	Requires referrals	Requires preauthorization	Pays for out-of-network care	Cost-sharing	Do you have to file claim paperwork?
HMO	Yes	Yes	Not usually required. If required, PCP does it.	No	Low	No
POS	Yes	Yes	Not usually required. If required, PCP likely does it. Out-of-network care may have different rules.	Yes, but requires PCP referral.	Low in-network, high for out-of-network.	Only for out-of-network claims.
EPO	No	No	Yes	No	Low	No
PPO	No	No	Yes	Yes	High, especially for out-of-network care.	Only for out-of-network claims

Source: Verywell

called into question. When insurance companies make the decision to allow or deny diagnostic testing and hospital admissions, the patient–physician relationship is further eroded, and the well-being of the patient becomes an issue.

> " "
>
> Although case law on MCO "corporate liability" is scanty, corporate liability claims could be made against MCO's on several potential grounds:
>
> - negligent credentialing of contracted providers,
> - negligent or excessive utilization review,
> - failure to implement specified quality assurance programs or redress identified deficits,
> - use of aggressive cost-control incentive designed to reduce utilization, or
> - denial of benefits or "bad faith" by the plan.
>
> Gillespie, K. (1997). *Perspectives: Malpractice law evolves under managed care.* The Robert Wood Johnson Foundation.

An MCO's in-network health care providers are typically compensated by a capitated rate, sometimes also known as "per member per month" (PMPM). The MCO, on behalf of all its members, contracts with various health care providers who make themselves available to provide care in exchange for a set fee per month. The fee represents the number of members in the provider's care. In some cases, physicians are employees of the MCO, and they work for a salary. In most cases, physicians are part of a larger network maintained by the MCO for the members' benefit.

Health Maintenance Organizations
HMOs are comprehensive health care delivery and compensation systems that provide physician and hospital services from participating providers. With the exception of emergencies, HMOs will not cover care provided by out-of-network providers. HMOs require that each member has a PCP who monitors the overall health of the member and provides referrals to specialist in accordance with the HMO's protocols. HMOs typically do not pay for specialist visits that have not been referred by the PCP. HMOs operate on the presumption that maintaining health and preventing illness is less expensive than the cost of treatment for the illness that would otherwise develop.

There are two main HMO provider payment structures: the prepaid group practice (PGP) and the individual practice association (IPA). Prepaid group practices are groups of physicians who agree to provide comprehensive health care services for a fixed prospective **per capita payment** to a definite population. The staff model and the group model

per capita payment pay equally according to the number of individuals

are two forms of PGPs. Under the staff model, the physicians are employees of the HMO, are salaried, and may at the end of the fiscal year receive a portion of any profit. In the group model, the physicians are organized as a partnership or corporation in a group practice. The group contracts with the HMO to provide care for HMO members, sometimes called subscribers. The group receives **capitation** payment and a share of the HMO's net income as a group and pays participating providers on a fee-for-service or salary basis.

In contrast, IPAs are groups of physicians who join together and enter into agreement with other organizations to provide medical services to a defined population. In this structure, the physicians practice in their own office on a fee-for-service or capitation basis. Comprehensive health benefits are provided to the designated population for a fixed periodic payment.

HMOs are regulated under the HMO Act of 1973 (42 *United States Code* section 300c-300e-17 [1976 and Supp. III 1979]). Under this Act, member physicians must agree to give at least one-third of their time to HMO subscribers. Employers with more than 25 employees must offer an HMO as an alternative choice to conventional health care coverage, if such a choice is available in the area.

In a continued effort to find the best combination of cost savings and quality care, MCO hybrids are routinely introduced. A point-of-service (POS) is a combination of a traditional fee-for-service plan and an HMO. Members are rewarded with lower costs when they choose to use their PCP as a gatekeeper but are not prohibited from choosing out-of-network providers. Members incur higher costs when they receive care from an out-of-network provider.

Preferred Provider Organizations

PPOs are groups of physicians and hospitals that contract with employers, health insurance companies, or third-party administrators to provide comprehensive medical services on a fee-for-service basis to subscribers. A PPO may be sponsored by a hospital, a physician, an employer, or an insurer, or it may be a **joint venture** between a hospital and a medical practice. The mechanisms used to control health care costs include **negotiated fee schedules** and **utilization reviews**. A PPO covers the cost of a preferred provider's care, as well as a reduced portion of a nonpreferred provider's care.

The PPO has emerged as the most commonly used form of health insurance coverage. Consumers like the freedom to choose their own providers, which is frequently cited as one of HMO's drawbacks. As you might expect, the member costs for a PPO is greater than for an HMO.

An exclusive provider organization (EPO) is a hybrid of a PPO and an HMO, where members can choose from a group of preferred providers. An EPO, however, will not pay any percentage of costs associated with a nonpreferred provider.

capitation payment in a lump sum to physicians, HMOs, and health care facilities to deliver health care to a segment of the population

joint venture a group of persons together performing some specific business undertaking that is limited in duration or scope

negotiated fee schedules the process of the submission and consideration of offers until an offer is accepted. Fee schedule refers to the amount an insurance company or other third-party payer will reimburse for a medical procedure.

utilization review a process by which hospitals review patient progress to efficiently allocate scarce medical resources

Accountable Care Organizations   The Affordable Care Act includes guidelines for ACOs and sets the stage for the increased popularity of ACOs. An ACO is a type of MCO that seeks to improve health care and reduce costs by using groups of physicians, hospitals, and other health care providers to coordinate cost-effective, quality health care and to reward positive patient outcomes by sharing cost-savings with providers. It functions similarly to an HMO but without the gatekeeper requirement, and out-of-network providers are covered at a reduced percentage.

Think of it as buying a television, says Harold Miller, president and CEO of the Network for Regional Healthcare Improvement and executive director of the Center for Healthcare Quality & Payment Reform in Pittsburgh. A TV manufacturer like Sony may contract with many suppliers to build sets. Like Sony does for TVs, Miller says, an ACO would bring together the different component parts of care for the patient – primary care, specialists, hospitals, home health care, etc. – and ensure that all of the "parts work well together."

The problem today, Miller says, is that patients are getting each part of their health care separately. "People want to buy individual circuit boards, not a whole TV," he says. "If we can show them that the TV works better, maybe they'll buy it," rather than assembling a patchwork of services themselves. "But ACOs will need to prove that the overall health care product they're creating does work better and costs less in order to encourage patients and payers to buy it."

Gold, J. (2011). *Accountable care organizations, explained.* Retrieved from http://www .npr.org/2011/04/01/132937232/accountable-care-organizations-explained

Health care providers and health insurance companies are forming ACOs for Medicare patients as well as for patients with private insurance. The ACOs created for Medicare patients include the Medicare Shared Saving Program (MSSP), the Advanced Payment system, the Investment system, the Pioneer system, and the Next Generation system. The variations in the ACO systems differ based upon characteristics such as the way patient outcomes are rewarded, how the providers are compensated, the subset of Medicare patients they serve, or the ACO's level of experience.

TELEMEDICINE

Telemedicine is a health care delivery system used when the patient is in one location and the treating physician is in another, possibly thousands of miles away. Telemedicine includes the use of video, as well as the transmission of electronically collected data to the remote physician from the patient. It is not new, though it is increasingly used in a variety of applications and settings, including:

- Children's Healthcare of Atlanta uses telemedicine for rural pediatric patients, including those who were the victims of sexual assault and who might not otherwise be able to get the specialized health care needed,
- an Arizona neurosurgical practice uses telemedicine so its patients can remember what was said during office visits. Patients have their consultation and follow-up visits videotaped, so the details are available,
- telepsychiatry services are being offered across the country to address the needs of psychiatric patients when psychiatric or emergency wards are full or other circumstances prevent the provider and patient from being face-to-face, and
- on-demand physician services. See Figure 1-1.

In health care's cost-sensitive environment, telemedicine has become prominent and its applications are many. It offers a way to provide quality care to patients in rural areas or to patients in need of specialized diagnostic evaluation.

9:22 p.m.	Recurrent sinus infection rises to the level where the patient can no longer tolerate the symptoms. She has been too busy all week to schedule an appointment with her primary care physician. It is now late in the evening on a Friday, and she does not want to be sick all weekend. She downloads a smartphone application for a national physician-on-demand service and creates an account. Insurance doesn't currently cover the cost of the visit, which is $40 for each 15 minutes. Her co-pay at her PCP is $25.
9:27 p.m.	Videoconferencing begins. The physician asks about patient's symptoms, history of sinus infections, and current medications. Physician concurs that the signs of a sinus infection are present and that an antibiotic is in order.
9:35 p.m.	Videoconference concludes and the physician electronically sends an antibiotic prescription to the patient's local pharmacy.
9:44 p.m.	Pharmacy calls the patient to report that the prescription is ready for pick up.
10:02 p.m.	Prescription is in the patient's hands, and she takes the first dose that night.
Three days later	Patient receives an email from the physician-on-demand company reminding the patient to follow up with her primary care physician if symptoms have not improved and that her treatment history is available in the smartphone application.

Figure 1-1 Timeline of physician-on-demand videoconference consultation

A physician in one state may, for example, "telepractice" treatment to a patient in another state. As with any new process, legal questions arise. For example, in which state or county is medicine being practiced—where the patient is ill or where the physician is located? Does the physician need a license to practice medicine in each state where he or she consults with a patient? Some issues affect the physician engaged in practicing. Others affect the medical profession as a whole:

> " "
>
> Telemedicine is a significant and rapidly growing component of health care in the United States. There are currently about 200 telemedicine networks, with 3,500 service sites in the US. Nearly 1 million Americans are currently using remote cardiac monitors and in 2011, the Veterans Health Administration delivered over 300,000 remote consultations using telemedicine. Over half of all U.S. hospitals now use some form of telemedicine. Around the world, millions of patients use telemedicine to monitor their vital signs, remain healthy and out of hospitals and emergency rooms. Consumers and physicians download health and wellness applications for use on their cell phones.
>
> American Telemedicine Association. (n.d.). *Telemedicine frequently asked questions (FAQs)*. Retrieved from http://www.americantelemed.org/main/about/telehealth-faqs-

The use of teleradiology is increasing dramatically and with international overtones. Hospitals contract with physician groups in India, for example, to read x-ray, computerized tomography, and magnetic resonance images. Likewise, some radiology groups have established branch locations in places like Hawaii to provide more round-the-clock service to health care providers in other time zones.

Another increasing use of telemedicine is in the field of home health care. More patients are being monitored at home to ensure their well-being. This may require the patient "reporting in" by computer, or it may be a device that sends signals to the medical provider without requiring the patient to do anything.

Across the United States, companies that provide physician-on-demand services are popping up to address the needs of patients in rural areas, patients who lack the ability to leave their homes, busy parents or professionals, and patients on vacation. Some of the physician-on-demand services come in the form of a house call by a physician and some provide care by videoconferencing. Currently, most health insurance companies do not cover the cost of a telemedicine consultation. As history shows telemedicine to be a cost-effective health care delivery system, you can expect to see health insurance companies entertain the idea of covering it. A handful of states already have laws that relate to telemedicine and health insurance coverage.

☑ SUMMARY

- The health care industry is a big business.
- What you do on the frontline matters.
- Understanding the laws that apply to a medical office is important for employees to protect themselves, their employer, and the patient.
- Because medicine is closely regulated by state and federal law, it is necessary for employees to be aware of statutes and regulations that define the procedures they are permitted to perform.
- Medical office professionals work in the delivery of health care and are held to a higher standard of care than laypersons without special knowledge and training.
- There are several types of legal entities, all of which are governed by state law.
- The Affordable Care Act made expansive changes to the way the health care industry does business.
- Managed care organizations include HMOs, PPOs, ACOs, and they all seek to reduce costs and deliver quality health care.
- Telemedicine is an alternative health care delivery system.

SUGGESTED ACTIVITIES

1. Find the website for your state's department of corporations. This is the department that registers businesses. Find a local business' registration material on the department of corporation's website. Can you tell what kind of legal entity it is? Can you tell what year it was created? What else does the business' online registration tell you?

2. What type of health insurance do you have? Is it an HMO, a PPO, an ACO, or some hybrid form of MCO? Are you familiar with your deductible? What other details about your health insurance are important to you?

STUDY QUESTIONS

1. Identify the major disadvantage of a sole proprietorship or a partnership.
2. How does a corporation differ from a partnership?
3. What conflicts exist when a MCO provides bonuses to physicians for providing fewer tests?

CASES FOR DISCUSSION

1. Dr. Webber joined the Gelder Medical Group, which was a medical partnership. Part of the agreement was that if for any reason his association with the group ended, he would not practice medicine for five years within 30 miles of the Village of Sidney, where the partnership was located. The agreement also provided that any member could be required to withdraw from the partnership upon a majority vote of the other members. Dr. Webber's work with the group turned out to be unsatisfactory to his partners, who felt he was an embarrassment to the group. Dr. Webber refused to withdraw from the association after he was terminated by the other physicians. Two months later, despite his earlier agreement, Dr. Webber opened a medical office in Sidney. The partnership brought suit to prevent him from carrying on his practice. Could they do this successfully?

2. Brackenridge Hospital admitted Plaintiff to its intensive care unit following a serious car accident. Medical resident Dr. Villafani and attending physician Dr. Harshaw performed a tracheostomy and inserted a breathing tube. Several days later, plaintiff experienced bleeding from the surgical wound. Dr. Villafani examined plaintiff but did not immediately share plaintiff's condition with Dr. Harshaw. Plaintiff went into cardiac and respiratory arrest resulting in permanent and severe brain damage. At the time of plaintiff's treatment, Dr. Villafani was enrolled in a general surgery residency program operated by St. Joseph's Hospital. Central Texas Medical Foundation, an institution participating with St. Joseph's placed Dr. Villafani at Brackenridge Hospital, and had a contractual agreement with St. Joseph's to do so. The Foundation and Brackenridge dictated the details of how and when Dr. Villafani performed his residency responsibilities while at Brackenridge. The contract between St. Joseph's and the Foundation prevented St. Joseph's from having any direct control over Dr. Villafani's work while at Brackenridge. Plaintiff sued several defendants, including St. Joseph's, who was found vicariously liable for plaintiff's injuries under the theory of respondeat superior. On appeal, the court reversed. Who, if anyone, should be held vivaciously liable for Dr. Villafani's treatment of plaintiff?

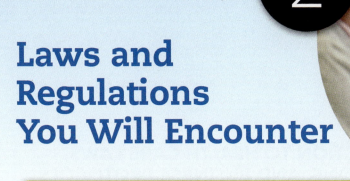

2

Laws and Regulations You Will Encounter

> "Law is an ordinance of reason for the common good, promulgated by him who has care of the community.
>
> *Thomas Aquinas*

OBJECTIVES

After reading this chapter, you should be able to:

1. Recognize the complexity of the government influence on the practice and licensing of medicine.
2. Describe the importance of understanding basic employment, discrimination, and harassment laws when hiring, promoting, and terminating employees.
3. Identify provisions of the Family and Medical Leave Act.
4. Recognize situations affected by the Americans with Disabilities Act (ADA).
5. Identify four social security benefits.
6. Recognize differences between Medicare and Medicaid.
7. Define the Employee Retirement Income Security Act (ERISA).
8. Recognize the importance of the Occupational Safety and Health Act (OSHA) regulations.
9. Define job descriptions, procedures, manuals, and employee handbooks.
10. Describe basic collection protocol.

BUILDING YOUR LEGAL VOCABULARY

Bargaining unit	Interstate commerce
Censure	Mitigating
Collective bargaining	Negligent per se
Disparate impact	Probable cause
Disparate treatment	Quality assurance
Facially neutral	Risk management
Inference	

INTRODUCTION TO HEALTH CARE LAWS, REGULATIONS, AND BUSINESS PROTOCOLS

In addition to the health care business framework discussed in Chapter 1, the laws and regulations that touch health care and those who work in the industry are also an important part of that framework. As a medical office professional, you will want to be aware of various medical practice laws and regulations, the nature of your employment, discrimination, sexual harassment, health care laws and regulations, and, in some situations, union membership and collective bargaining. In addition, it is helpful to remember that you work in a field that is highly regulated by federal and state legislation. Ignorance of a law or a regulation does not excuse a medical office professional's violation. You are a professional and expected to know the laws and regulations that govern your profession.

Although the professional status of medical assistants has grown during the past few years, many state laws and regulations, including medical practice acts and nursing practice acts, either do not acknowledge the existence of the medical assisting profession or do not authorize the delegation of administrative and clinical duties to medical assistants.

GOVERNMENT REGULATION OF HEALTH CARE PROVIDERS

Medical Practice Laws

Medical practice laws control the practice of medicine. State legislatures establish state medical boards with the authority to control health care provider licensing. In all states, individuals who are not physicians are prohibited from practicing medicine, yet not every state defines what "practicing medicine" means. When there is no definition of medical practice and a disagreement arises between a health care professional and a licensing board, the matter may be taken to court on a case-by-case basis.

Medical practice acts may include nursing practice acts, or the two may exist independently. The requirements for other health care professionals and their licensure depend on individual state law.

Licensure statutes were originally required to exclude incompetents from the practice of medicine. In *Hawker v. New York* (170 U.S. 189 [1898]), the U.S. Supreme Court extended physician licensure decisions to include standards of behavior and ethics, holding that in a physician, "character is as important a qualification as knowledge."

Licensing boards not only grant licenses but also renew and revoke licenses. They may fine, reprimand, and **censure**. In so doing, the board must follow due process. Due process requires that a practitioner be put on notice that there is a pending suspension or revocation, be given an opportunity for a prompt hearing, and be given the rights to confront the accuser, prepare an effective defense, retain counsel, and cross-examine any witnesses.

censure a formal statement of disapproval

One ground for the revocation or suspension of a medical license is permitting unlicensed personnel to perform medical procedures normally restricted to physicians. Physicians should consider the consequence of loss of license when assigning procedures to nonphysicians.

State Board of Registration Licensing statutes regulate a state's Board of Registration, which could be known by other names, such as Board of Healing Arts. Complaints about physicians are brought to the board's attention by anonymous communications, newspaper articles, patients, hospitals, other physicians, insurance companies, and employees. The board has the power to perform investigations and adjudications according to its rules. The board may have access to records involving the health care provider's practice—prescriptions, hospital records, reimbursement claims—as long as the patient's identity is withheld.

Mandatory Reports Physicians are required to submit reports to various governmental agencies under certain circumstances. To whom and when the reports are submitted are factors that vary from state to state. Certain reports are required by all practicing physicians, and these include births, deaths, and communicable diseases. Generally, physicians are required to report injuries and suspicious or "unnatural" deaths to the local coroner or medical examiner. In many states, failure to report certain injuries or deaths may result in misdemeanor charges.

Controlled Substances Acts Controlled substances acts restrict the distribution, classification, sale, and use of certain drugs, often defined as *controlled substances*. These acts cover everyone from criminals who are not involved in health care delivery to physicians, who have the license to write prescriptions. Not every drug that is controlled is considered to have the potential to be abused. Because different states have vary-ing prescription and over-the-counter drug regulations, a federal Con-trolled Substances Act of 1970 (CSA) was implemented. Most states have enacted the Uniform Controlled Substances Act, which is very similar to the CSA.

Statistically, malpractice suits involving drugs usually involve pre-scriptions. This is important for medical office professionals because phy-sicians, physician's assistants, and nurse practitioners (in some states) are allowed to write prescriptions, whereas medical assistants are not.

Abuse   Physicians, nurses, and other health care professionals are required in most states to report the abuse of children, elderly, and patients. The Child Abuse Prevention and Treatment Act requires that states meet certain uniform standards to be eligible for federal assistance in setting up programs to identify, prevent, and treat prob-lems caused by child abuse and neglect. It also protects the reporter of abuse against liability and includes a penalty clause that permits the prosecution of professionals who have knowledge of but do not report abuse.

Medical assistants should remember that they are agents of the physician. A suspected case of child abuse should be carefully docu-mented. Office policy should be closely followed regarding the handling of such a case.

Elder abuse is handled at the state and national level, and virtually every state has some form of elder abuse law. Exactly who is protected and from what the legal protection is provided varies from state to state. Federal acts that seek to protect various forms of elder abuse include The Elder Justice Act of 2009, The Older American Acts, and Elder Abuse Victims Act of 2009. See Chapter 4 for a more detailed discussion of elder abuse.

> ❝ ❞
>
> Approximately 1 in 10 Americans aged 60+ have experienced some form of elder abuse. Some estimates range as high as 5 million elders who are abused each year. One study estimated that only 1 in 14 cases of abuse are reported to authorities...
>
> Abusers are both women and men. In almost 90% of elder abuse and neglect incidents, the perpetrator is a family member. Two-thirds of perpetrators are adult children or spouses.
>
> National Council on Aging. (n.d.). *Elder abuse facts*. Retrieved from https://www.ncoa .org/public-policy-action/elder-justice/elder-abuse-facts/

EMPLOYMENT LAW

Laws to protect employees often have both positive and negative effects. Years ago, hospitals were thought of as "charity" employers. They would hire individuals who were otherwise unemployable—the aged, handicapped, and homeless—off the street. Often there was housing within the hospital structure that completed the employment picture, offering the employee a bed to lie in, food for the stomach, and a place in society. By offering this employment package, hospitals not only acted like today's social service agencies but also kept the price of hospitalization down by paying employees less than prevailing wages.

This hiring pattern set the stage for present health care employment. Tradition dies slowly. The paternalistic attitude of hospital employers, particularly large-city teaching hospitals, combined with low wages provides fertile fields for the development of employee unions. Recently, there has been an increase in the organization of health care workers at all levels, from the unskilled to the professional.

Hiring Process

Interviewing   Discrimination law has made many changes in the employment interview situation necessary. Employers are not allowed to ask interview questions involving race, religion, age, or whether a woman is pregnant. Because of the importance of the employment interview in getting the job, there is considerable dissension among employment specialists as to the handling of these matters. For example, *The Wall Street Journal*, on February 13, 1990, ran the following on the front page:

Title VII of the Civil Rights Act of 1964 bars companies from asking applicants about family plans. But Felice Schwartz, president of Catalyst, suggests women confront the issue in job interviews: Open discussion of child-rearing plans, she contends, moves an interview "from insistence on the rights women had achieved...to a partnership with an employer..."

She's right, some say. But many protest... Marnee Walsh, employment manager at Boston Edison Co., believes volunteering information could be "career suicide. It's an outrageous question for an interview that has nothing to do with a woman's capabilities on the job." Madelyn Jennings, senior vice president of personnel at Gannett Co., ventures "employers might as well start asking men if they have a family history of heart attacks." Besides, says Betty Bessler, vice president at Mary Kay Cosmetics, Inc., "Personal plans change."

The Wall Street Journal, p. 1 (1990, February 13)

Preemployment Testing   Employers are allowed to test potential employees as part of the hiring process, but such tests must be carefully constructed, usually by experts, to ensure that they only measure the skills and abilities necessary to do the job. In *Griggs v. Duke Power Company*, a landmark case in discrimination law, the U.S. Supreme Court established a strict standard, called the business necessity test, for business practices that have an adverse impact on various minority groups. Some forms of testing were determined to be a subtle means of discrimination:

Duke Power Company, a large power-generating corporation in the Carolinas, for years limited blacks to the labor department, the lowest-paying area of the company, and refused to approve requests for transfers to other departments. When Title VII was passed, the company instituted a policy which stated that employees who wanted transfers from the labor department had to present a high school diploma or pass a high school aptitude test. Black employees sued, contending that the company was trying to lock them into their jobs as laborers by imposing unnecessary transfer requirements that they would be unable to meet because of unequal educational opportunities.

The U.S. Supreme Court found that the transfer policies were unlawful because neither the high school completion requirement nor the aptitude test was shown to bear a demonstrable relationship to successful performance of the jobs for which it was used. Under Title VII, the Court declared, "practices, procedures, or tests, neutral on their face, and even neutral in terms of intent, cannot be maintained if they have a discriminatory impact on minorities and are unrelated to measuring job capability." Selection practices that are fair in form but discriminatory in operation can be used only if they are justified by a "business necessity."

Griggs v. Duke Power, 401 U.S. 424 (1971)

Drug Testing   Another area of preemployment testing in which the Supreme Court has made decisions relates to drug testing. Because many hospital employees have responsibilities that directly affect patient care, an argument could be made that drug testing is needed to ensure the public's safety. On the issue of safety, *National Treasure Employees Union v. Von Raab* could be analogous to the situation of health care workers. The Court determined in this decision that mandatory drug tests for applicants and employees seeking promotions to sensitive positions in the U.S. Customs Service were constitutional and permissible. The Supreme Court had previously ruled that drug testing of employees is a "search and seizure" within the realm of the Fourth Amendment, and that each case must be resolved on a case-by-case basis using a balancing test between individual rights and public safety. The *Von Raab* decision considered public policy with public safety outweighing concerns about employees' rights to privacy. Preemployment drug testing is now considered routine in many health care settings, particularly hospitals. The law specifically requires tests that provide "qualitative data" on the presence of drugs or alcohol. The intent of the law is to determine whether the employee is fit for duty.

Equal Opportunity Employment

In the United States, there is a myth that everyone has an equal opportunity to be hired for a job and, after hired, to be president of the company. Realistically, everyone cannot reach the highest rung on the corporate ladder, but, according to the Civil Rights Act of 1964, the opportunity to do so cannot be denied employees on the basis of race, color, religion, sex, or national origin.

Title VII of the act prohibits employment discrimination and applies to all employers of 15 or more employees whose business involves **interstate commerce**, to labor unions of 15 or more members, to employment agencies, as well as to state, local, and federal employees. The Equal Employment Opportunity Commission (EEOC) administers and enforces Title VII. Illegal discrimination may be shown by either **disparate treatment** or **disparate impact**.

interstate commerce the movement of goods and services, or services that rely on the movement of goods, which cross state borders within the United States

disparate treatment a marked difference between two things

disparate impact the force of impression of one thing on another

Disparate Treatment   The most obvious form of discrimination occurs when an employer treats similarly situated employees differently because of their race, sex, religion, or national origin. Because of the difficulty in proving a disparate treatment situation, courts allow plaintiffs to prove disparate treatment indirectly. **Inferences** may be drawn from the acts of the employers. In other words, if an act looks discriminatory, it may well be discriminatory. If an employer has been shown to discriminate in the past, the inference will be stronger that the present act involves conscious discrimination.

Inference a process of reasoning by which a fact is deduced as a logical consequence of other facts

Disparate treatment cases are proven by the plaintiff establishing a prima facie case, the elements being (1) the plaintiff must be a member of one of the groups protected by Title VII, (2) the plaintiff must be capable of doing the job, and (3) he or she must have been discriminated against.

Disparate Impact   Some employment policies are **facially neutral**, in that they appear to treat all employees equally, but have a "disparate" or "adverse" impact on a particular protected group. For example, a minimum height requirement may discriminate against women, or a maximum weight requirement may discriminate against men.

facially neutral on the surface the matter is impartial, or does not take an active part in either side

An employer, faced with the charge of disparate impact, may counter that the policy is justified by business necessity and is related to job performance. In the following case, an employer's business necessity defense was upheld by the court:

Gregory Backus, RN, requested placement as a full-time registered nurse in the labor and delivery section. The hospital refused the request on the basis that it did not employ male RNs on the obstetrics and gynecology units and gave as a reason their concern for female patients' privacy and personal dignity. Backus filed a sex discrimination complaint with the EEOC, alleging that the hospital's refusal to transfer him to the labor and delivery section was discriminatory based on sex.

Testimony in the hospital's defense relied on its policy of recognizing and respecting the privacy rights of its patients. Hospital policy required that catheterizations be performed by individuals of the same sex as the patient. The hospital's policy of restricting nursing positions in labor and delivery came from the fact that obstetrical patients continually have genitals exposed and that there are few duties that a nurse performs that are not sensitive or intimate in nature.

The court decided against Backus and found merit in the hospital's argument that the majority of women patients would object to intimate contact with a member of the opposite sex in the labor and delivery room. The court commented that "in addition to offending patients, a male nurse would necessitate the presence of a female nurse to protect the hospital from charges of molestation... The court refused to consider a male nurse analogous to a male doctor because the doctor, and not the nurse, had been chosen by the patient."

It follows that it is reasonably necessary to the normal operation of the hospital's business that delivery room nurses be female.

Backus v. Baptist Medical Center, 510 F. Supp. 1191 (1980)

Genetic Information Nondiscrimination Act of 2008   Health care insurers and group health care plans may not deny coverage or charge higher premiums based solely on an individual's likelihood of developing a disease in the future. The Genetic Information Nondiscrimination Act of 2008 (GINA) also prohibits employers from using genetic information when hiring, firing, training, or promoting employees. Recent amendments to GINA include requirements that employee wellness programs be voluntary and that the wellness programs cover spousal participation.

Sexual Harassment Sexual harassment is unwanted sexual attention from anyone the victim may interact with on the job in which the victim's response may be restrained by fear of reprisals. This can include peers, subordinates, supervisors, customers, and clients. The range of behavior includes verbal comments, subtle pressure for sexual activity, leering, pinching, patting, and other forms of unwanted touching as well as rape and attempted rape. Some harassers identify their own behavior as flirting, but there is a distinction between flirting and sexual harassment. Flirting is often described as instinctual and natural between genders, whereas sexual harassment has elements of premeditation and persistence. Flirting offers pleasure to both parties, whereas in most cases, harassment occurs against the victim's wishes. The looks between the parties engaged in flirting attract and complement, whereas the look or stare of a harasser makes the victim feel invaded, shamed, and naked. Flirting is a mutual interaction between the parties, whereas sexual harassment involves obscene suggestions and hints, often followed with pinches, pats, and grabs.

Sexual harassment has always been a problem for women at work. In the past, it was kept quiet because women who were in the workplace desperately needed their jobs and there was no support for their position as the victim. *Cosmopolitan* magazine, in a 2015 national survey of 2,235 employed women, found that one out of three respondents had experienced sexual harassment at work. Of those who experienced harassment, 70 percent did not report it.

Sexual harassment was painfully brought to the nation's attention in confirmation hearings regarding the appointment of Supreme Court Justice Clarence Thomas. Anita Hill, an attorney who worked for Thomas earlier in his career, accused her former boss of sexually harassing her. All of the elements of a sexual harassment case were brought before the public on national television in the Senate confirmation hearings. Anita Hill was a credible witness, and Clarence Thomas, the epitome of a respected nominee. Someone had to be lying. The 98 percent male Senate confirmed Clarence Thomas for the position of Supreme Court justice. The majority of working women believed in their hearts that Anita Hill was telling the truth.

College Campuses have reported an increase in the number of reported instances of sexual harassment and sexual assault. The Association of American Universities 2015 Campus Survey on Sexual Assault and Sexual Misconduct reported that the "incidence of sexual assault and sexual misconduct due to physical force, threats of physical force, or incapacitation among female undergraduate student respondents was 23.1 percent, including 10.8 percent who experienced penetration." Of those who were assaulted, only 5 percent to 28 percent reported the incidents. The survey also showed that "[t]he most common reason for not reporting incidents of sexual assault and sexual misconduct was that it was not considered serious enough."

Sexual harassment is not a problem confined to the United States alone:

A nursing home employee in Quebec alleged that she missed five weeks of work because of depression and stress caused by "sexist remarks, insistent and vicious looks, and unwanted touching" by a security guard at work.

Quebec's Worker Compensation Board originally ruled against her claims but decided after a review that there appeared to be no other cause for her depression aside from her encounters with the guard.

The Board ruled that she had a period of extreme stress provoked by the climate of work. It also ruled that Quebec's law defines an accident to include any event which occurs at work and causes injury, illness, or death. It said the woman was entitled to benefits for a work-related accident.

The Wall Street Journal, p. 1 (July 1982)

RN Magazine addressed the issue with the following:

A well-known surgeon at a Chicago hospital tells off-color jokes to nurses and anyone else within earshot. He's been doing it for years. Some nurses avoid him entirely and others pretend not to hear, but no one ever tries to stop him.

Then one night, following surgery, when he and an OR nurse are alone, joking progresses to groping and grabbing. As she struggles to break free, her uniform rips.

Screaming she runs to her supervisor's office and reports the incident. When confronted with the allegation, the surgeon admits to the transgression and the hospital slaps him with a six-month suspension.

Horsley, J. E. (January 1990). Legally speaking: Don't tolerate sexual harassment at work. *RN*, 69

Filing with the EEOC Most EEOC actions begin with the filing of a Charge of Discrimination by an individual who believes he or she has been discriminated against. A Charge of Discrimination must be filed within 180 days following the incident, unless the facts warrant an exception that extends the period to 300 days. After a Charge of Discrimination is filed, the EEOC will conduct an investigation.

If the EEOC finds **probable cause** and that Title VII may have been violated, attempts are made to mediate the matter. If the parties

probable cause having more evidence for than against

are not able to reach agreement, the EEOC issues a Right to Sue Letter to the complaining party, who is free to pursue the matter in a court of law. Under certain conditions, the EEOC may initiate a federal lawsuit.

FAMILY AND MEDICAL LEAVE ACT

The Family and Medical Leave Act of 1993 (FMLA) requires employers of 50 or more people to provide up to 12 weeks of unpaid leave each year for the "serious health condition" of an employee or member of the employee's immediate family or for the birth or adoption of a child. The FMLA covers:

- all public employers,
- private employers who have 50 or more employees on the payroll during each of 20 or more calendar workweeks in either the current or preceding calendar year, and
- employees who have been employed for at least 12 months and who have worked at least 1,250 hours in the 12 months preceding commencement of the FMLA leave.

In 2010, the Department of Labor clarified the FMLA definition of "son and daughter" to "ensure that an employee who assumes the role of caring for a child receives parental rights to family leave regardless of the legal or biological relationship." In 2015, the Department of Labor issued a final rule that amended the regulatory definition of "spouse" under the FMLA. The amended definition makes clear that "eligible employees in legal, same-sex marriages will be able to take FMLA leave to care for their spouse or family member, regardless of where they live. This will ensure that the FMLA will give spouses in same-sex marriages the same ability as all spouses to fully exercise their FMLA rights."

AMERICANS WITH DISABILITIES ACT

The ADA covers physical as well as mental disabilities in employment, public services, public accommodations, and telecommunications. A *disability* is defined as a physical or mental impairment that substantially limits one or more of the major life activities of an individual, or a record of such impairment, or being regarded as having such an impairment. The ADA covers conditions ranging from infection with the AIDS virus to cancer to mental retardation, but excludes certain antisocial conditions such as kleptomania, pedophilia, and active illegal drug addiction.

Title I of the act prohibits employment discrimination and places the burden on an employer to prove that the requirements of a specific job could not be changed to accommodate a disabled applicant.

Titles II and III of the act, in part, guarantee the disabled access to the workplace. Professional offices of health care providers are in the public sector and, as such, require an employer to make "reasonable modifications" for the disabled to gain access.

Title IV requires all telecommunications carriers to provide a relay system that will allow the hearing impaired to communicate with a hearing individual by wire or radio. The ADA required the availability of telecommunications devices for the deaf (TDD) by 1995. Among the services provided by public safety agencies is the 911 telephone response service. Title IV requires that "telephone emergency response services, including 911 services, provide direct access to people who use TDDs and computer modems." Maintenance of this equipment is also mandated by the ADA.

The EEOC has issued detailed guidelines defining *disability* under the ADA. The employee may have a past impairment or simply be "regarded as" having an impairment. The guidelines provide examples of conditions that are not impairments—for example, pregnancy, physical characteristics like hair or eye color, common personality traits, and normal deviations in height or weight. Perhaps the most significant example of these conditions is found in the *Cook* case:

Bonnie Cook, 5'2" tall and weighing more than 200 pounds, was turned down for a job as an institutional attendant for the mentally retarded at the Ladd Center, a residential facility for retarded persons. Ms. Cook had passed the Ladd Center's physical examination, and the Center acknowledged that she was capable of performing the job adequately despite her "morbid obesity." However, the center worried that Ms. Cook's morbid obesity would hinder her ability to evacuate residents in an emergency and put her at greater risk of developing future serious ailments which would result in her being absent from work and possibly filing workers' compensation claims. At trial, Ms. Cook claimed that, regardless of whether "morbid obesity" is a "handicap," the Ladd Center "regarded" her morbid obesity as a handicap. The jury agreed and awarded her $100,000.

Cook v. Rhode Island, 10 F.3d 17 (1st Cir. 1993)

Under the ADA, an employer has a duty to provide reasonable accommodation to the known mental or physical limitations of a qualified individual with a disability. In the following case, the court upheld an employer's right to fire an employee whose handicap, major depression, kept the employee out of work for months with no clear indication of when he could return.

Mr. August requested, as accommodations, permission to work part-time, to miss some morning meetings, and to report late for work. His employer refused. The court suggested that, in some cases at least, an employer might be obliged to provide such "reasonable accommodations," but that in Mr. August's case it was not clear that he would have been able to perform capably even with these accommodations.

August v. Offices Unlimited, Inc., 981 F.2d 576 (1st Cir. 1992)

In *Griece Mills v. Derwinski*, 967 F.2d 794 (2d Cir. 1992), a hospital was not required to accommodate the request of a head nurse suffering from depression to report to work at 10:00 a.m., as such accommodation would have imposed "undue hardship" on the hospital. In defining *undue hardship*, the ADA requires consideration of the following factors:

- the nature and cost of the accommodation needed,
- the overall finances of the facility,
- the overall resources of the covered entity, and
- the type of operation or operations of the covered entity.

Notably, an employer is obligated only to accommodate "known" physical or mental limitations of a disabled worker.

The administration of a hospital learned that Doe [a pharmacist] was infected with HIV and sought to bar him from preparing IV or hyperalimentation solutions, citing the risk of transmission. Condemning the job restriction as unnecessary and detrimental to his career, Doe filed suit. In finding that Doe did not present a significant risk to others in the workplace, [the court ruled in Doe's favor].

[A nurse was found to be a significant risk to others in the workplace.] The court found that IV's, catheterizations, and dressing changes...are invasive procedures and because AIDS is fatal, even a minute risk is unacceptable.

Kelasa, E. V. (January 1993). HIV vs. a nurse's right to work. *RN*, 63

In another AIDS case, a dentist who refused to treat two patients who were HIV positive paid $120,000 under the ADA in a settlement with the Justice Department. The dentist argued that the AIDS patients posed a "significant risk" and required specialized dental care beyond his expertise. But a U.S. District Court found that he had engaged in "blatant discrimination." There is no such thing as a "specialist for the purposes of cleaning teeth," the court said. The dentist "would not have refused these persons but for their disability" (*United States v. Morvant*, 843 F. Supp. 1092 [E.D. La. 1994]).

FEDERAL AGE DISCRIMINATION ACT

The Federal Age Discrimination in Employment Act of 1967 (FADA) covers age discrimination and protects the rights of older workers. It provides that workers over the age of 40 years cannot arbitrarily be discriminated against because of age in any employment decisions. This includes hiring, discharge, layoff, promotion, wages and other terms and conditions of employment, referrals by employment agencies, and membership in and activities of unions.

The FADA applies to employers with more than 20 employees, and to public and private employers, including state and local governments and their agencies. States individually may have separate laws further protecting workers. The act is administered by the EEOC.

EQUAL PAY ACT

Violations of the Equal Pay Act are a form of sex discrimination actionable under Title VII. The act was passed in 1963 to end the practice of paying women less than men for the same job. Equal work is defined as work requiring substantially similar "skill, effort, and responsibility." It does not mean equal pay for comparable work. The comparable worth theory is based on the premise that particular jobs have been traditionally underpaid because they have been held primarily by women. The 2009 Lilly Ledbetter Fair Pay Act ensured that victims of unequal pay would have enough time to commence a lawsuit. The Act made clear that the 180-day statute of limitations for filing an equal-pay lawsuit begins with each paycheck issued.

FAIR LABOR STANDARDS ACT

State and federal laws regulate employees' wages, hours, and working conditions. The Fair Labor Standards Act (FLSA) establishes a federal minimum wage, mandates extra pay for overtime work, regulates the employment of children, and is administered by the Department of Labor.

Under the FLSA, Congress periodically adjusts the minimum wage rate. The minimum wage applies to all employers who are involved in interstate commerce but exempts executives, administrators, professional employees, outside salespersons, state employees, and agricultural workers. Overtime is considered to be any hours worked in excess of 40 hours per week and must be compensated at one and one-half times the employee's regular rate of pay.

Medical offices are often confronted with issues involving overtime pay. Overtime must be paid for work permitted but not necessarily required. For example, an employee may voluntarily work overtime without being required by the employer to put in extra hours, or it may be necessary for an employee to work through lunch or after hours to complete the job. In either case, the employee is entitled to overtime pay. Supervisory and professional employees are exempt from the law. In December 2016, a new rule will take effect that will change the requirements under which an employee must receive overtime. The new rule is intended to be more inclusive in that it expands the definition of covered employees, so more workers are entitled to overtime.

WORKERS' COMPENSATION

Workers' compensation laws are administered by state governments and create a mandatory insurance system that reimburses employees for losses sustained because of work-related injury or disease, regardless of fault. Losses include the cost of medical care, lost income, and rehabilitation expenses. It also provides continuing payments to the spouses and/or children of workers who die of occupational disease or injury. The law applies to all industrial, service, private, state, and local government employees and is paid for by the employer.

SOCIAL SECURITY

Social security includes several related programs: retirement, disability, and dependent's/survivor's benefits. Each part has its own set of rules regarding who is qualified to receive benefits and has its own schedule of payment of benefits. Benefits are paid to the retired or disabled worker and/or the worker's dependent or surviving family. The amount paid is based on the worker's average wages while working in employment covered by social security during his or her working life.

To receive social security benefits, an individual must accumulate a predetermined number of work credits in qualified employment. Work credits are measured in quarters of a year (three months) during which time the individual was employed earning the required minimum wage or more.

Retirement Benefits

Retirement benefits require a total of 40 quarters or 10 years of work credit from covered employment. An individual becomes eligible for retirement benefits at age 62 years. If the person chooses to retire at 62 years of age, the monthly benefit payment will be considerably less than if retirement takes place at 65 years of age. Under new regulations, retirement benefits will not be available until 67 years of age.

Disability Benefits

Disability benefits are paid to individuals who are disabled. Any medical condition that prevents an individual from being gainfully employed may be considered a disability, particularly if it is included on the list of disabling conditions found on the Social Security Administration's list. There are special provisions for people who are blind.

Dependent's Benefits

Certain dependents of a retired or disabled worker are eligible for monthly dependent's benefits if the worker is eligible for retirement or disability benefits.

Survivor's Benefits

Surviving family members of a deceased worker may be entitled to survivor's benefits. To ensure fair and equitable distribution of survivor's benefits, the Social Security Administration lists survivors who are eligible.

MEDICARE

Medicare is a federal insurance program for people who are entitled to Medicare from their social security contributions and payment of premiums. Everyone 65 years of age or older, rich or poor, is entitled to Medicare coverage, as are some people on social security disability and everyone with permanent kidney failure.

Medicare Hospital Insurance, known as Part A, provides basic coverage for inpatient hospitalization and posthospital nursing and home health care. In addition, it provides limited coverage for rehabilitation in nonacute care hospital facilities. There is a yearly deductible.

Medicare Medical Insurance, known as Part B, pays 80 percent of "reasonable" charges for physicians' fees, outpatient hospital and laboratory work, medical equipment and supplies, home health care, therapy, and so on. A monthly premium is charged for Part B.

In 2005, in response to rapidly increasing costs of prescription drugs, Congress passed a significant expansion to Medicare, creating Part D, coverage for many medications that was effective January 1, 2006. Enrollment is voluntary; there is a deductible, a co-payment, and a "doughnut hole": As of 2008, the patient must meet a $275 deductible; when that has been met, the patient must pay a co-payment of 25 percent of costs up to $2,510. At that point, coverage ends and patients will not receive coverage for their prescriptions again until they reach a threshold of $5,726 in total drug expenditures. Then 100 percent coverage begins. Part of the Obama administration's agenda for health care reform includes reduction of the size of the doughnut hole.

MEDICAID

Medicaid is a program jointly administered by the federal government and state government. For that reason, rules vary from state to state. Medicaid is provided for low-income individuals and is obtainable through local social services or welfare departments. Medicaid reimburses for Medicare deductibles and for the portion of "reasonable charges" not paid by Medicare (20 percent) for elderly beneficiaries receiving Medicare coverage. States can, and do, change both the eligibility requirements and the reimbursement rates in response to changing budget realities. This frustrates both beneficiaries and providers alike. Indeed, many physicians will not accept Medicaid patients because the reimbursement is so low.

EMPLOYEE RETIREMENT INCOME SECURITY ACT

The Employee Retirement Income Security Act (ERISA) protects and regulates pensions. A pension is an agreement between an employee and an employer under which each contributes a certain amount of money while the employee works for the employer. These contributions create a fund from which the employee is paid a certain amount of money upon retirement, usually at the age of 65 years.

In the past, many employers and employees contributed to pension plans, but employees often did not collect or benefit at retirement for the following reasons: People changed jobs and had to leave their pension rights behind; workers were "let go" just before they reached retirement age; and pension plans, or whole companies, went out of business.

Since the passage of ERISA in 1974, some of the abuses of pensions have been controlled. The act sets minimum standards for pension plans guaranteeing that a worker's pension rights cannot be unfairly denied.

HEALTH INSURANCE PORTABILITY AND ACCOUNTABILITY ACT OF 1996

The Health Insurance Portability and Accountability Act of 1996 (HIPAA) is an expansion of ERISA and an outgrowth of managed care. HIPAA amends ERISA by guaranteeing renewal and transferability of health insurance coverage to those who already have coverage and to their dependents. One of the HIPAA's mandates has been to prohibit discrimination in issuing health insurance coverage. The HIPAA nondiscrimination provision generally prohibits group health plans and group health insurance issuers from discriminating against participants or beneficiaries based on any "health factor."

In forming its patterns for analyzing discrimination, HIPAA used the term "similarly situated" to identify different groups: full-time versus part-time, northerners versus southerners, male versus female, those with diabetes versus those without, different occupations, and so forth. An example of illegal discrimination is a group health insurance plan that excludes individuals who participate in certain recreational activities, such as motorcycling. As in any legislative act, there are clauses that require further interpretation on administrative appeal or litigation in court, and the wording regarding insurance eligibility promises these types of issues. For example:

NEWS

The Act prohibits medical underwriting: it bars health insurers from using, as rules of eligibility, an individual's health status, medical or mental conditions, claims experience, medical treatment history, genetic information, disability or evidence of insurability. Health insurers may, however, select in a non-discriminatory basis, the coverage and benefits they wish to offer. For example, a health insurer may exclude benefits for AIDS or cancer in its policies, but cannot deny coverage to an individual with AIDS or cancer when its policies otherwise offer AIDS or cancer coverage.

Roverner, J. (1996). Analysis of the provisions of the Health Insurance Portability and Accountability Act of 1996. *The Health Lawyer, 9*(3), 1

HIPAA has many rules, and compliance is required for Medicare reimbursement. Compliance is mandatory for all health care organizations that send or receive standard electronic transactions for health claims or other health plan information. Emphasis is placed on patient privacy regulations (covered more completely in Chapter 10) and staff training. Regulations regarding health care are increasing at the state and federal level, with the most significant being the Health Information Portability and Accountability Act of 1996 (HIPAA).

HITECH ACT

The Health Information Technology for Economic and Clinical Health Act (HITECH) encourages and requires the use of various methods of health care technology with improved health care as the objective. The Act requires the use of electronic health records (EHRs), but the adoption of the new process has taken more time than expected. Financial incentives were offered to health care providers establishing EHRs. There remains a portion of health care providers, typically solo and small practices, who have not yet made the switch to EHR. Consequently, the Centers for Medicare and Medicaid Services (CMS) announced that some deadlines have been extended until 2017 to ensure all have the opportunity to comply. Nonetheless, there has been a significant increase in the use of EHRs.

OCCUPATIONAL SAFETY AND HEALTH ACT

Congress enacted the Occupational Safety and Health Act (OSHA) in 1970. This act now is in effect in hospitals and other health care facilities. The OSHA rules and regulations are intended to prevent injuries and promote job safety, and OSHA is authorized to enforce its standards through complaint, inspection, and investigation.

The OSHA places employers under the general duty to provide a workplace free from "recognized hazards"—for example, undue exposure to toxic substances, inoperable safety equipment, poor air quality, and excessive noise levels. In addition, OSHA requires detailed records of job-related injuries and may conduct unannounced workplace inspections to assess an employer's compliance.

OSHA can assess penalties of up to $1,000 for each violation and as high as $10,000 for repeated or willful violations. Although OSHA protects employees' rights, it also imposes responsibilities on employees. Employees may not be discharged or discriminated against for filing a complaint or testifying against an employer due to violations of OSHA regulations.

Right-to-Know Laws

Right-to-know regulations, originated by OSHA for the protection of industrial workers, now extend to cover health care workers. The right-to-know legislation grew directly out of concerns about hazardous substances and their health effects. The underlying purpose of the law is to make certain that all employees have an opportunity to know what chemicals they are handling, the potential health effects of those chemicals, and ways to prevent or reduce health risks.

These regulations give each employee the right to (1) a complete list of all hazardous chemicals used in the workplace, (2) the contents of every product and the hazards involved in its use, (3) education about hazardous chemicals with which an employee may come in contact, and (4) protective equipment to use when handling dangerous chemicals.

The law addresses toxic and poisonous chemicals, corrosive irritants, flammable materials, and carcinogens. It requires that each product be labeled. There are three types of labels: written labels with extensive information about the chemical; an encoded label with fire, reactivity, and health hazards categories coded 1–4 for severity; and symbolic labels.

Material Safety Data Sheets (MSDSs) on every product must be made available to each employee upon request. These sheets list every ingredient in the product. Every medical office should have an MSDS notebook, which is updated regularly.

Special regulations regarding chemical spills prevent workers from cleaning up a spill until the MSDS has been checked to determine whether there are any hazards or necessary precautions. Each spill requires an incident report listing the name of the chemical and the details of the spill—where it took place, the time, the date, who was involved, and what was done to clean it up.

Regulations for Blood-Borne Pathogens

The AIDS epidemic has focused the health care industry's safety concerns on blood-borne infections, including HIV and hepatitis B. Approximately 5.6 million employees who "reasonably could be expected" to come into contact with human blood or other potentially infectious material are affected by these regulations. The regulations cover both administrative and clinical aspects of practice.

The regulations order employers to offer hepatitis B vaccines free of charge to every employee who can be reasonably anticipated to have skin, eye, mucous membrane, or parenteral contact with blood or other potentially infectious materials.

Potentially infectious materials, in addition to products made from human blood, include semen, vaginal secretions, cerebrospinal fluid, synovial fluid, pleural fluid, pericardial fluid, saliva in dental procedures, any body fluid that is visibly contaminated with blood, and all body fluids in situations where it is difficult or impossible to differentiate between body fluids.

Regulations require universal precautions: a written exposure control plan; a list of all job classifications in which employees have occupational exposure; engineering and work practice controls; procedures for disposal of waste and sharps; availability of protective equipment, including gloves; a written schedule and method for housecleaning and decontamination, including laundry; postexposure evaluation processes; and employee training. Orange-red or fluorescent orange warning labels with the Biohazard legend must be affixed to containers of regulated waste, to refrigerators and freezers containing infectious materials, and to containers used to transport them.

UNIONS AND HEALTH CARE WORKERS

The history of the organization of health care workers dates back to 1919, when the first known attempt to organize hospital employees took place in San Francisco. The issues were shorter hours and improved working conditions. In 1936, the American Federation of Labor organized engine room, laundry, and dietary employees; nurse's aides; and orderlies in three San Francisco hospitals. Since 1946, the ANA (American Nurses' Association) has supported **collective bargaining**, and most registered nurses have chosen their state nurses' association as their collective bargaining representative. In August 1974, Public Law 93-360 amended the National Labor Relations Act (NLRA) to include nonprofit hospitals and health care institutions. By bringing hospitals, convalescent homes, HMOs, health clinics, nursing homes, and extended care facilities under the NLRA, Congress set the stage for the collective bargaining relationship between management and employees in these institutions.

collective bargaining procedural attempt to achieve collective agreements between an employer and accredited representative of a group of employees, to improve the conditions of employment

People join unions for many reasons, primarily because of dissatisfaction with wages, benefits, or working conditions. The job you hold determines the **bargaining unit** you may join. When a union is organized, the employer and the union are obligated to bargain in good faith with one another.

Among nurses, collective bargaining is relatively well established but still is a controversial and emotional subject. Unions have had mixed results in organizing hospital clerical personnel. Health maintenance organizations and other alternative health delivery systems offer a fertile field for union organizers. Whether to join a union is a personal decision that depends on an individual's philosophy. It requires considerable self-examination and a weighing of the positive and negative aspects of union membership.

bargaining unit the labor union, or group of employees with similar interests, authorized to conduct negotiations on behalf of the employees who are members of the union or group

WORKING CONDITIONS

The working conditions in a medical office should be defined in individual job descriptions, an office handbook, and procedure manuals.

Job Description

Every position in an office should have a job description. Some job descriptions are divided into two parts: the responsibilities required of each employee and the listing of tasks to be performed by each employee. Examples include the following:

The front desk personnel will:

- answer the telephone,
- make appointments for new and returning patients,

- collect co-payments and other payments for services,
- greet patients and others who enter the office, and
- complete other tasks as assigned.

The clinical personnel will:

- take patients' vital signs and update the medical chart before they see the physician,
- assist in preparing patients for examination,
- prepare and administer medications as directed by the physician,
- collect and prepare laboratory specimens, and
- complete other tasks as assigned.

The administrative personnel will:

- interview patients and obtain insurance plan and identification numbers;
- complete all third-party billing forms;
- transcribe letters dictated by the physician;
- maintain, control access to, and file patients' medical records; and
- complete other tasks as assigned.

Although the preceding lists are just examples, remember that job descriptions are an essential part of written standard office procedures and establish authority and responsibility for carrying out procedures.

Procedures Manual

In addition to the job description, each office should have a procedures manual. A procedures manual describes in detail the manner in which a task in the job description should be carried out. It is important as an educational tool for new employees, as well as a resource for substitutes when a regular office employee is ill or on vacation. Written standard office procedures help maintain high standards of patient care, protect against the omission of important steps, ensure compliance with government and third-party regulations, and decrease the possibility of a malpractice action. They aid in achieving the **risk management** goals for the office as well as maintaining **quality assurance**.

If a patient is injured during a procedure and the guidelines for performing the procedure as written in the procedures manual were not followed, the health care employee could be **negligent per se** without **mitigating** circumstances. If an employee is injured during the performance of a procedure and the guidelines for performing the procedure were not followed, the employee could be guilty of contributory negligence. In contrast, following the procedures manual conscientiously could absolve the employee and/or the physician of any fault, particularly if it is shown that some other factor caused the patient's injury.

risk management the practice of considering the risk of actions taken and taking steps to minimize the risk associated with them

quality assurance responsibility to uphold the quality of care patients receive

negligent per se conduct that is against common knowledge that, by its act, without argument, can be declared negligence

mitigating make less severe due to considerations of fairness and mercy

The importance of a procedures manual is illustrated in the following Georgia case involving a nurse at a Kaiser call center working without written protocol. Medical call centers are identified as nurse-triage lines, demand management call centers, or nurse-on-call centers and function 24 hours a day to allow patients an opportunity to make informed, cost-effective health care choices.

A nurse received a call from a family with an infant with a 104-degree fever. She recommended that the child be driven to a network hospital forty-five minutes from home. The parents drove part way and circled back to the nearest hospital emergency room. The infant suffered circulatory collapse and lost both hands and most of both legs. The family sued alleging that the nurse's bad advice caused delay in treatment which in turn caused circulatory collapse and loss of limbs. On February 2, 1995, a Fulton County jury found Kaiser negligent and awarded the family in excess of $45,000,000 in damages.

Kearney, K. A. (1996). Legal liability and risk considerations for a medical call center. *The Health Lawyer, 9*(3), 20

Employee Handbook   The Employee Handbook usually provides personnel policies and related instructions. It includes information about work hours, sick leave, pension benefits, evaluation procedures, and so on. If the company is unionized, the handbook cannot be changed without negotiating with the union, whereas if the employees are not protected by a union, handbook changes are usually placed in a prominent place to put employees on notice prior to company policy change. Some courts consider the handbook an extension of the employment contract, whereas other courts hold the opposite. In either situation, the handbook is an important document whose contents should be reviewed and understood early in the employer–employee relationship.

COLLECTIONS

Overdue Accounts

Every business has overdue accounts. Some patients do not pay because they do not have the money, but others are habitual delinquents. Office personnel who are on top of collection problems keep in contact with patients and update addresses and phone numbers.

The first step in collection is to contact the individual and determine whether there is a valid reason for the failure to pay. The second step is to set up a pay schedule. If a patient owes the physician, that patient probably owes many others as well. In all instances, if your office has a protocol that differs from what is described herein, follow your office protocol.

Some physicians prefer to handle all collections through the mail and make use of colored stickers that are available to place on an overdue bill to emphasize the matter. Because the debt is "incurred primarily for family or household purposes," attempting to collect the due amount is subject to a number of federal and state regulations. The medical assistant should know and follow office policy and procedure when trying to collect overdue accounts. If a physician's staff members or their agents engage in overly vigorous collection activity, they risk being sued for defamation, invasion of privacy, intentional infliction of emotional distress, or other torts.

The federal Fair Debt Collection Practices Act (FDCPA) prohibits many different collection practices—for example, threats of violence, use of abusive language when trying to collect the debt, harassment by means of phone calls, and deception and unfair methods of collection (e.g., threatening to deposit a postdated check before the date of the check, intentionally causing the debtor's other checks to be dishonored).

Collection Practice

A typical office policy regarding collections will generally be to notify the debtor in writing of the amount due. Typically, a phone call may precede a letter to serve as a "friendly reminder," for example at 30 days. At 60 days, a letter would be sent; followed by another letter at 90 days. Typically, a medical office will not send the account to a collection agency until the account is 120 days past due. If the collection agency is unsuccessful with its techniques, the account may move to the legal arena.

A typical collection suit begins with the filing of a small claims action in civil court. If uncontested, a judgment will be entered for the plaintiff (creditor). If contested, the judge makes a ruling on the facts as presented by the parties before the court, and issues an order or a judgment. Once the judgment is issued, and if the debtor fails to pay, there are follow-up procedures to ensure that the judgment is satisfied.

Bad Checks

A check tendered for services rendered that is returned unpaid by the bank, for whatever reason, is grounds for a criminal complaint. In some states, creditors are allowed to simultaneously pursue both criminal and civil actions to secure payment; in others, the creditor must choose the venue. A criminal suit cannot be used to settle a civil action.

Collection of physicians' fees is complicated because of third-party reimbursement. Regardless of the insurance coverage, the patient is responsible for the payment of the fee unless the physician has entered into an agreement to accept the insurer's rate of payment as payment in full.

Bankruptcy Bankruptcy is the process by which a financially troubled individual or business is declared by a bankruptcy court to be incapable of paying his or her debts, the debtor's available assets are distributed to creditors as required by bankruptcy law, and the debtor is granted a discharge from liability for most of the remaining unpaid debts. There are three major kinds of bankruptcy proceedings: liquidation, business reorganization, and repayment plans for debtors with regular income. After an individual initiates bankruptcy proceedings, the creditor (e.g., a physician's office) may not seek payment from the debtor patient. The creditor may only communicate with the court-appointed receiver.

Letter to Terminate Delinquent Patients

When a patient refuses or is unable to pay a medical bill, the physician must make a decision about whether to continue to treat that patient. If the physician decides to terminate the patient, the following procedures should be followed to avoid abandoning the patient:

1. Write a letter to the patient stating that the bill is overdue and has been overdue for a defined period of time. Often offices will have templates for these types of letters, so you will not have to start your letter from scratch.

2. Check the contents and form of the letter with the physician's attorney to make certain that the procedure complies with all local and federal laws.

3. Allow the patient a reasonable amount of time during which payment will be accepted (30 days). Inform the patient that the physician–patient relationship will be terminated after that date.

4. Mail the letter first-class, certified mail, return receipt requested. In addition, send another copy of the letter regular first-class mail. Many times patients will not pick up certified mail at the post office but will open or at least accept a first-class letter at the door. First-class mail is not returned to the office unless the person is no longer at the address.

5. The return of the certified mail with notification of the first-class mailing on the bottom of the letter will document that the letter has been mailed.

6. Keep records of the letter and the return postal receipt in the patient's chart.

7. Keep detailed notes in the patient's chart of any further communication the patient has with the office.

8. If your employer has different procedures in place, follow your employer's procedures.

☑ SUMMARY

- Because medicine is closely regulated by state and federal law, it is necessary for employees to be aware of laws and regulations that define the procedures they are permitted to perform.
- Discrimination is an issue in the hiring and promotion of employees.
- Sexual harassment is defined as a form of discrimination, and it is a serious problem for women in the workforce.
- The ADA regulates the hiring and promotion of physically and mentally disabled individuals. The FADA protects the rights of older workers. The Equal Pay Act prevents the practice of paying women less than men for the same job. The FLSA establishes a federal minimum wage, mandates extra pay for overtime work, and regulates the employment of children. The ERISA involves pensions. The OSHA affects health care workers, particularly with regulations involving right-to-know laws and blood-borne pathogens.
- Workers' compensation and Social Security affect every employer and employee.
- Medicare and Medicaid are government-sponsored health care delivery and compensation systems.
- Procedures manuals, job descriptions, and employee handbooks are all part of the business side of a medical practice, as are laws affecting collection procedures.

SUGGESTED ACTIVITIES

1. Sexual harassment is a problem in almost every workplace. To determine your level of sophistication about harassing behaviors, answer the following questionnaire. Discuss your answers with your classmates.

---

1. What percentage of the female workforce is affected by sexual harassment? _____ percent

	AGREE	DISAGREE
2. Only young and attractive women are harassed.	❐	❐
3. Bosses are the only ones who have the power to sexually harass.	❐	❐
4. The way a woman dresses influences whether or not she is harassed.	❐	❐

5. Sexual harassment is only a problem between people. ☐ ☐

6. We have laws to protect people against sexual harassment. ☐ ☐

7. There is an equal amount of sexual harassment of men as of women. ☐ ☐

8. Ignoring sexual harassment is the best way to handle it. ☐ ☐

9. Sexual comments and advances should only be considered as sexual harassment if they are repeated more than once. ☐ ☐

(Adapted from Massachusetts State Department of Education, Sexual Harassment Survey)

2. Find the website for a cleaning product you like. Does it have an MSDS posted anywhere on the website? Do they have a number to call if you want the product's MSDS?

STUDY QUESTIONS

1. Construct a hiring interview for a woman you suspect is pregnant.
2. What Act would you reference if a coworker asked you if she would be able to take time away from work for several weeks to care for her child?
3. One of the medical assistants receives a needle stick. As office manager, what would you do?
4. Write a letter requesting payment on an overdue account of a friend of the physician.

CASES FOR DISCUSSION

1. Joan Leikvold was hired by Valley View Community Hospital as an operating room supervisor in 1972. She did not have a contract for a specific duration, nor was she told that the hospital would not discharge her except for cause. She was provided with a policy manual and told that the policies were to be followed in her employment relationship with the hospital. In 1978, she became the director of nursing. In October 1979, she requested a transfer back to her former position in the operating room. The chief executive officer (CEO) felt that it was inadvisable for someone who had been in a managerial position to take

a subordinate position. Leikvold withdrew the transfer request but was subsequently fired. Her personnel record indicated "insubordination" as the reason for discharge.

Leikvold was an at-will employee. *At-will* means that there is a contract made for an indefinite duration and either party, employer or employee, may terminate the contract at any time for any reason, or without reason, provided the reason is not discriminatory. Can the CEO fire Leikvold?

2. Plaintiff Raymond Vadnais alleged that, in 1986, he visited [a physician] at Beth Israel Hospital's ear, nose, and throat clinic complaining of ear pain. After antibiotics failed to relieve the pain, [the physician] recommended surgery. However, after [the physician] learned that the plaintiff was infected with HIV, he refused to perform the operation. Should the physician be required to perform the operation?

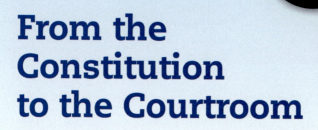

From the Constitution to the Courtroom

 The powers not delegated to the United States by the Constitution, nor prohibited by it to the States, are reserved to the States respectively, or to the people.

Tenth Amendment to the Constitution of the United States (1791)

OBJECTIVES

After reading this chapter, you should be able to:

1. Differentiate between federal and state law.
2. Differentiate between the origins of statutory, administrative, and common law.
3. Understand what makes up a federalist government.
4. Identify the steps necessary for the passage of federal and state legislation.
5. Distinguish between the appellate paths of the federal judicial system and the state judicial system.
6. Identify three administrative law agencies involved in the regulation of the medical office.
7. Identify the parties to a lawsuit.
8. Explain basic trial procedures.
9. Identify the stages of an appeal.
10. Demonstrate techniques that aid in being a good witness.

BUILDING YOUR LEGAL VOCABULARY

Adjudicate	Interrogatory
Arbitration	Judgment
Assault	Mediation
Battery	Misdemeanor
Beyond a reasonable doubt	Motion
Cert. denied	Negligent act
Civil	Negotiation
Common law	Perjury
Concurrent	Plaintiff
Contingency	Preponderance of evidence
Criminal	Pretrial conference
Cross-examination	Reformation
Defendant	Restraint
Deposition	Retribution
Deterrence	Standard of proof
Direct examination	Strict liability
District attorney	Tort
Enumerate	Writ of certiorari
Felony	

IT ALL STARTS WITH THE CONSTITUTION

The American system of government and its legal system flow from the Constitution. The Constitution determines whether federal or state law is applicable and enforceable. Federal, state, statutory, administrative, and common law all recognize the Supremacy Clause of the U.S. Constitution. The legal system dictates how disputes are resolved in courts. Once a dispute exists, the process is predictable but not always enjoyable. Testifying as a witness in a lawsuit can give you knots in your stomach, a sense of self-doubt, and sleepless nights. Knowledge is the best antidote.

When the U.S. Constitution was enacted in 1787, it included a Preamble and seven statements, called Articles, which broadly described how the new nation would function. Since then, 27 Amendments to the Constitution have been added. The Preamble, the Articles, and the Amendments make up the Constitution that provides the structure for federal and state government in the United States.

The Constitution's first three Articles address the separation of powers, which expressly separates the federal government into three distinct branches: the executive (president), the legislative (Congress), and the judicial (federal courts). It is this separation of powers that allows for a system of "checks and balances," where no one branch of government is more powerful than another. The system of checks and balances prevents abuse of power by ensuring that the powers of each branch of government can be reviewed by another branch of government.

The concept of "federalism" arises in the Constitution's next three Articles. Federalism is a system of government that, in the United States, recognizes two **concurrent** government structures: the federal and state governments, where each has specific powers. Some of these powers are overlapping. The states govern a majority of everyday legislation and services pursuant to the Constitution. The Supremacy Clause, discussed later, ensures that the federal government can legislate certain matters that fall under one of its enumerated powers, including interstate commerce and foreign relations.

concurrent happening at the same time

Article I, Section 8 of the Constitution and subsequent Amendments **enumerate** the federal government's powers and responsibilities. These powers and responsibilities are referred to as enumerated powers. The Tenth Amendment clarifies that "[t]he powers not delegated to the United States by the Constitution, nor prohibited by it to the states, are reserved to the states respectively, or to the people."

enumerate to list a number of things

The first ten Constitutional Amendments (also referred to as the "The Bill of Rights") define issues of social liberty and justice afforded to the U.S. citizens. The remaining 17 Amendments further define issues of social liberty and justice, government structure and protocol, and powers of the federal government. You can find a copy of the Constitution and the Bill of Rights at https://www.archives.gov.

The Supremacy Clause

A fundamental part of the U.S. federalist structure is Article VI, Clause 2 (also referred to as "the Supremacy Clause"), which reads, "[t]his Constitution, and the laws of the United States which shall be made in pursuance thereof; and all treaties made, or which shall be made, under the authority of the United States, shall be the supreme law of the land; and the judges in every state shall be bound thereby, anything in the Constitution or laws of any State to the contrary notwithstanding." Consequently, when there is a conflict between federal and state law, the Constitution tells us that federal law will govern. There are exceptions to this rule.

Enumerated Powers

The Constitution enumerates the federal government's powers, as well as concurrent powers shared with the states. States may legislate issues that have been constitutionally reserved for the federal government provided the state laws do not conflict with the federal laws.

The Constitution could not expressly define every enumerated power the federal government needs to govern effectively. As a result, disputes arise that challenge the federal government's authority to enact or implement a law. In these instances, courts use legal analysis to decide whether the disputed action by the federal government falls within its enumerated powers.

The Interstate Commerce Clause   The Commerce Clause (Article I, Section 8, Clause 3) describes enumerated powers found in the U.S. Constitution. The clause states that the U.S. Congress shall have the power "[t]o regulate commerce with foreign nations, and among the several states, and with the Indian tribes." The Interstate Commerce Clause specifically refers to the federal government's power to legislate "among the several states."

When an act of commerce involves more than one state, the Interstate Commerce Clause is often used as legal authority for Congress to exercise legislative power over state activities. Over many years and many different lawsuits, courts have expanded the definition of "commerce" as it pertains to whether Congress may legislate. A narrow definition of "commerce" is a business transaction. The broad definition includes many types of interaction, both of a business and a social nature.

The Necessary and Proper Clause (Article 1, Section 8, Clause 18) is frequently used together with the Interstate Commerce Clause to further justify Congress' authority to make certain laws. The Necessary and Proper Clause states that Congress is authorized to "make all laws which shall be necessary and proper for carrying into execution the foregoing powers, and all other powers vested by this Constitution in the government of the United States, or in any department or officer thereof." As a result, the Necessary and Proper Clause gives Congress the power to pass laws that are "necessary and proper" to carry out its express powers, which can be interpreted in many ways.

Executive Branch

The president and the president's cabinet make up the executive branch. The president appoints the cabinet members, who are then confirmed by the Senate. The cabinet is an advisory committee comprised of the vice president and the heads of 15 federal agencies (each head, with a few exceptions, holds the title of "Secretary"). The federal agencies represented in the cabinet are Department of State, Department of the Treasury, Department of Defense, Attorney General, Department of the Interior, Department of Agriculture, Department of Commerce, Department of Labor, Department of Health and Human Services, Department of Housing and Urban Development, Department of Transportation, Department of Energy, Department of Education, Department of Veterans Affairs, and Department of Homeland Security. The executive branch is responsible for carrying out and executing laws made by Congress.

Congress

Congress is made up of the House of Representatives and the Senate, who together pass legislation. See Figure 3-1, *How an idea becomes a law*. Legislation is also referred to as statutory law or Statutes. Article I, Section 8 of the Constitution enumerates all of Congress' express powers, including the power to tax and to spend those taxes for the citizens' welfare, to borrow money, to create money, to declare war, to regulate immigration, among many others.

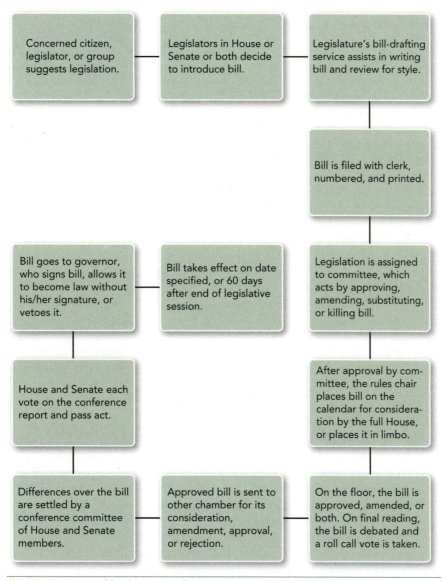

Figure 3-1 How an idea becomes a law

Congress has 535 voting members, including 435 Representatives and 100 Senators. Each state has two senators elected to serve six-year terms. The members of the House of Representatives are each elected for a two-year term, and there may be no more than 435 at any one time. Each House of Representative member represents a specific geographical district, which is determined proportionately by the number of people living in the district. Each state must have at least one representative in the House.

The Judiciary

The objective of the federal judicial branch is, in part, to interpret whether laws are Constitutional. As part of the checks and balances system of federalism, the judiciary reviews laws passed by Congress and the president to ensure the laws are Constitutional.

There are judicial branches of government in both the federal and state systems, and they operate very similarly. There are many rules related to jurisdiction that determine whether a lawsuit belongs in the federal court or a state court. Federal courts are the appropriate forum for lawsuits arising from federal law. In some instances, lawsuits arising from state law are decided in federal court if the plaintiff and defendant reside in different states. When the plaintiffs and defendants are in the same state, lawsuits arising from state law are typically decided by state courts.

The structures of the federal and state legal systems are comparable. There are usually three levels of courts: the trial court, the mid-level appellate court, and the highest level appellate court. See Figure 3-2, *Federal and state appellate processes*. The federal court system divides the United States into Circuits representing certain regions of the country, and within each Circuit are several Districts. In the federal system, the trial court is referred to as the "District Court," the mid-level appellate court is the "Circuit Court," and the highest court in the land is the "U.S. Supreme Court." There is but one Supreme Court, located in Washington, D.C.

HEALTH CARE: FEDERAL OR STATE LAW?

Health care professionals today regularly face a confusing mix of federal and state law. But, this was not always the case. For the most part, in United States' early years, the federal government did not legislate health care. The Constitution does not contain any express federal powers or rights related to health care. The enumerated powers, including the Interstate Commerce Clause, the Supremacy Clause, and the Necessary and Proper Clause have, however, played a part in allowing the federal government to legislate health care.

State Appellate Process

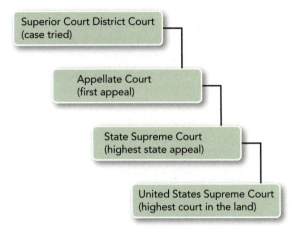

Federal Appellate Process

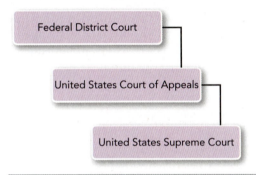

Figure 3-2 Federal and state appellate processes

After the Great Depression in the early 1930s, President Franklin D. Roosevelt instituted The New Deal programs focused, in part, on citizen welfare, including Social Security. The spirit of these programs was continued when President Lyndon B. Johnson created additional federal programs related to health care in the 1960s. Medicare was created then as a federal program that assists retirement age and disabled citizens with health insurance. Medicaid was, and still is, a joint federal and state effort to provide health care to low income mothers and children, disabled citizens, and the elderly. In addition, President Johnson enacted several programs focused on health through nutrition, including Food Stamps and school lunch programs. Often, the funding of health care programs is a federal matter and the states administrate the programs in accordance with a mix of state and federal regulations.

Over the past 60 years, the federal government's involvement in health care matters has fluctuated depending on the then-current president's view of federalism. Some presidents believed that the federal government should be less involved with health care matters and that the states should be more involved, while other presidents sought to increase the federal government's involvement and lessen the state's involvement. The tension between the federal and the state governments is a hallmark of federalism. As a result, the federal and state governments have become increasingly intertwined in health care funding and regulation.

The Affordable Care Act (ACA) raised a highly contested debate between the federal and state governments regarding the constitutionality of requiring all citizens to purchase health insurance. Congress passed the ACA and contended that the Interstate Commerce Clause, among others, provided the authority. Opponents argued that the Interstate Commerce Clause could not provide the authority to Congress because the failure to purchase insurance was not "commerce." The federal government also took the position that its authority came from its enumerated power to tax.

After the ACA was signed into law in March 2010, 26 states filed a lawsuit against the federal government in a Florida district court and alleged that the requirement to purchase insurance was unconstitutional. In January 2011, the district court judge ruled that Congress did not have the power to require the purchase of health insurance. The court also ruled that the rest of the ACA could not stand without the insurance provision, so he struck down the entire Act. The Department of Health and Human Services appealed the decision. In August 2011, a panel of three judges from the 11th Circuit Court of Appeals agreed with the lower court and affirmed the decision to strike the insurance requirement. At the same time, the appellate court ruled that the ACA could stand on its own and reversed the part of the lower court decision that struck the entire ACA. The department of Health and Human Services then petitioned the Supreme Court to hear the case, which is referenced as *National Federation of Independent Business v. Sebelius*, 567 U.S. (2012).

Supreme Court Chief Justice Roberts wrote the part of the decision related to the insurance requirement and said, "The Affordable Care Act's requirement that certain individuals pay a financial penalty for not obtaining health insurance may reasonably be characterized as a tax. Because the Constitution permits such a tax, it is not our role to forbid it, or to pass upon its wisdom or fairness." A majority of the Supreme Court justices also held that another controversial part of the Act that expanded Medicaid was unconstitutional as it would force states to decide between accepting the expansion and risking the loss of current Medicaid funding from the federal government.

The Health Insurance Portability and Accountability Act of 1996 (HIPAA) is another example health care-related federal law. HIPAA ensures that patients have the same right of privacy across the United

States, and that insurance companies and health care providers have the same obligations to protect patient health information regardless of the state of their location or business. At the same time, states have enacted laws that mirror HIPAA and are sometimes more stringent. Medical care professionals should be aware of the federal HIPAA regulations, as well as the regulations of the state where they work.

Some aspects of health care, such as the regulation of physicians, are largely handled by the state. Medical practice acts and health care licensing regulations directly affect health care professionals. All states have nursing practice acts, and some have medical assistant practice acts. As health care becomes increasingly specialized and more expensive, there has been more cross-training among professionals and other medical office professionals have assumed more specialized duties, and regulation of those who work in health care has expanded.

ADMINISTRATIVE LAW

Administrative law governs the activities of administrative agencies of government. Both federal and state governments have administrative law. To enable the federal government to exercise its authority and enforce the law, Congress delegates authority to administrative agencies. Administrative agencies then make rules and regulations pertaining to the agency's specialty. Congress may give certain agencies power to **adjudicate** disputes involving the application of those rules to particular parties under certain circumstances. In carrying out their responsibilities, agencies usually perform one or more of the following functions: (1) rule making, (2) adjudication, (3) prosecution, (4) advising, (5) supervision, and (6) investigation. Examples of federal agencies include the Federal Aviation Administration, Centers for Disease Control and Prevention, Federal Emergency Management Agency, Drug Enforcement Agency, among many hundred others.

adjudicate to hear and resolve a lawsuit by a judicial process

COMMON LAW

Common law is different, but no less valid, from law enacted by Congress (statutory law) and administrative law. Common law is judge-made law that arises, in part, from judges' interpretation of statutory or administrative law. Judges wishing to be fair and consistent in the administration of justice decide cases by looking to the past and basing their decisions on similar past decisions when the facts are substantially the same. This has given rise to the principle of *stare decisis*, which is Latin for "let the decision stand." *Stare decisis* gives stability and predictability to the court system yet allows for flexibility when there are new or different facts.

common law law created by judge's decisions and by customs

THE DISTINCTION BETWEEN CRIMINAL AND CIVIL LAW

criminal the system of law concerned with crimes against the state or someone who has been proven guilty of such an offense

civil the system of law concerned with lawsuits between individuals or between an individual and the state where the case does not relate to the violation of a criminal statute

plaintiff one who brings a court action against another

defendant a person or party against whom a plaintiff's allegations are brought

felony a crime more serious than a misdemeanor and punishable by imprisonment for more than one year or death

misdemeanor an offense less serious than a felony and which may be punished by a fine or sentence to a local prison for less than one year

assault any deliberate attempt or threat to inflict bodily injury on another person and with apparent ability to do so

battery illegal touching of another person

reformation the rehabilitation of a criminal; changed behavior

restraint restriction of liberty

retribution something given or demanded in payment or as a punishment for criminal wrongdoing

deterrence punishment used to discourage crime

In both the federal and the state court systems, there are two major divisions of law: **criminal** and **civil**. In a criminal case, the state is the **plaintiff**; the person charged with the crime is the **defendant**; and the defendant may face imprisonment. Later in this chapter, illustrations of direct examination and cross-examination use the actual testimony of Anne Capute, a nurse on trial for knowingly giving an overdose of morphine to a terminally ill patient.

A crime is defined as the performance of an act forbidden by law or the omission of an act required by law. In either case, the criminal defendant is punished by society. Crimes are divided into felonies and misdemeanors. A **felony** is a crime punishable by death or imprisonment. A **misdemeanor** is a crime punishable by imprisonment in jail for less than one year or a fine. See Figure 3-3, *The criminal case process*. State and federal legislatures define conduct that determines whether an act is a crime and, if so, whether it is a felony or misdemeanor. In a criminal case, the defendant is found guilty or not guilty. In a civil case, the defendant is found liable or not liable.

It is also possible to have a civil case arising from a criminal act. A defendant in a civil case, however, does not face the possibility of imprisonment. In a civil case, if a defendant loses the case, the defendant usually has to pay the victim money damages. For example, in an **assault** and **battery** criminal prosecution, the state tries a defendant for the crime of assault and battery. A defendant that is found guilty is then punished by the state. The victim in such a case is neither a plaintiff nor a defendant in the criminal case. The purposes of punishment are **reformation**, **restraint**, **retribution**, and **deterrence**. In some instances, the victim may then attempt to collect damages from the defendant by bringing a civil lawsuit for assault and battery. In some cases, a defendant who is not guilty of a criminal charge can be found liable for damages in a subsequent civil suit. See Figure 3-4, *The civil case process*.

The case of O.J. Simpson provides a good example. Simpson was accused and found not guilty of murdering his ex-wife Nicole and her friend Ron Goldman. Even though Simpson was found not guilty, the Goldman family members sued Simpson in civil court for the wrongful death of their son and were awarded damages of $33.5 million. The reason a civil jury could find Simpson liable and the jury in the criminal case found him not guilty is because of the difference in the **standard of proof** required in each type of case. The standard of proof in a civil case is **preponderance of the evidence**. The higher standard in the criminal case—**beyond a reasonable doubt**—prevented the jury from finding Simpson guilty.

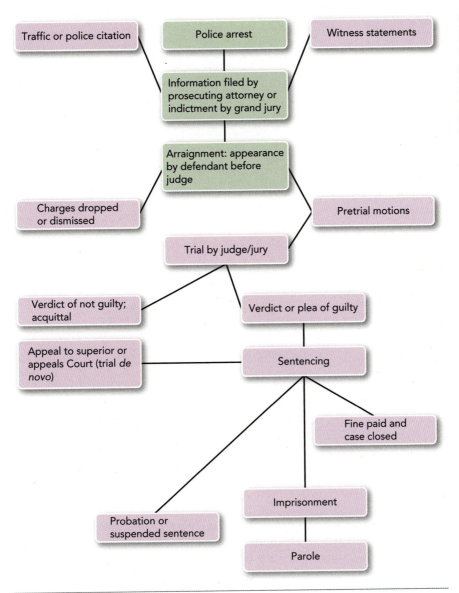

Figure 3-3 The criminal case process

standard of proof level of proof required, which is established by considering all evidence

preponderance of the evidence the greater weight of the evidence that is more likely than not

beyond a reasonable doubt evidence so strong and credible that it leaves no more than a remote possibility that there is another explanation for what happened

tort a private wrong or injury, other than breach of contract, for which the court will provide a remedy

negligent act failure to take reasonable precautions to protect others from the risk of harm

strict liability responsibility of a seller or manufacturer for any defective product unduly threatening personal safety

The most common civil lawsuit in the health care industry is an action known as a **tort**. Tort liability is based on one of the following grounds: intentional acts, **negligent acts**, or **strict liability**. Intentional torts may be actions toward property or a person. Negligence may be the result of the performance of an act on a patient without using due care or the failure to do something that is required. Strict liability is imposed on a seller or manufacturer for physical harm caused to a

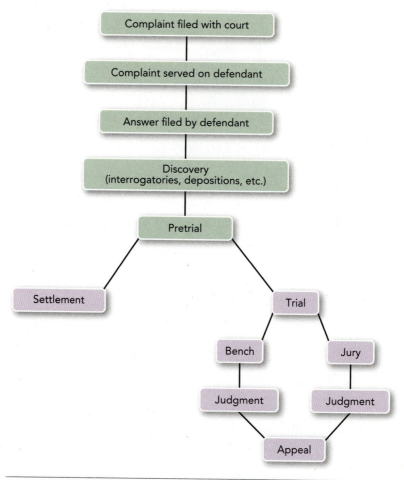

Figure 3-4 The civil case process

user or consumer when a product is in a defective and unreasonably dangerous condition. Although common law once included both criminal and civil law, most crimes have now been defined by state or federal statute. Of interest to medical office professionals is medical malpractice, which is a civil law tort.

INTO THE COURTROOM

Now that you have some background as to the different types of laws and lawsuits, it makes sense to talk about trial. Chapter 6 contains an in-depth discussion of Medical Malpractice cases, and the next section is a summary of the process and what might happen should you be named as a party in a lawsuit or a called as a witness.

What Happens During a Lawsuit

Medical malpractice attorneys estimate that fewer than 10 percent of the malpractice lawsuits that are filed actually go to trial. It is also estimated that of those that go to court, only 10 percent result in a final **judgment**. The remaining cases are settled out of court either by agreement, **arbitration**, or **mediation**. Settling may take place at any time, including before a case is filed, after judgment, or during or after an appeal. Medical malpractice lawsuits follow the same steps as other civil litigation lawsuits and pass through the phases described in the following sections.

Phase I   The first phase is the time period in which the alleged negligence occurs. The patient becomes aware that he or she has been injured or that something is not quite right and complains to the physician or another professional. Insurance companies require their insured to file an incident report at the earliest possible time. These reports collect facts but do not admit fault. Sometimes professionals deny there is a problem and fail to file an incident report. Sometimes they try to shift the burden of guilt onto the patient. Anger can become a significant problem. The patient is angry, the relatives are angry, and the professional becomes angry. If the physician is unable to smooth over the incident, a medical assistant or other member of the office staff may be able to dissipate the anger and head off litigation.

Office personnel can work to make this happen by improving the relationship between the physician and the patient. In a book by R.M. McGraw, *Ferment in Medicine*, the following psychological factors are found to be at the root of many malpractice cases: "the need to be noticed, the need to be thought worth something, and the need to be loved." Recent studies of quality control experts reaffirm the importance of the patient–physician relationship. There is a high correlation between satisfaction with health care and the development of a trusting relationship between the professional and the patient. A professional office staff can complement the physician in all these areas. Many times a patient is more comfortable and finds it less intimidating to ask medical office professionals questions. You should always document these conversations and place them in the patient's file.

Phase II   When the patient seeks the advice of an attorney regarding the alleged harm, the second phase begins. The first thing an experienced medical malpractice attorney will do is obtain a copy of the patient's medical records. This may be done by asking the patient to obtain personal records or by having the patient sign an authorization to allow the physician to release the records to the attorney. Physicians and health care facilities often charge for providing the medical records to authorized parties other than the patient.

judgment a court's decision regarding the rights and obligations of the parties in a dispute

arbitration a hearing held between two or more parties who disagree on an issue but agree in advance to abide by the decision of an impartial third person

mediation a neutral party meets with the plaintiff and defendant with the intent of persuading them to settle their dispute

The original medical records should *never* be released. You should only release a copy of a patient's medical records after verifying that a signed release form is in the patient's chart. Always document who received what records and when, how the records were delivered, and the amount paid. This should show as a charting entry with the initials (or name) of the person who gave the documents to the requestor. It is also good risk management policy to require at least 24 hours for requests to be processed and to allow for discussion and review with the physician. The fees charged for the medical record copies must be reasonable and customary, and only those documents specifically requested should be duplicated and provided. Ask the requestor to identify a specific period of time for which records are sought.

The patient's lawyer will have one or more experts review the records and may have an independent physician examine the patient. At this point, the patient will, within the legal system, be referred to as a plaintiff. Plaintiff's attorneys most often only take malpractice cases on a **contingency** basis, which means that the lawyer will not be paid unless the plaintiff recovers monetary damages. If the plaintiff does not recover any monetary damages, the lawyer is not owed any fees.

During the second phase, the insurance company, the physician, and the attorney for the patient may negotiate a settlement. If these **negotiations** do not result in a settlement, the patient's attorney files a "Complaint," which details the facts of the case and the allegations of what went wrong, who is to blame, and how the plaintiff has been hurt. When a Complaint is filed, the patient officially becomes the plaintiff and the physician or health care facility becomes the defendant. The defendant then provides a response to the plaintiff's Complaint, which is called an "Answer." Often the parties will meet with the judge assigned to the case, where they will create a schedule for the rest of the case. At this point, the parties will begin "Discovery," which is a name for the various ways that the parties collect factual information regarding the case. Discovery includes **depositions**, **interrogatories**, **motions**, and witness identification, among others.

The end of the second phase of the lawsuit comes when discovery is complete, a **pretrial conference** is held, and the judge declares the case is ready for trial.

Phase III

A trial is a means of settling a dispute between two parties before a judge and jury. A jury determines what facts are credible, and the judge determines what specific laws are involved in the matter. A bench trial is one where the judge takes the place of the jury. The plaintiff presents the facts of the case as he or she sees them, and the defendant has the opportunity to present the facts of the case as he or she sees them. The finder of fact—the jury, or the judge, if it is a bench trial—determines what facts are credible. The judge oversees the trial and makes decisions about the relevant law. Rarely is a trial as dramatic and colorful as those portrayed on television and in the movies.

contingency something that may occur but is dependent on an uncertain future event

negotiation exchange and consideration of offers until parties agree on a solution that is acceptable to both

deposition a prior sworn statement by a witness to be used in court as testimony taken under oath and subject to cross-examination

interrogatorie written questions about a case addressed to one party by another

motion the application to a court or judge for a ruling in favor of the one applying

pretrial conference the first court conference of parties involved in a dispute

The attorneys are just people trying to make a living by presenting their clients' cases. The judge is trying to offer both parties a fair hearing, as well as keep cases moving through the court. The witnesses are ordinary people who have been subpoenaed, voluntarily or involuntarily, to provide testimony about what they observed. Frequently, one or both sides will present evidence through the use of an expert witness. This is someone who has special knowledge of the issues involved that are not commonly known to a layperson. Testimony of an expert can go beyond the facts of the case and can include matters of medicine that affect the condition of the plaintiff or the treatment by the defendant. The members of the jury are trying to listen attentively, so that they may render a fair decision.

At the start of a trial, the attorneys for both parties make opening statements, which tells the fact finder their theory of what happened. Then the plaintiff presents evidence through witnesses, documents, and expert opinions. The defense then presents its defense of the case through witnesses, documents, and expert opinions. Once the defense concludes the presentation of the defense case, a plaintiff may be provided with the opportunity to rebut certain aspects of the defense case. Then, both parties have an opportunity to present a closing statement, which summarizes the evidence presented. If there is a jury (rather than a bench trial), the judge will read the jury instructions, which tell the jurors about how they are to deliberate and the applicable law.

Once the jury concludes its deliberation, the verdict, also called the decision or the judgment, is announced in the courtroom. After the verdict is announced and damages, if any, are awarded, the lawsuit moves to Phase IV.

Phase IV   Either side has the right to appeal the decision provided there is a legal basis to do so. Usually the losing party pursues an appeal. There is a long list of legal basis that will allow an appeal. What does not constitute a legal basis for appeal, however, is that one of the parties did not like the outcome of trial and wants a "do over." The chart in Figure 3-2, *Federal and state appellate processes*, indicates the route of an appeal for most civil lawsuits tried in the state court system. The appeal of lawsuits tried in the state court system will be heard in the respective state's court of appeals. In the federal judicial system, appeals go to the Federal appellate courts, also called the Circuit Courts. The highest court in the United States is the Supreme Court, who reviews the requests and accepts fewer than 2 percent of cases it receives from lower appellate courts.

When you review Supreme Court decisions, some will be marked **"cert. denied."** This means that the Supreme Court received a **writ of certiorari** from the party appealing the decision and refused to hear the case, letting the law stand as is. According to *Black's Law Dictionary*, a writ of certiorari is an order by an appellate court that is used when the court has discretion to decide whether to hear an appeal.

cert. denied when the United States Supreme Court refuses to hear a case on appeal

writ of certiorari an order used by the United States Supreme Court to indicate the cases it wishes to hear

You as a Witness

Most lawsuits are won outside of the courtroom. The preparation of the attorney and the witnesses is crucial to winning a lawsuit. When considering your testimony, look at both sides and see where you fit into the total picture before you get to the hearing. Try to anticipate what defense the other side will offer to your remarks. Try to be objective about your strong points and weak arguments, and follow the instructions given to you by your attorney.

- Pay attention. Trials sometimes become very boring, and it is hard to follow what is happening. If you are testifying or going to be testifying, it is important to recognize that the judge and jury are looking at you, trying to determine whether you are a credible witness. The way you behave is being observed at all times. If you give deposition testimony, everything you say is being recorded and can be used against your trial testimony to test your credibility. In some cases, where the witness has a valid reason for not being able to attend trial to give testimony, the witnesses' deposition may be read into the record at trial. So, deposition testimony is extremely important. If you feel tired while you are testifying, ask for a recess. Do not daydream and mentally remove yourself from the situation. It is important that you concentrate on the proceeding.

- Behave in a professional manner. The people who are listening to you testify do not know you. The way you look and present yourself is very important when assessing your credibility. Respond clearly and in your own language to the questions. Sit up straight and do not chew gum, tap your fingers, or twirl your thumbs or hair. Dress in a manner consistent with the competent professional that you are. The opposing party's attorney will be evaluating not only your words but also how you present yourself. In some lawsuits, one witness can make or break a case.

- Answer the question and only the question. Do not offer information if it is not requested. When someone asks you a question, do not give flippant, offhand responses. Do not make a joke or answer quickly in an attempt to conclude the proceeding quickly. Think about what you are saying. If you are given something to read, make certain that you read it thoroughly. In addition, if you do not know an answer or do not understand the question, say so. Do not make up any answer and always be truthful.

- Cooperate with your attorney. If your attorney objects to a question, do not answer anyway because you think it will not hurt you. Confer privately with your attorney during a recess about any disagreements or questions.

- Honesty is the best policy. Remember, you are testifying under oath, and any false statement, no matter how small, may ruin your credibility as a witness. Lying under oath is **perjury**, which is a crime.

perjury a false statement under oath

Criminal and civil procedures are covered in volumes of material and take at least two semesters to study in law school and years to perfect in the courtroom. The material covered in this chapter will provide you with a good idea of how you generally fit into the picture if you must testify in a lawsuit.

The Art of Examination

The method used to present the facts to the judge and jury is adversarial. This means that both the plaintiff and defendant try to win their case by interviewing their own witnesses and cross-examining witnesses from the opposing side. Asking questions in an attempt to reveal certain information is an artistic endeavor. A witness should be prepared for both **direct examination** and **cross-examination**, which require different questioning techniques by the attorney and responses from the witness. Questions on direct examination will be open-ended and narrative. Questions on cross-examination are called leading questions. This is because the lawyer will usually ask questions in the form of a statement that leads the witness to agree or disagree with the statement.

direct examination the first interrogation of a witness by the party for whom the witness has been called on behalf of that party's claim

cross-examination interrogation of a witness by a party other than the direct examiner

The following is an excerpt from *Fatal Dosage*, a book written by Gary Provost involving the true story of a nurse on trial for murder. The defendant in this case is on trial for knowingly giving an overdose of morphine to a terminally ill patient. The **district attorney** is prosecuting the case for the Commonwealth of Massachusetts. Attorney Pat Piscitelli is defending the nurse, Anne Capute. In addition to providing an example of the techniques of *direct* and *cross-examination*, this section was chosen to show the importance of medical record documentation and the extent to which an individual may be required to testify to support a medical record. Mrs. Costello, Anne Capute's supervisor, is testifying about record-keeping practices at the hospital. The district attorney, Mr. Pina, in the direct examination, is trying to emphasize the number of times and the amount of morphine injected into the patient:

district attorney the official prosecutor of a judicial district

> 66 99
>
> MR. PINA: What did you discuss about that notation, 10:15 on Saturday night?
>
> MRS. COSTELLO: We discussed Anne's understanding. Again we discussed Anne's understanding of the presence of apnea.
>
> MR. PINA: What did she say?
>
> MRS. COSTELLO: She indicated to me, as I previously testified, her understanding of apnea.
>
> MR. PINA: Was what?
>
> *(Continues)*

(Continued)

MRS. COSTELLO: Absence of respiration.

MR. PINA: Did you discuss anything else about the 10:15 notation?

MRS. COSTELLO: I don't remember specifically that we did.

MR. PINA: What did you discuss next?

MRS. COSTELLO: We discussed the "11:15 morphine sulfate, forty-five milli-grams, sect, in right arm, nail beds are bluish, extremities warm, apnea ten to fifteen seconds in duration. Not responding. Condition very poor. Valium ten milligrams, IM times two at 6 p.m., and 9:45."

MR. PINA: Would you tell us what that discussion was?

MRS. COSTELLO: I asked Anne to describe to me the effects of that dose, forty-five milligrams, on the patient…and Anne stated to me that it would kill her. "My God, it would be enough to kill an elephant." After this discussion Anne acknowledged to me, "I must have killed her."

Provost, Gary, *Fatal Dosage*, pp. 196–197 (1986)

In this direct examination, the questions to the witness (Mrs. Costello) are open-ended and she is able to answer freely and in her own words. The work of the plaintiff (in this case, the district attorney) is to get the facts of the case into the record and prove the elements of the case. In a criminal case, the prosecution must prove its case beyond a reasonable doubt. What follows is the cross-examination of Mrs. Costello by Attorney Pat Piscitelli. He is trying to discredit Mrs. Costello's testimony and the hospital's procedure for document-ing medication.

66 99

The hospital's procedure for documenting medication had been criticized. Its procedure for the narration of nurses' notes had been criticized. Nursing care policies were often in conflict with other policies. One physician did not write progress notes until after the patient had been discharged. Another was using a rubber signature stamp on case histories and physicals.

ATTY. PISCITELLI: Was there a deficiency noted that telephone and verbal orders were not used sparingly and were not initialed by the physician as soon as possible?

MRS. COSTELLO: That's correct.

ATTY. PISCITELLI: Was there also a deficiency to the effect that there was no listing of nurses qualified to administer intravenous medication?

MRS. COSTELLO: That's correct.

ATTY. PISCITELLI: Was there a deficiency concerning the policy of reporting adverse effects of drugs?

MRS. COSTELLO: That's correct.

ATTY. PISCITELLI: Was it also noted that 696 records were not completed and filed within fifteen days?

MRS. COSTELLO: Yes.

The assault continued. Pat pulled out volumes of nurses' notes showing that all the minor mistakes Anne had made were being made almost daily by dozens of nurses.

Pat showed no mercy. He pointed out four and five mistakes at a time. Before long it grew into hundreds, hundreds of stupid little mistakes of the type that Anne had been criticized for. And Costello, as emotionless as a computer, was helpless. All she could do was sit there and say that Pat was correct.

Provost, Gary, *Fatal Dosage*, pp. 200–202 (1986)

The answers given by Mrs. Costello are short and controlled by Attorney Piscitelli as he works both to discredit the record keeping of the hospital and to build sympathy for his client, Anne Capute, by showing that everyone makes mistakes. That is the job of the defense attorney.

A witness on cross-examination should not try to explain his or her responses. Instead, the witness should let his or her lawyer follow up with questions to clarify after the attorney conducting the cross-examination is finished. A witness on cross-examination should simply and precisely answer the question.

☑ SUMMARY

- All law in the United States flows from the Constitution.
- The federal government concurrently exists with state government, which is the basis for a federalist system of government.
- Federal and state governments each regulate different aspects of the health care industry. In some instances, both governments regulate. The Supremacy Clause tells us that if there is a conflict between federal and state law, that federal law will govern.

- The federal government is divided in to three branches: the executive, the legislative, and the judiciary.
- The judicial branch of law, both in the federal and state governments, is responsible for settling legal disputes.
- Only a small percentage of the malpractice lawsuits go to trial.
- Each lawsuit that does go to trial follows certain phases of development. From the time the alleged negligence occurs to the time the case actually goes to trial, both sides are involved in discovery, which is a form of legal investigation.
- The outcome of the investigation may be to decide that there is no case, to settle, or to take the matter to a judge or a judge and jury. After a case has been tried, the matter may be appealed by either side.
- It is important that an individual who is a party or a witness in a trial undertake extensive preparation. Time should be spent with counsel preparing the questions and answers that the attorney will ask, as well as anticipating those of the other side. Attention also must be paid to the dress and demeanor of the witness.

SUGGESTED ACTIVITIES

1. Research the name and background of the current Secretary of Health and Human Services for the federal government. Who is the lead official on health and human services in the state where you will work?
2. Watch the short video (available online) "I'm Just a Bill" by Schoolhouse Rock, which summarizes the law-making process in an unforgettable way.
3. Research the names of the Federal Circuit Court and District Court in which your office is located.
4. Negotiation is an art and a part of everyday life. Think of an incident you have negotiated within the past week. Document the original differences between the parties, the steps that led to a solution, and the final agreement. Review the feelings you had about the experience. Practice negotiating the following situations:
   - A child wants to stay with his or her mother and not come with you to the examining room;
   - An elderly patient refuses to remove clothing for an electrocardiogram;
   - You contact a customer service representative regarding a service or product you paid for but are not satisfied with;
   - You want a raise but your employer says the company does not have the money; and

- Your employer's daughter calls and wants to speak to her mother right away. This is the fourth call within an hour and your boss does not wish to speak with her daughter again. You wish to remain on speaking terms with the child and obey your employer's wishes.

5. Watch the movie *The Verdict* with Paul Newman, an excellent portrayal of a medical malpractice cause of action. It accurately demonstrates legal procedures, the problems of the legal profession, the agony of the plaintiff, the role of the judge, the effect of politics on the court, and an example of a "real-life witness" who is involved in a malpractice action in a position similar to that of a medical assistant.

6. While watching *The Verdict*, rate the witnesses as excellent, adequate, or poor on the following items:
   - The attention span of the witness;
   - Whether the manner of the witness matched the part that was being played;
   - Whether the witness answered the questions directed to him or her; and
   - Whether the witness was cooperative.

7. Incident reports are an important part of the defense of a case. An incident report should be clear, concise, and truly objective. Practice your skills in writing such a report by observing something that happens in your school, office, or home. Document the incident in such a manner that it is truly an objective report.

8. Find a recent court case, preferably one with medical involvement, and prepare to role-play the parts of witness, plaintiff's attorney, and defendant's attorney. Practice being a credible witness, forming and answering direct examination questions, and forming and answering cross-examination questions. This will give you some idea of how it feels to be a witness and how to answer the different types of questions.

STUDY QUESTIONS

1. What are the three branches of government? Why is it necessary to separate the government in this way?

2. What are the three levels of the judiciary? And, what is the name of the highest court in the United States?

3. Can federal agencies make their own rules and prosecute those who violate the rules?

4. Explain the major distinction between criminal and civil law.

4

Criminal Acts and Intentional Torts

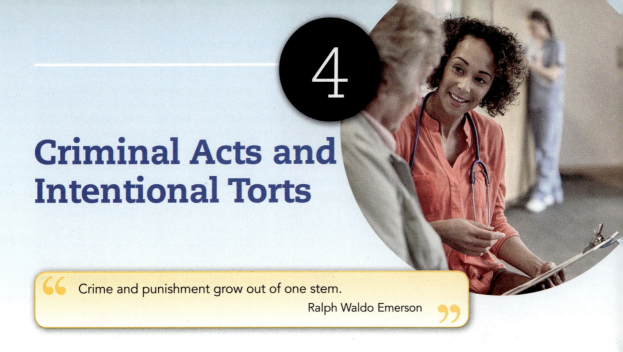

> " Crime and punishment grow out of one stem.
>
> Ralph Waldo Emerson "

OBJECTIVES

After reading this chapter you should be able to:

1. Summarize the various felonies described in the text.
2. Identify behavior that is classified as criminal.
3. Recognize some of the indicators of an abused child or elderly person.
4. Explain what types of abuse mandates reporting.
5. Distinguish between criminal and civil causes of action.
6. Describe the various types of fraud.

BUILDING YOUR LEGAL VOCABULARY

Conspiracy
Euthanasia
Larceny
Malice
Manslaughter
Murder

Qui tam lawsuit
Respectable minority
Robbery
Theft
Wanton

CRIMINAL ACTS

Criminal acts are an unfortunate reality in a health care setting. From euthanasia to the theft of prescription drugs to reporting child or elder abuse, a health care professional will encounter issues associated with crimes along the way.

There are two classifications of crimes, which depend on the severity of the crime. A misdemeanor is an offense classified lower than a felony and generally punishable by a fine or imprisonment other than in a penitentiary. A felony is defined as a crime of grave or more serious nature than those designated as misdemeanors. Under federal law and many state statutes, it is any offense punishable by imprisonment for a term exceeding one year or death. The crimes discussed in the following sections are classified as felonies.

Robbery

robbery the forcible stealing of the personal property of another either from his or her person or in the immediate presence of the victim

theft stealing property without consent of the owner

Law and medicine interact in many different ways. An individual is guilty of **robbery** if, while carrying out **theft**, the victim is physically injured or has been threatened and put in fear of bodily injury. Robberies in a health care setting are rare, but they do happen. Often the perpetrator is looking for prescription drugs or prescription pads.

Ferndale police said [the suspect] was shown on a surveillance tape putting a mask on his face and pulling out a handgun before he entered and robbed the office of a doctor's office…

The suspected pointed his gun at a receptionist and Dr. Ahmad Salahuddin and demanded money, police said. Both told the suspect they had no money and he left after stealing only a prescription pad, police said.

McConnell, M. (2014, April 21). Man suspected in armed robbery of Ferndale doctor's office arrested. *The Daily Tribune*. Retrieved from http://www.dailytribune.com/article/DT/20140421/NEWS/140429953

Murder

murder an act done with intent to kill the victim

An act done with intent to kill the victim constitutes **murder**. The state must prove guilt beyond a reasonable doubt in a criminal case. Anne Capute, described in Chapter 3, the nurse who injected "enough [morphine] to kill an elephant," was also tried for murder. In her case, the question was not whether her acts killed the patient but whether she had performed the acts with the intent to kill. In the element of intent, the jury could not find her guilty beyond a reasonable doubt.

"Anne, do you know the effects of that dosage on a patient?" asked the supervisor. "My God, it would be enough to kill an elephant," responded Anne. "Why did you give her all this medication, Anne?"

"I wanted to keep her comfortable."

Provost, G. (1986). *Fatal dosage* (pp. 196–197).

This is a conversation that took place at Morton Hospital in Taunton, Massachusetts, when a nursing supervisor first interviewed a nurse later accused of willfully and intentionally killing her patient. The interview was reconstructed in Chapter 3. The facts in this case were not disputed. Approximately a year and a half after the incident, the nurse, Anne Capute, heard the foreperson of the jury bring back the verdict of "not guilty."

A Milwaukee criminal case involving a medical laboratory that had been accused of misreading Pap smears of two women tested the question of whether a corporation can be charged with murder. The matter was brought into the courts after the deaths of the two women were reviewed by an inquest jury. The jury recommended criminal charges against the physician in charge of the lab, a lab technician, and the lab itself. As a result, the physician and technician agreed to practice restrictions. The AMA stated that this was the first case in which a medical lab had been charged with a crime because of an error. In the past, charges involving the misreading of a Pap smear were tried as malpractice cases.

Attempted Murder

An attempt to commit a crime is itself a crime. To prove that a defendant is guilty of an attempt, three things must be proven beyond a reasonable doubt: that the defendant had a specific intent to commit that particular crime; that the defendant took an overt act toward committing that crime, which was part of carrying out the crime, and came reasonably close to actually carrying out the crime; and that the defendant's act did not result in a complete crime.

Security cameras in the Vanderbilt University Medical Center parking garage spotted Dr. Ray Mettetal on August 22 in a wig, false beard, and shoes with lifts. He was seized by the campus police, who became suspicious because of his shabby disguise, and he has been held without bail since then. When he was arrested, a large syringe that investigators said contained a lethal solution of salt water and boric acid was found in the pocket of his padded trench coat.

(Continues)

Euthanasia

euthanasia an intentional action or lack of action causing the merciful death of someone suffering from a terminal illness or incurable condition

Unlike the Nurse Capute murder case, mercy killing differs in that there is intent to kill. Mercy killing is known as **euthanasia**. According to *Black's Law Dictionary*, euthanasia is the act or practice of painlessly putting to death someone suffering from incurable and distressing disease as an act of mercy. While suicide is not a crime in many states, helping someone commit suicide can have criminal implications. With the exception of a handful of states that allow for physician-assisted suicide or those who have no relevant statute, it is a criminal act to help someone end their life. Notably, penalties for acts of euthanasia tend to be more lenient than for murder. Euthanasia is further discussed in Chapter 12, Death and Dying.

Manslaughter

manslaughter an unpremeditated taking of a human life

malice an unjust intention to commit an illegal act to injure someone

wanton done with reckless disregard of another's rights or needs

respectable minority a minority acceptable to its peer group

Manslaughter is defined as the unlawful killing of another without **malice**. For there to be a conviction for manslaughter, it is necessary to prove that there is **wanton** or reckless conduct. Every physician makes errors in judgment at some point in his or her career, but an error in judgment is not necessarily wanton or reckless conduct. A misdiagnosed condition or error in treatment, so long as the judgment had some recognizable foundation in medicine, may result in civil liability but will not be considered criminal conduct.

Manslaughter is the charge when a physician does not practice in good faith, uses a form of treatment not accepted by at least a **respectable minority** of the medical profession, or practices under the influence of drugs or alcohol, causing death to a patient. In the following case, former physician Conrad Murray was convicted of manslaughter in the death of famed entertainer Michael Jackson.

Conrad Murray was a physician hired by Michael Jackson to serve as his personal physician for the "This Is It" tour in 2009. Mr. Murray was a cardiologist with a specialty in internal medicine. While in rehearsals for the tour, Mr. Murray would arrive at Mr. Jackson's home every night to, among other things, ensure Mr. Jackson was able to sleep. As part of his care of Mr. Jackson, Mr. Murray used a spectrum of prescription drugs, some of which are not typically used outside of a hospital setting, including: Propofol, Benoquin, Lorazepam, Midazolam, and Lidocaine. At trial, the evidence showed that almost every night for two months before Mr. Jackson's death, Mr. Murray administered Propofol. The prosecution showed that the bedroom did not have the requisite monitoring devices normally used with Propofol, an anesthesia. On the night of Mr. Jackson's death, he returned from rehearsals and was unable to sleep. Throughout the night, Mr. Murray administered several doses of valium, Lorazepam, Midazolam, and at some point Propofol. The subsequent autopsy showed that Mr. Jackson had a number of drugs in his system at the time of his death, including Propofol, Lidocaine, Valium, Ativan, Midazolam, and Ephedrine. The coroner concluded that Mr. Jackson's death was caused by Mr. Murray's administration of Propofol and benzodiazepines; that the treatment administered was not medically indicated; Propofol should not have been used for insomnia; and that the use of an anesthesia in a non-hospital setting was inappropriate.

People v. Murray, unpublished decision (Cal App. 2014)

Conspiracy

A **conspiracy** is defined as a scheme between two or more people formed for the purpose of committing, by their joint efforts, some unlawful or criminal act, or some act that is lawful in itself but becomes unlawful when done by the concerted action of the conspirators. A conspiracy is a separate crime. To prove a defendant guilty of the crime of conspiracy, three things must be proven beyond a reasonable doubt: that the defendant joined in an agreement or plan with one or more other persons; that the purpose of the agreement was to do something unlawful; and that the defendant joined the conspiracy knowing of the unlawful plan and intending to help carry it out.

conspiracy an agreement among conspirators

Larceny

Larceny is stealing. It is the wrongful taking of the personal property of another with the intent to permanently deprive that person of such property.

larceny stealing or removing someone's personal property to convert it illegally or deprive the owner of its possession; larceny is a felony

To prove the defendant guilty of larceny, three things must be proven beyond a reasonable doubt: that the defendant took and carried away the property; that the property was owned or possessed by someone other than the defendant; and that the defendant took the property with the intent to permanently deprive that person of the property. An example of larceny in a health care setting would be office employees stealing drug samples or medical supplies.

ABUSE

Three types of abuse may involve medical office professionals with criminal investigating agencies: child abuse, elder abuse, and domestic violence.

Child Abuse

There were an estimated 702,000 individual incidents of child abuse in 2014. Out of every 1,000 children in the United States, 9.4 were the victims of substantiated or likely abuse.

Key findings in the 2014 report included:

- The national estimates of children who received an investigation or alternative response increased 7.4 percent from 2010 (3,023,000) to 2014 (3,248,000).
- The number and rate of victims of maltreatment have fluctuated during the past 5 years.
- Comparing the national estimate of victims from 2010 (698,000) to 2014 (702,000) show an increase of less than 1 percent.
- Three-quarters (75.0%) of victims were neglected, 17.0 percent were physically abused, and 8.3 percent were sexually abused.
- For 2014, a nationally estimated 1,580 children died of abuse and neglect at a rate of 2.13 per 100,000 children in the national population.

Children's Bureau (Administration on Children, Youth and Families, Administration for Children and Families), U.S. Department of Health and Human Services. (2014). *Child maltreatment 2014*. Retrieved from http://www.acf.hhs.gov/ programs/cb/resource/child-maltreatment-2014

Legislative Response   Responding to the concerns of the public, Congress passed the Federal Child Abuse Prevention and Treatment Act, which requires the reporting of instances of physical and mental "injury…

under circumstances which indicate that the child's health or welfare is harmed or threatened." In addition, every state legislature has made child abuse a crime, and physicians have been listed in the statutes as mandated reporters.

Supporting this role for the physician, Susan Black, M.D., president of the Massachusetts Academy of Family Physicians, commented:

> [P]hysicians in a community are well known for handling families in crises… The physician knows where the power is in the house: she or he knows who's got the authority, who's got the love, and who's got some personal issues that may prevent the victim from regaining health. Family physicians also have tremendous credibility in a court…and are often the only professional that family members are willing to talk with.

Mandated Reporters of Abuse   Teachers, nurses, and other licensed health care providers are also identified as mandated reporters under state statutes. At times, mandated reporting may cause personal conflict to the physician and other members of the health care team who have been caring for an entire family. But the child, not the parent, is the patient, and it is universally held that confidentiality in the patient–physician relationship does not exist when parents abuse children. At the same time, it is important for reporters to maintain interpersonal relationships with the family in spite of the possibility of being expected to produce evidence against them. In private life, anyone—family, neighbor, or concerned adult—may file a child abuse complaint with a protective agency. In the physician's office within the scope of employment, unless listed as a mandated reporter, medical office professionals should file a complaint only when delegated that task by the physician.

A physician's failure to report child abuse is a matter being addressed by medical societies across the country. It is also being addressed by district attorneys:

A woman took her daughter, then under age 14, to see Zucco in August 2011 and reported that the girl had been sexually assaulted by a family member. Zucco did not perform a medical exam and told the girl that reporting the incident would result in her name being printed in a newspaper. The mother took her daughter to county Child Protective Services, which contacted authorities and investigated, county Prosecutor Gregg Marx said.

Lane, M. B. (2013, April 11). Doctor to serve jail time for not reporting abuse of child. *The Columbus Dispatch.* Retrieved from http://www.dispatch.com/content/stories/local/2013/04/10/doctor-sentenced-for-not-reporting-abuse.html

Because of Dr. Zucco's failure to report child abuse, the court sentenced him to serve 10 days in jail and 200 hours of community service, placed him on five years of probation, and ordered him to pay a $250 fine in addition to court costs.

Filing a Complaint   Procedures for reporting suspected child abuse begin by telephoning the child protective services agency in your state. Be prepared to give the following information:

> ❝ ❞
>
> 1. The name(s), address, present whereabouts, date of birth or estimate of age and sex of the reported child(ren) and of any other children in the household.
> 2. The names, addresses, and telephone numbers of the child's parents or other persons responsible for the child's care.
> 3. The principal language spoken by the child and the child's caretaker.
> 4. Your name, address, telephone number, profession, and relationship to the child. (Nonmandated reporters may request anonymity.)
> 5. The full nature and extent of the child's injuries, abuse, or neglect.
> 6. Any indication of prior injuries, abuse, or neglect.
> 7. An assessment of the risk of further harm to the child, and if a risk exists, whether it is imminent.
> 8. If the above information was given to you by a third party, the identity of that person, unless anonymity is requested.
> 9. The circumstances under which you first became aware of the child's alleged injuries, abuse, or neglect.
> 10. The action taken, if any, to treat, shelter, or assist the child.
>
> National Center for Child Abuse and Neglect Specialized Training

Child protective agencies screen the complaint after a report has been filed. Agency social workers determine whether the child is "at risk," monitor care for the child at home or in foster placement, escort the complaint through the legal system, and establish criteria to achieve the goal of the child's return home. The substantiation, or confirmation, of abuse is critical to the well-being of the child and family. Nationwide, about 40 percent of all reports are substantiated.

The agency also decides whether to refer the complaint to the district attorney. When the case is referred to the district attorney, the matter becomes criminal, and the penalty for the abuser may be prison.

Other Reporting   Federal, state, and local statutes, as well as office or hospital protocols, require that you report certain incidents. Some reporting is mandated by law and some reporting is based upon protocols found in your office manual. In all instances, it is imperative that the reporting be accurate, complete, timely, and as detailed as possible.

Every state has statutes that set forth the mandatory reporting of certain health matters, including births and deaths, venereal and other communicable diseases, injuries resulting from violence such as stab and gunshot wounds, child and elder abuse, blindness, immunological proceedings, requests for plastic surgery to change a person's fingerprints, and cases of industrial poisoning, among others. The method for reporting will vary with each state, but will generally include the type of information required for suspected child abuse. Medical assistants should be aware of the health matters in their home state that require mandatory reporting and the method for reporting.

In addition, you may encounter a scenario where you observe an illegal activity in the health care setting and must report it by following proper protocol. In such an instance, consult your office manual for detailed instructions. Most offices and hospitals will have a written protocol that includes the following steps:

1. Write down the facts of the illegal activity and the people involved.

2. Follow office protocol in contacting the appropriate person or department (often called Quality Assurance). Identify yourself and the purpose of your call (to report an illegal activity).

3. Confirm that you will not be penalized for reporting the illegal activity and request information about protocol should you experience retaliation.

4. Provide detailed information about the illegal activity and ask how the process works, what type of response you can expect, and when you can expect it. Ensure you do not violate any patient privacy statutes or rules by disclosing patient information that would otherwise require a patient's authorization.

5. Take detailed notes about the questions you ask and the responses provided to you.

6. If you do not receive a response within the time you were told, follow up with the appropriate person or department and make notes about the questions asked and responses given.

7. Retain your notes so you have evidence that you made the report and that you followed protocol in your reporting.

Sometimes an error in patient care requires reporting, as well. In such an instance, consult your office manual for detailed instructions. Most offices and hospitals will have a form for recording an error in patient care (sometimes called a "patient incident report" or "incident report") and a written protocol that includes the following steps:

1. Provide a detailed report to a supervisor or other person as directed by your office manual.

2. Obtain the appropriate form for reporting an error in patient care.

3. On the patient incident report, record the patient's status before the incident and complete the section that discusses the incident with as much detail as possible.

4. Complete all other sections of the patient incident report including all people involved in the incident; how the incident was corrected; any related policies, procedures, or protocols; observations about patient or family reaction to the incident. Sign and date the incident form and obtain any other required signatures. Forward to risk management for review.

When you are making a report of any incident, ensure that you keep your detailed notes of the event that required reporting, the people involved, and the steps you took in reporting the event. If your notes include patient information protected by federal or state privacy statutes, ensure your notes are disclosed to third parties only with proper authorization.

Legal Process   Cases that reach the courts are known as petitions for care and protection. Many attorneys are involved in care and protection proceedings. When the petition is presented in court, the child is identified by the attorney representing the protective agency. Additional attorneys are appointed for the child, the parents (often individually), and possibly the grandparents, as well as a court investigator and/or guardian ad litem. The guardian ad litem serves in the best interest of the child, whereas the attorney appointed for the child advocates for the position of the child. The court investigator serves as an extension of the court and investigates the family's history: educational, economic, medical, and psychological. The attorneys for the other members of the family represent and advocate only in their clients' interests.

The Medical Record   In any court procedure, evidence must be offered to the trier of fact in an effort to convict or defend the defendant. In child abuse cases, the medical record often holds critical information that is used in determining whether a child is returned to the parents. Physical examinations document the physical injuries, psychological examinations document the extent of mental abuse and the effect of the family dynamics on the child, and therapists' progress notes are critical in determining whether the family is motivated to change to meet the standards set by society.

Confidentiality   Every attorney wants, but is not necessarily entitled to, every medical report. Access to medical records is protected by patient–physician confidentiality statutes, and the patient holds the privilege to withhold or release the records. Usually parents hold the right to exercise the patient–physician confidentiality privilege for their children, but when the family is involved in a child abuse investigation, the patient–physician privilege is held by the protective agency, and permission for release of information about the child must be received from the agency. The parents still maintain the right to withhold or release their own medical records.

Sections of the medical record may cover the issue of fault. Usually the physician will ask a child, "How did this happen?" and the physician will document the answer. It is common practice for an emergency room staff to separate caretaker from child on arrival at the hospital to interview each person individually. The staff members then compare notes before determining whether the child is at risk and whether it is necessary to place the child in emergency protective custody. This information becomes part of the medical record but may not be given as much weight as documented injuries because of the lack of experience of the interviewers in ascertaining truth.

Access to Child Abuse Records   The records of a minor in any situation are confidential. In a child abuse case, all medical, school, court, department of social services, and department of youth services records are covered by Health Insurance Portability and Accountability Act of 1996 (HIPAA). These records cannot be released by anyone to anyone without proper authorization. The final course of action available to access a record involves the filing of a complaint seeking a court order compelling the release of the record.

Behavioral Indicators of Child Abuse   Children who are abused physically or emotionally display certain types of behavior. Many of these are common to all children at one time or another, but when they are present in sufficient number and strength to characterize a child's overall manner, they may indicate abuse:

- Overly compliant, passive, undemanding behaviors aimed at maintaining a low profile, avoiding any possible confrontation with a parent that could lead to abuse.

- Extremely aggressive, demanding, and rageful behaviors, sometimes hyperactive, caused by the child's repeated frustrations at not getting basic needs met.

- Role-reversed "parental" behavior, or extremely dependent behavior. Abusive parents have been unable to satisfy certain of their own needs appropriately and so turn to their children for fulfillment, which can produce two opposite sets of behavior in children.

- Lags in development. Children who are forced to siphon off energy, normally channeled toward growth, into protecting themselves from abusive parents may fall behind the norm for their age in toilet training, motor skills, socialization, and language development.

Physical Indicators of Child Abuse

- Bruises and welts
- Burns
- Lacerations and abrasions
- Skeletal injuries
- Head injuries
- Internal injuries caused by blows to midline of abdomen

Elder Abuse

> **66 99**
>
> When the available evidence is taken into consideration, an estimated overall prevalence of elder abuse of approximately 10% appears reasonable. Thus, a busy physician caring for older adults will encounter a victim of such abuse on a frequent basis, regardless of whether the physician recognizes the abuse.
>
> Lachs, M. S., & Pillemer, K. A. (2015, November 12). Elder abuse.
> *The New England Journal of Medicine, 373*, 1947–1956.

As the population of the United States grows older and lives longer, opportunities for elder abuse increase.

Elder Abuse Defined   The World Health Organization defines elder abuse as "a single or repeated act or lack of appropriate action, occurring within any relationship where there is an expectation of trust which causes harm or distress to an older person."

Types of Abuse   This book will deal specifically with all of these subjects except psychological abuse.

1. Passive Neglect
   Esther, approximately 85 years of age, brings her sister, Martha, into the medical office for a visit with the physician. For the past several weeks, Martha has not been eating well, has been vomiting a bit, and appears generally run down. The medication that the physician prescribed six months ago has been depleted, and no one has renewed the prescription. Martha's clothes are rumpled, her hair is stringy, and she appears unkempt, as does Esther. Prior to this time, Esther has been able to adequately take care of Martha but apparently can no longer do so. Martha is an example of a passively neglected elder.

2. Active Neglect

The case of Anne Capute (described in Chapter 3) at Morton Hospital in Taunton, Massachusetts, could be interpreted as a matter of active neglect.

3. Financial Abuse

Other dimensions of abuse involve money. For example: "You won't believe what happened," reiterated a distraught woman. "My husband's aunt was at home. Sure, she was a bit confused but not ready for a nursing home. Last Friday, Almeida and her daughter, cousins of the aunt, arrived and the next day Auntie was in the hospital. Three days later she was admitted to a nursing home. This morning, the postman stopped and asked if anyone had been to see Auntie lately. He was just there and water was trickling out the front door.

I went to the home, let myself in, and found water everywhere. Someone had left the water faucet on in the second-floor bathtub. Two days later, all of Auntie's bank accounts were depleted and the cousins were off to their home, 1500 miles away."

This is known as "rape of the estate." A relative arrives on the scene, usually at the death of the aged person, takes every article in sight and leaves before the sun comes up, never to be seen again. In this case, the relatives could not wait for the aunt to die. As part of their plan, they implicated a physician in the hospital and nursing home admission process. The court unknowingly cooperated and issued a temporary guardianship to the cousins. The abusive relatives left a legal entanglement that survived the death of the aunt and enriched the pockets of several attorneys. This type of abuse can be identified as financial on the part of the cousins and passive neglect on the part of the physician.

4. Physical Abuse

The following involves physical abuse and is viewed from the perspective of the employee abuser. "I've been fired," she cried over the telephone, "and it's so unfair. This patient...he hit me...he kicked me...I was only protecting myself. It wasn't my fault his leg got broken. I want to sue..."

Joanne had been taking care of an elderly patient in a local nursing home. He was a difficult patient, cantankerous at times, verbally abusive, and, lately, physically abusive. Joanne was getting him ready for bed at night and he "kicked" her. She stated that she grabbed his foot while he was in bed and pushed against it toward his body with her body to protect herself. She heard a "snap," then a "scream" from the patient, and then remembered nothing but confusion. The next day Joanne was called into the supervisor's office and fired for elder abuse.

The abuse was physical in nature. Joanne caused the breaking of the man's leg. This incident took place in Massachusetts, where the law requires the reporting of each incident of elder abuse. Joanne was worried, when she talked with her lawyer, that she would not be employable as a nurse's aide ever again and that her sole skill for maintaining herself financially would be taken from her because of this "accident." In fact, that is what happened. Her attorney contacted the state registry of abusers and found that Joanne had been reported two previous times for abusing residents in nursing homes. The registry board would not give her another chance.

Legislation and Penalties   Laws regarding reporting and penalties for failure to report abuse vary from state to state. All 50 states have reporting laws as well as agencies designated in one way or another to monitor and investigate allegations of abuse. Every state has a hotline for reporting and some procedure for investigating complaints of elder abuse.

Nurses can lose their licenses to practice, be fined from $25 to $1,000, be imprisoned from ten days to six months, and encounter civil liability for damages, for failure to report abuse. Medical assistants fall under the heading of health care providers and, as such, may or may not be penalized, depending on the reading of the state statute.

For information on your state statute, go to the National Center of Elder Abuse's Web site, https://ncea.acl.gov.

Domestic Violence

Domestic violence is not simply one partner hitting another. A man or woman who brutally beats his or her spouse or intimate partner is committing domestic violence. A person who threatens to harm his or her spouse or intimate partner is also committing domestic violence. The United States Department of Justice defines domestic violence as follows:

> 66 99
>
> …a pattern of abusive behavior in any relationship that is used by one partner to gain or maintain power and control over another intimate partner. Domestic violence can be physical, sexual, emotional, economic, or psychological actions or threats of actions that influence another person. This includes any behaviors that intimidate, manipulate, humiliate, isolate, frighten, terrorize, coerce, threaten, blame, hurt, injure, or wound someone.
>
> **Physical Abuse:** Hitting, slapping, shoving, grabbing, pinching, biting, hair pulling, etc. are types of physical abuse. This type of abuse also includes denying a partner medical care or forcing alcohol and/or drug use upon him or her.
>
> **Sexual Abuse:** Coercing or attempting to coerce any sexual contact or behavior without consent. Sexual abuse includes, but is certainly not limited to, marital rape, attacks on sexual parts of the body, forcing sex after physical violence has occurred, or treating one in a sexually demeaning manner.

Emotional Abuse: Undermining an individual's sense of self-worth and/or self-esteem is abusive. This may include, but is not limited to constant criticism, diminishing one's abilities, name-calling, or damaging one's relationship with his or her children.

Economic Abuse: Is defined as making or attempting to make an individual financially dependent by maintaining total control over financial resources, withholding one's access to money, or forbidding one's attendance at school or employment.

Psychological Abuse: Elements of psychological abuse include—but are not limited to—causing fear by intimidation; threatening physical harm to self, partner, children, or partner's family or friends; destruction of pets and property; and forcing isolation from family, friends, or school and/or work.

Domestic violence can happen to anyone regardless of race, age, sexual orientation, religion, or gender. Domestic violence affects people of all socioeconomic backgrounds and education levels. Domestic violence occurs in both opposite-sex and same-sex relationships and can happen to intimate partners who are married, living together, or dating.

Domestic violence not only affects those who are abused, but also has a substantial effect on family members, friends, co-workers, other witnesses, and the community at large. Children, who grow up witnessing domestic violence, are among those seriously affected by this crime. Frequent exposure to violence in the home not only predisposes children to numerous social and physical problems, but also teaches them that violence is a normal way of life—therefore, increasing their risk of becoming society's next generation of victims and abusers.

The United States Department of Justice. (n.d.). *What is domestic violence?*
Retrieved from https://www.justice.gov/ovw/domestic-violence

In 1994, the Violence Against Women Act (VAWA) was passed by Congress as an act incorporated into the Crime Bill. The VAWA provided $1.6 billion to confront the national problem of gender-based violence. The VAWA recognizes that there is no place—home, street, or school—where women are spared the fear of crime. Under Title I, Safe Homes for Women, the bill addresses the right of women to be free from domestic violence specifically through the interstate enforcement of protection orders. Prior to the passing of the VAWA, the majority of states did not give full faith and credit to protection orders issued in other states. According to *Black's Law Dictionary*, the full faith and credit clause of the United States Constitution (Article IV, §1) provides that the various states must recognize, with some exceptions, legislative acts, public records, and judicial decisions of the other states within the United States. Without full faith and credit statutes, a state may only protect victims of domestic violence within its boundaries, limiting the protection afforded victims if they leave the state issuing the protective order.

The passing of the VAWA offered women two avenues of protection from domestic violence: the state courts and the federal courts. The original petition for protection against domestic violence is filed in the state courts and through the state court system. The federal courts enter when there is an interstate violation of a protection order and the matter becomes a federal offense, as is shown in the following:

In January of 1995, the U.S. Attorney for the Southern District of West Virginia charged a man in the first federal domestic violence case. Christopher Bailey was indicted on January 4, 1995, by a grand jury for interstate domestic violence and federal kidnapping after bringing his unconscious wife to a Kentucky hospital. Bailey faces up to life imprisonment and $500,000 in fines. The FBI has been involved in the investigation and has alleged that Christopher Bailey seriously injured his wife in their home in West Virginia and then travelled through West Virginia, Kentucky and Ohio for six days with his wife sometimes tied up in the trunk. Because the federal domestic violence law is untested, Bailey is also charged with federal kidnapping since that crime is "tried and true."

> Klein, C. F. (1995, Summer). Full faith and credit interstate enforcement of protection orders under the Violence Against Women Act of 1994. *Family Law Quarterly, 29*(2), 253–272.

In addition, the Violent Crime Control and Law Enforcement Act of 1994 makes it a federal crime to possess a firearm and/or ammunition while subject to a protection Order or after conviction of a qualifying misdemeanor crime of domestic violence.

The magnitude of the problems rooted in and affected by domestic violence is evidenced in the facts that follow:

2015 NATIONAL STATISTICS

- Every 9 seconds in the US, a woman is assaulted or beaten.
- On average, nearly 20 people per minute are physically abused by an intimate partner in the United States. During one year, this equates to more than 10 million women and men.
- 1 in 3 women and 1 in 4 men have been victims of [some form of] physical violence by an intimate partner within their lifetime.
- 1 in 5 women and 1 in 7 men have been victims of severe physical violence by an intimate partner in their lifetime.
- 1 in 7 women and 1 in 18 men have been stalked by an intimate partner during their lifetime to the point in which they felt very fearful or believed that they or someone close to them would be harmed or killed.

- On a typical day, there are more than 20,000 phone calls placed to domestic violence hotlines nationwide.
- The presence of a gun in a domestic violence situation increases the risk of homicide by 500%.
- Intimate partner violence accounts for 15% of all violent crime.
- Women between the ages of 18–24 are most commonly abused by an intimate partner.
- 19% of domestic violence involves a weapon.
- Domestic victimization is correlated with a higher rate of depression and suicidal behavior.
- Only 34% of people who are injured by intimate partners receive medical care for their injuries.

National Coalition Against Domestic Violence. (2015).
Domestic violence national statistics fact sheet. Retrieved from
http://ncadv.org/files/National%20Statistics%20Domestic%20Violence%20NCADV.pdf

Physicians' offices, emergency rooms, and ambulatory care clinics offer victims of domestic violence an opportunity to receive help not only in the treatment of current wounds but also in the prevention of future incidents. Recently, the AMA has made physician assistance in the reduction of domestic violence a priority.

Sexual Assault

The United States Department of Justice defines sexual assault as "Sexual assault is any type of sexual contact or behavior that occurs without the explicit consent of the recipient. Falling under the definition of sexual assault are sexual activities as forced sexual intercourse, forcible sodomy, child molestation, incest, fondling, and attempted rape." Health care professionals encounter victims of sexual assault when a victim seeks treatment in medical facilities following a sexual assault or when a patient is sexually assaulted by personnel providing medical care within the facility. The following case is unique and deals with the issues:

A former physician already charged with sexually assaulting a patient is now being charged with committing sexual acts on as many as five women, at least four of whom were patients, in Riverside County, according to court documents…

(Continues)

(Continued)

McGuire is now charged with 26 counts, all of them felonies. They include three counts of rape by force or fear, six counts of sexual battery involving a restraint and three counts of sexual battery. He has a sentencing enhancement for use of a firearm, and another sentencing enhancement for committing sexual acts on patients.

Groves, A. (2016, April 6). Temecula: Physician charged with
additional felonies in amended complaint. *The Press Enterprise*.
Retrieved from http://www.pe.com/articles/mcguire-786778-acts-sexual.html

The patient–physician relationship is determined to be a fiduciary relationship, which means that the physician is held to the highest standard of trust. According to *Black's Law Dictionary*, the term *fiduciary* refers to a duty to act for someone else's benefit. It is the highest standard of duty implied by law. Such relationships arise whenever confidence is reposed on one side and domination and influence result on the other. Although rape is a crime whenever it is committed, it is a particularly heinous one when committed by a physician in the patient–physician relationship. Patients must be able to trust physicians. Public policy demands that patients be protected from abuse of power and breach of trust. This policy is intended to cover all persons involved in the care of the ill, children, and the elderly.

Although all states require that physicians report evidence of the rape of a minor child or of an elderly person, not all states require a physician to report treating an adult rape victim. In *Rape and Sexual Assault Reporting Requirements for Competent Adult Victims*, attorney Teresa P. Scalzo reports that not all states have laws that require medical professionals to report that they have treated an adult rape victim. Of the laws that do exist, Ms. Scalzo indicates that laws "requiring medical personnel to report that they have treated a competent, adult rape victim can be broken down into the following categories: (1) laws that specifically require medical professionals to report treatment of a rape victim to law enforcement; (2) laws that require the reporting of injuries that may include rape; (3) laws relating to other crimes or injuries which may impact rape and sexual assault victims; and (4) laws regarding sexual assault forensic examinations which may impact rape and sexual assault reporting."

FRAUD

The high cost of fraudulent claims has given rise to an interagency "Strike Force" led by the U.S. Department of Justice in conjunction with the Department of HHS. The government has the capacity to do "real time" analysis of Medicare billings to ensure that hospitals, laboratories, health maintenance organizations, and physicians' offices are complying with billing and service requirements.

On June 18, 2015, Attorney General Loretta E. Lynch and Department of Health and Human Services (HHS) Secretary Sylvia Mathews Burwell announced the largest takedown in Strike Force history. The announcement stated that it was the largest takedown "both in terms of the number of defendants charged and loss amount," and it resulted in "charges against 243 individuals, including 46 doctors, nurses and other licensed medical professionals, for their alleged participation in Medicare fraud schemes involving approximately $712 million in false billings. In addition, the Centers for Medicare & Medicaid Services (CMS) also suspended a number of providers using its suspension authority as provided in the Affordable Care Act...

The defendants are charged with various health care fraud-related crimes, including conspiracy to commit health care fraud, violations of the anti-kickback statutes, money laundering and aggravated identity theft. The charges are based on a variety of alleged fraud schemes involving various medical treatments and services, including home health care, psychotherapy, physical and occupational therapy, durable medical equipment (DME) and pharmacy fraud. More than 44 of the defendants arrested are charged with fraud related to the Medicare prescription drug benefit program known as Part D, which is the fastest-growing component of the Medicare program overall.

U.S. Department of Justice, Office of the Attorney General.
(2015, June 18). Press release.

Fraud can take many forms. It includes "upcoding" procedures to more expensive ones than were actually performed, kickbacks for referrals, filing false information, and billing for services not provided. It can even include "renting patients," in which patients are recruited for procedures they do not need. The provider then splits the reimbursement with the patient. The government's net is wide when it investigates and prosecutes for fraud.

False Billing

In 2009, four medical workers were convicted of fraud after filing $5.3 million in false HIV-therapy claims to Medicare, including two medical assistants employed by physicians. Clinics owned and operated by the two physicians were paid for bogus HIV treatments. Physicians manipulated the blood samples, prescribed obsolete drugs, and falsified medical records.

Four employees of the clinic…including the executive director, the medical director, the medical director, a social worker and a supervising therapist, were charged with grand larceny, conspiracy and filing false documents. According to the indictment, the four defendants filed more than 3,000 reimbursement claims with the state from May 1990 to December 1993 falsely indicating that therapists had provided individual psychotherapy sessions in excess of 30 minutes to dozens of Medicaid recipients when, in fact, the visits were far shorter, were for less expensive group sessions, or never occurred at all… The indictment also alleged that to conceal the fraud, the defendants "doctored" patients' medical records to make it appear that individual therapy sessions over 30 minutes had been provided.

Officials said that under applicable Medicaid regulations, [the clinic] is reimbursed $30 for each individual therapy session lasting 15 to 29 minutes and $60 for a session lasting more than 30 minutes… All four defendants surrendered to the police and pleaded not guilty. If convicted of all counts, they could each face up to 23 years in prison.

Four at a clinic are accused of Medicaid fraud. (1995, February 8).
The New York Times, B2.

Billing for Services Not Authorized or Warranted

A recent case of billing fraud involved radiologists providing diagnostic tests not ordered by primary care physicians and then billed for procedures not supported by the medical records. These physicians entered into a settlement with the government by paying $2 million and agreeing to a five-year integrity agreement.

Billing for Unnecessary Services

Fraud frequently involves providing unnecessary medical services to patients who are not aware they are healthier than their physicians have told them. In a 2007 case, a physician routinely found his patients had skin cancer, performed unnecessary surgeries, and billed Medicare.

Nearly every patient who had a biopsy was told he or she had skin cancer and needed surgery. According to court testimony, one former patient said that she became so accustomed to Rosin finding cancer that she would schedule surgery before he gave her the biopsy results.

Because Rosin could bill Medicare for each layer of skin he removed, many patients were subjected to unnecessary removal of layers, leaving some permanently disfigured. Others, like Hillenbrand, underwent surgery many times.

Brown, E. (2007, November). Diagnosis Medicare fraud. *AARP Bulletin Today.*

Although it may seem that government strike forces are the only ones interested in fraud, that is far from the truth. Many of the cases come from the government sector because it is such a large payer for so many people. Health insurance executives, in a recent article in *The New York Times*, accused physicians of regularly writing erroneous diagnoses for patients who then collect for noncompensated care. Dr. Paul Parker, in an article in *Medical Economics*, related his experience while having his teeth cleaned by a dental hygienist:

As I opened wide in a dental chair not long ago, my hygienist set me straight about her favorite OBG specialist: "He's a doll. Chronic cervicitis. Vaginitis. Dysmenorrhea. I don't even have to ask, and he puts down a diagnosis…"

"Don't you know that putting down a false diagnosis is illegal?" I responded. "Maybe," she said. "But it's not such a big deal." She smiled slyly. "Dentists do it, too."

Parker, P. *Medical Economics.*

Delegation of Duties

Health care delivery by proxy is another area that sets the trap for Medicaid and Medicare billings. Even though a paraprofessional can legally perform a given service under the terms of a state's medical practice act, it does not mean that Medicare will pay for the service. This is an area that has particular significance for medical assistants. In Massachusetts, for example, Blue Cross/Blue Shield regulations have been promulgated as follows:

Rule 2. To be eligible to receive payment for services from Blue Shield, a participating provider must personally perform those services. Blue Shield will, however, pay a participating provider for services which are performed by his/her assistant who has been approved by and registered with Blue Shield in accordance with this Rule.

Generally, Blue Shield will pay a participating provider for services performed by an assistant: (a) who is a salaried employee of that provider and who works a certain number of regular hours per week for that provider, regardless of the number of patients seen; (b) who is registered, licensed

(Continues)

(Continued)

or qualified under Massachusetts law to perform such services; (c) who performs the services under the direct, personal and continuous supervision of a Blue Shield participating provider who practices in the same or related field...

"Direct, personal and continuous supervision" under this Rule means that the participating provider must perform or participate in an initial examination or evaluation of the patient and actively participate in the continuing management of the patient's treatment. While the provider need not be in the room where the assistant renders his or her services, that provider must be on the same premises and immediately available to provide personal assistance and direction. Availability by telephone or other electronic communication does not constitute direct, personal and continuous supervision. The participating provider must also document his/her supervision of assistants in the clinical record of the patient.

Forgiving Copayments

In an August 18, 2015, article entitled "Healthcare Fraud Shield's Latest Article: Patient Cost Forgiveness—Why is it a problem?" physicians were warned that "In addition, routinely waiving patient copays could also be construed as fraud... Providers who waive copays are exposed to HIPAA risk because, arguably, the provider is misstating his or her charge to the commercial plan. For example, assume a $100 total charge where the patient has an 80/20 plan. If the provider waives the patient's obligation to pay 20%, then, again arguably, the commercial plan owes only 80% of $80." Notably, each state has different laws and policies regarding insurance fraud. In some states, the waiver of copayments may qualify as fraud. So, be aware of your state's regulations, and review your policies and procedures.

Kickbacks

The Medicare-Medicaid Antifraud and Abuse Amendments contain a provision that makes it illegal for a person or institution to make or receive payment of any kind in return for obtaining or introducing the referral of Medicaid or Medicare patients. Criminal penalties will be imposed on anyone who knowingly and willfully solicits or receives any kickback, bribe, or rebate in return for referring a patient to a physician, physical therapist, pharmacy, and so on, or for referring to a patient any item or service that may be paid for in full or in part by Medicare or Medicaid.

Medco Health Solutions, the largest U.S. pharmacy benefit manager, agreed to pay $155 million to settle fraud allegations brought by the federal government and several former company employees, the *Newark Star-Ledger* reports (Silverman, *Newark Star-Ledger*, October 24, 2006).

The allegations, which involve mail-order prescriptions provided to members of the Federal Employees Health Benefits Program, include most of a complaint filed by two former company employees under the False Claims Act (*Kaiser Daily Health Policy Report*, May 8, 2006). The federal government in 2003 amended the complaint. According to the complaint, Medco cancelled and destroyed prescriptions to avoid penalties, sought kickbacks from pharmaceutical companies to promote their medications and paid kickbacks to health insurers in exchange for their business.

Wisenberg, B. (2006, October 24). PBM Medco Health Solutions agrees to settle Medicare fraud, kickback allegations for $155 million. *News-Medical.net*. Retrieved from http://www.news-medical.net/?id=20754

Penalties

The government has established an office—the Office of the Inspector General (OIG) in the U.S. Department of HHS—to police the entire realm of fraud and mispayments. The government no longer needs to show intent—only that the physician knew or should have known that the charges were improper.

For every claim that OIG finds was not provided as reported, the physician may be fined and held liable for as much as double the amount claimed for each item or service. There is also the possibility of criminal prosecution and sanctions involving suspension from the program. Sanctions have a serious impact on a physician who has built a practice at least in part on income from Medicare patients.

Informants

An investigation is usually triggered by a tip. Tips come from Medicare carriers, peer review organizations, state licensing boards, whistle-blowing physicians, ex-staff members, and patients. Investigators make their case through beneficiary or patient interviews, documentation within the medical record, and interviews of other physicians and nurses. Some cases are easy, as in the following: "We had an ophthalmologist who had his machine repossessed for nonpayment by the manufacturer, and for a year after that he was still billing Medicare for procedures performed by the machine. He pleaded guilty and is serving time."

The government provided an incentive to those who know of fraudulent provider behavior by recognizing their right to bring a lawsuit on behalf of the government in exchange for generous rewards. This **qui tam lawsuit** has been popular since the mid-1990s and provides significant disincentive to cheat the system because it empowers virtually anyone with knowledge to sue the provider.

qui tam lawsuit whistleblower brings suit and receives share of recovery as reward

Medical assistants, as indicated previously in the bogus HIV treatment case, may be considered co-conspirators with the physician in fraud. The gist of a conspiracy is to agree to disobey or disregard the law. Two types of intent must be proven: intent to agree and intent to commit the substantive offense. When an assistant bills for a physician and consents to mark the insurance form in any manner that does not reflect the true situation, the assistant may be found guilty of conspiring to commit fraud. A defendant, of course, may be guilty of participation in a criminal conspiracy without actually profiting from or having any financial stake in it.

Health Insurance Portability and Accountability Act of 1996

On August 21, 1996, President Clinton signed into law the HIPAA, also known as the Kassenbaum-Kennedy Health Insurance Reform Bill. Included in the HIPAA is a provision requiring every health plan and provider to maintain "reasonable and appropriate" safeguards to ensure the confidentiality of health information. The safeguards are intended to protect the disclosure of "individually identifiable information" that refers to any information that (1) identifies the individual; (2) relates to the individual's physical or mental health—past, present, or future—or payment for health care; or (3) is created or received by a health plan, provider, or employer.

Any health plan provider, or other person, who knowingly obtains or discloses "individually identifiable information" in violation of the Act is subject to a fine of $50,000 and a year in prison. If the information is obtained or disclosed through false pretenses, the fine increases to $100,000 and 5 years in prison. If such information is obtained or disclosed with the intent to sell, transfer, or use it for commercial advantage, personal gain, or malicious harm, the fine becomes $250,000 and 10 years in prison.

Individuals and organizations may request the U.S. HHS Inspector General to issue fraud alerts to inform the public that certain practices are considered suspect or of concern to the Medicare and Medicaid programs. As a requirement of the Act, the HHS, in consultation with the attorney general, will issue advisory opinions, within 60 days of request, to determine whether these activities are prohibited by fraud and abuse provisions.

These decisions are an attempt to address unsettled areas of past law, whether a waiver of coverage or deductibles or the transfer of items or services for free or for less than market value is "remuneration," and other matters of similar concern. Such waivers will be legal only when they are not used to solicit patients, are not routinely waived by the provider, and are waived only because of a patient's financial need.

Under the Act, health care fraud is made an independent federal crime and includes knowing and willful schemes to defraud any health care benefits program, not just Medicaid and Medicare. Penalties include fines and up to 10 years in prison, which may become 20 years if the crime results in serious bodily injury and life imprisonment if the crime results in death.

The Act establishes the Medicare Integrity Program for private investigations and audits, encourages individuals to report fraud, and allows for rewarding individuals who report fraud. In addition, the Act requires the HHS to establish a national data bank to record information about providers and suppliers that have committed health care abuse.

Since the enactment of HIPAA, the HHS has developed a large number of sweeping regulations, especially affecting the privacy of patient information.

Embezzlement

Embezzlement occurs in the medical office when the assistant handling the payments from patients takes the money and uses it for his or her own purposes. To have embezzlement, (1) there must be a relationship, such as employment, between the individual who embezzles and the owner of the money; (2) the money must come into the hands of the embezzler because of the relationship; and (3) there must be intent to fraudulently misappropriate the money.

Illegal Sale of Prescription Drugs

The number of medical professionals arrested for illegally selling prescription drugs is on the rise. To be found guilty of this offense, the substance in question must be a controlled substance; the individual being charged must have a perceptible amount of the substance on his or her person or have distributed some perceptible amount of that substance with the intent to distribute it to another person or persons; and the individual must have done so knowingly or intentionally:

Michael Troyan, a physician assistant who operated two urgent care clinics on the east end of Long Island was arrested this morning pursuant to a grand jury indictment with conspiring to illegally distribute oxycodone, a highly addictive prescription pain medication. Also this morning, a search warrant was

(Continues)

(Continued)

executed at the East End Urgent and Primary Care in Riverhead by the DEA's Long Island Tactical Diversion Squad which is comprised of agents and officers of the DEA, Nassau County Police Department, Rockville Centre Police Department, and Port Washington Police Department. The Long Island Tactical Diversion Squad was also assisted by agents and officers of the Department of Health & Human Services, the Southampton Town Police Department, and the Suffolk County District Attorney's East End Drug Taskforce…

The indictment and public filings allege that between November 2011 and October 2015, Troyan, a physician assistant with authority to prescribe controlled substances, issued prescriptions for thousands of oxycodone pills to co-conspirators for the purpose of illegally re-selling the pills for cash. Troyan was captured on video in an undercover operation writing phony prescriptions for oxycodone and receiving large quantities of cash at his Riverhead medical office for prior illegal sales. Troyan was receiving half of the profit from the sale of the oxycodone pills…

If convicted, the defendant faces a maximum sentence of 20 years' imprisonment and a $1 million fine."

Office of the Attorney General, Eastern District of New York. (2015, November 4). Riverhead physician assistant arrested for conspiracy to illegally prescribe oxycodone. *United States Department of Justice.* Retrieved from https://www.justice.gov /usao-edny/pr/riverhead-physician-assistant-arrested-conspiracy -illegally-prescribe-oxycodone

One of the defenses available to the defendants in the preceding case charges the investigators with illegal search and seizure, discussed in the following section.

Search and Seizure

The Fourth Amendment of the U.S. Constitution protects an individual against unreasonable searches of person, house, office, or vehicle and unreasonable seizure of person, papers, and effects. The amendment further provides that no warrant shall issue except upon probable cause supported by oath or affirmation and, particularly, a description of the place to be searched and the persons or things to be seized. It is generally accepted that police may not enter a person's home without a search warrant. In the following case, the defendant attempted to extend the expectations of privacy in his home to his hospital room:

On October 18, 1977, at approximately 11 p.m., the defendant was stopped, identified, and searched by a Sacramento police officer on the corner of Sixth and T streets. At the time, the defendant, although male, was dressed in women's clothing and carrying a handbag. The officer observed that he was carrying certain matchbooks, a sharp steak knife (six or seven inches long), and a broken crescent wrench. After a warrant check on the defendant proved negative, he was given a certain green card and released. Defendant walked in the direction of nearby Southside Park.

Sometime between 12:15 and 12:45 on the morning of October 19, defendant was seen with an unidentified male in the doorway of the women's restroom in Southside Park. About 8:45 that morning the Sacramento police homicide department was summoned to the scene, where a dead male had been found.

The autopsy revealed the victim had been dead from six hours prior to 10:00 a.m. and it could have been as long as 16 hours. It also revealed the victim had been stabbed…the wounds were made by a knife or knife-like instrument. The coroner opined to police officers that the killing had homosexual overtones.

On October 19, the defendant readmitted himself to Sutter Hospital. On readmission, two nurses had observed blood on his shoes and stockings. While in his hospital room, an officer observed a pair of shoes in an open closet with what appeared to be a great deal of caked blood on them. On the way to the station, the defendant requested permission to return to his apartment for his purse and a check. When the officer opened the defendant's purse to check for weapons, he observed blood on the purse and inside a three-by-five green card similar to the one given to defendant by the officer making the stop the previous night. The purse and its contents were seized as evidence. The defendant attempted to suppress this evidence by claiming that his Fourth Amendment rights had been violated.

The contents of the purse were not suppressed because the searching of the purse occurred during a pre-arrest search, which is necessary for the safety of the officers. The question of expectation of privacy and violation of the Fourth Amendment focused on the officer's view of the blood-caked boots in the hospital room. The court determined that no Fourth Amendment violation occurs when a nurse permits an officer to enter a patient's hospital room for purposes unrelated to a search, the patient does not object to the visit, and the officer then sees evidence in plain view.

People v. Brown, 88 Cal. App. 3d 283, 151 Cal. Rptr. 749 (1979)

Individuals who are arrested for driving while intoxicated are asked to take breathalyzer tests and provide blood samples for laboratory analysis. The U.S. Supreme Court has upheld the admissibility of blood tests by a physician using standard medical procedures in which the blood was taken from a conscious person who did not consent but who offered no physical resistance. Other incidents of search and seizure are found in medical treatment situations. For example:

⚖️

A gun battle between the police and three armed men occurred following the robbery of a supermarket. One policeman and one robber were killed; another robber was shot but escaped. A few weeks later, the police picked up an individual they suspected was the robber who got away. He was taken to the hospital, where X-rays indicated metallic fragments in his buttocks. The police obtained a search warrant, and a surgeon removed the metal while the suspect was under local anesthesia. The metal fragments were identified as parts of police bullets and used as evidence against the defendant. He was convicted of the policeman's murder. He appealed the conviction and the Indiana Supreme Court held that such an extensive intrusion into his body had constituted a sufficiently unreasonable violation of his constitutional rights to require reversal of his conviction.

Adams v. State of Indiana, 229 N.E.2d 834 (Ind. 1973)

CIVIL CAUSES OF ACTION— INTENTIONAL TORTS

Civil law covers all bad acts except criminal actions. Most cases in medical malpractice law fall within the civil law of torts. A tort is a private wrong or injury, other than breach of contract, for which the court will provide a remedy. To have an action in tort, there must exist a legal duty between the plaintiff and the defendant, a breach of that duty, and injury as a result of the breach. Tort liability is classified as intentional, negligent, or liability without fault. For a tort to be intentional, the defendant must intend to commit the act. An intentional tort differs from negligence. In negligence, injury to the patient occurs because the defendant fails to exercise the degree of care required in doing what is otherwise permissible.

The importance of intentional torts for the patient or plaintiff lies in the ability of the victims to receive damages for injury. In a criminal case of assault and battery, for example, the victim may get back money, if robbed, but cannot sue for emotional distress, pain and suffering, diminished employability, and so on. This is processed in the courts by the plaintiff filing two complaints: one criminal and the other civil. The criminal complaint functions to punish the perpetrator. The civil complaint functions to make the victim whole. This is an equitable remedy under which a person is restored to his or her original position prior to the loss or injury.

Intentional torts against the person include assault, battery, intentional infliction of emotional distress, false imprisonment, invasion of privacy, and defamation of character. Defenses available to defendants include privilege, consent, self-defense, the defense of others, and error.

Assault and Battery

Assault is defined as any willful attempt or threat to injure another person with the apparent ability to do so. Battery is nonconsensual touching. A physician may be charged with assault and battery because of failure to obtain informed consent to treatment. Occasionally, the charge of battery is filed against a health care provider who has acted in anger. For example:

> An injury occurred to a four-year-old child that required sutures. When the patient returned with her mother to have the sutures removed the defendant suggested that the child should lie on the examining table and the mother was directed to hold her down. The child began to cry and tried to sit up. This behavior hindered the doctor in removing the sutures and he spanked her quite hard. The bruises remained visible on the child's buttocks for approximately three weeks. The mother immediately removed the child from the doctor's office and took the child to another physician who removed the sutures without incident. The mother then sued the physician for assault and battery and the jury returned a verdict in her favor.
>
> *Burton v. Leftwich*, 123 So. 2d 766 (La. 1960)

Invasion of Privacy

The United States Supreme Court has recognized that privacy is a constitutional right. Independence in making certain kinds of important decisions is a privacy interest. For example, *Roe v. Wade*, a case decided by the Supreme Court in 1973, determined that a woman's decision to have an abortion was a right of privacy.

This right of privacy, whether it be founded in the Fourteenth Amendment's concept of personal liberty and restrictions upon state action…or in the Ninth Amendment's reservation of rights to the people, is broad enough to encompass a woman's decision whether or not to terminate her pregnancy.

Roe v. Wade, 410 U.S. 113, 93 S. Ct. 705, 35 L.Ed.2d 147 (1973)

The individual's right to expect privacy in situations of medical care must be respected by medical assistants and other health care deliverers. It has been established for many years that the admission of nonessential persons during treatment without the consent of the patient constitutes a violation of the right of privacy. The following is a case from 1881 that is still good law today:

A doctor was called to the home of a woman in labor to deliver her baby. He took a friend with him who was not a physician. The friend was present throughout the delivery and held the woman's hand while she was experiencing labor pains. The doctor did not tell the patient that his friend was not another physician. The patient sued for violation of her right to privacy and the court held that she had a legal right to privacy at the time that her child was born.

DeMay v. Roberts, 9 N.W. 146 (Mich. 1881)

In the following case, the court held that a medical office staff was guilty of violating a patient's family's privacy by continuing to contact the family:

A female patient was hospitalized and died during the period of hospitalization. Approximately one month after her death, a notice was sent to her by her family physician's office with an appointment for her periodic check-up. Her husband wrote to the physician explaining that she had died and that he and his children found the notice upsetting. Shortly thereafter, he filed a wrongful death action against the family physician, apparently for failure to diagnose her illness. Two additional check-up letters were received, the second being addressed to her daughter. The family sued for invasion of privacy and harassment. The court was of the opinion that sending two more letters after being informed that a malpractice suit had been filed against the physician was an invasion of privacy.

McCormick v. Haley, 307 N.E.2d 34 (Ohio 1973)

False Imprisonment

The tort of false imprisonment is defined as intentionally confining a person without the legal right to do so or without his or her consent. Examples of false imprisonment are found where patients have been kept in a hospital for failing to pay their bills or have been committed to a mental hospital when there was no probable cause to commit, as in the following case:

⚖️

A 79-year-old woman was tricked into going into a mental hospital by being told that she was going into a regular hospital for treatment. She signed herself in, but as soon as she found out where she was, she tried to sign herself out. She was denied the right to leave. In spite of her age and physical infirmities, she climbed out a second floor window, ran to a telephone, and called her lawyer. Within an hour he had a court order releasing her. The hospital did not raise the argument that she was incompetent. They did not ask for a civil commitment. The court found that the patient had been falsely imprisoned and did not accept the hospital's defense that the patient must try to escape or is assumed to consent.

Geddes v. Daughters of Charity, 348 F.2d 144 (1965)

False Claims Act

The Department of Justice civil fraud section follows provisions of the False Claims Act (FCA) to recover funds in the health care area. The government needs to prove only a deliberate (i.e., reckless but not intentional) false claim and may obtain a fine or penalty of $5,000–$10,000 per claim plus multiple damages. The most difficult aspect of the FCA is to determine the "knowledge" standard, or what one must "know" to be held liable under the act.

The FCA defines *knowing* and *knowingly* to mean that a person "(1) has actual knowledge of the information; (2) acts in deliberate ignorance of the truth or falsity of the information; or (3) acts in reckless disregard of the truth or falsity of the information" (31 U.S.C. §3729[b]). There is "no proof of specific intent to defraud" requirement. The importance of the FCA for medical office personnel is involved with billing procedures.

The Affordable Care Act added amendments to the False Claims Act, including, among others, redefining "obligation" under the False Claims Act to include retention of any overpayments and reporting requirements when an overpayment occurs, and the federal Anti-Kickback Statute, which criminalizes the act of soliciting, receiving, offering or paying for money in exchange for patient referrals for services paid by the government. The Anti-Kickback Statute makes clear that, "a person need not have actual knowledge…or specific intent to commit a violation." So, "not knowing" is not a defense.

Defamation of Character

Violation of a patient's right to privacy may result in the charge of defamation of character being filed against a health care employee. Defamation of character occurs when one person communicates to a second person about a third in such a manner that the reputation of the person about whom the discussion was held is harmed. Such a written communication is termed libel, whereas spoken defamation is slander. Charges against physicians for defamation of character are closely interwoven with charges of invasion of privacy or disclosure of confidential information. The following is a case against a nurse for slander:

A woman who was employed by a caterer had a condition which brought about false positive Wasserman tests. She did not have and had never had syphilis. There was no diagnosis of syphilis by the physician treating the woman. The doctor's nurse attended a social affair, which was catered by the patient's employer. The nurse told the hostess that the employee was being treated by the physician for syphilis. This information affected the patient's employment and the employer's business. The court held that there was a good cause of action for slander against the nurse.

Schessler v. Keck, 271 P.2d 588 (1954)

Public versus private interest is a consideration of the court in the preceding case. In 1920, there was no cure for syphilis and it was a dreaded contagious disease. The courts determined that public interest outweighed private interest.

Mr. Simonsen visited Dr. Swensen with symptoms that were compatible with syphilis. The doctor diagnosed plaintiff Simonsen's case as syphilis before obtaining the results of lab tests. He told Simonsen to move out of his hotel, where he was a resident, until a definite diagnosis could be made, to prevent the spread of the disease.

The next day after the visit, the doctor learned that the plaintiff was still at the hotel. He called the owner of the hotel and informed him that Mr. Simonsen had a contagious disease. The owner forced Simonsen to move. The Wasserman test came back negative and Simonsen sued Dr. Swensen. The court determined that under these circumstances, the doctor had a duty to disclose this information.

Simonsen v. Swenson, 177 N.W. 831 (Neb. 1920)

Intentional Infliction of Emotional Distress

The intentional infliction of emotional distress is sometimes referred to as the tort of "outrageous conduct." This term distinguishes it from insults, indignities, threats, or annoyances. It is a tort that is usually tried before a jury because conviction depends on whether an average member of the community would consider the conduct outrageous.

The plaintiff was permitted to sue a hospital on a claim of intentional infliction of emotional distress, among others, after she was sexually assaulted by another patient when she was an inpatient in a psychiatric ward. Delk was admitted to the Columbia Peninsula Center for Behavioral Health due to her bipolar condition. Delk's medical history included mood disorders and hospitalizations, and long term psychiatric problems that arose after multiple episodes of sexual assault. As a result, she was considered to be a high risk to herself and was deemed to require full time supervision and surveillance. Delk claimed that during her hospitalization, a male patient, who was believed to be HIV positive, entered her room and sexually assaulted her. The nursing staff "observed and documented the presence of this unauthorized adult male in [Delk's] room, no further actions occurred from the staff or management of… No notation was made in [Delk's] medical records regarding the sexual assault." She alleged that, as a result of "[d]efendant's extreme, reckless, outrageous and intentional infliction of emotional distress," she "suffered severe mental, emotional and physical trauma."

The court noted that a claim for intentional infliction of emotional distress requires proof "by clear and convincing evidence, that: the wrongdoer's conduct is intentional or reckless; the conduct is outrageous and intolerable; the alleged conduct and emotional distress are causally connected; and the distress is severe. A plaintiff must allege each of these elements with the requisite degree of specificity." The court held that Ms. Delk pled sufficient facts, which if proven at trial, would allow a finding that the defendants acted recklessly because it is common knowledge that HIV can develop into AIDS, a fatal disease; Mrs. Delk was exposed to HIV as a result of the sexual assault; and, the hospital failed to tell her about her attacker's HIV positive status so she could prevent transmission of the disease to her family members.

Delk v. Columbia Healthcare Corp., 523 S.E.2d 826 (Va. 2000)

☑ SUMMARY

- There is a difference as to the severity of misdemeanor and felony crimes.
- Intent makes the difference as to whether the behavior is labeled criminal or civil, intentional or negligent.
- If a patient is injured from an act performed with premeditation and malice, it is determined that the defendant is a criminal.
- If the patient is injured because of an aggressive act by the defendant carried through without premeditation or malice, the defendant is accused of an intentional tort. If the patient's injury simply happened, the defendant is alleged negligent.
- Statutes are, in part, laws made by legislatures defining which acts are criminal felonies or misdemeanors and which acts are civil torts. In addition, there are common law crimes: murder, manslaughter, rape, fraud, sodomy, robbery, larceny, arson, burglary, and mayhem.
- Most cases in medical malpractice fall within the civil law of torts. Civil actions differ from criminal actions in that in a civil action, one party is suing the other party for damages because of an injury committed by the other party. These are private, civil claims rather than public claims filed by the state against an individual.
- Torts include the intentional torts of assault and battery, false imprisonment, invasion of privacy, defamation of character, intentional infliction of emotional distress, and negligence. The defenses available to defendants accused of intentionally injuring patients include privilege, consent, self-defense, the defense of others, and error.

SUGGESTED ACTIVITIES

1. Visit the local district court. Make arrangements with the clerk of the court before attending and request an interview with one of the judges about philosophy regarding criminals and criminal activity. Try to get to court early to see arraignments, trials, and dispositions. While in the court, keep your eyes on the lawyers and clients in the hall. This is where most of the court's business occurs. When the lawyers come before the judge, an agreement has usually been reached. Defendants in a district court who are indigent are usually represented by public defenders or local bar advocates. Ask the clerk of the court to arrange for a judge to spend some time with the class. Prepare questions in advance and write them down.

2. Criminal law makes the headlines every day in the local paper. Search the paper and review the reported criminal actions. After reading the accounts of the crime, determine whether a medical office may be involved in any aspect of the case and how.

STUDY QUESTIONS

1. Murder is a crime. How does murder differ from euthanasia? Do the courts treat the two differently?
2. How is the medical office affected by statutes and regulations on child and elder abuse?
3. A patient who has not paid a bill has come to the emergency room for medical treatment. While there, a medical assistant notices a large amount of money in her purse. The medical assistant tells the security guard. The guard stands at the patient's room and refuses to let her leave until she pays some money toward her bill. Can the patient file charges against the hospital? If so, what will the proper complaint read?

CASES FOR DISCUSSION

1. In most states, physicians are mandated to report child abuse. Following are four hypothetical cases involving child abuse. Determine whether you would report any of these cases as child abuse:

   • The dirty house case: Mr. and Mrs. Jones and their two preschool children, John and Mary, live in a decrepit house with three large dogs and a number of cats. Mr. Jones works as a laborer. Mrs. Jones is not employed outside the house and does nothing inside either. There is trash all over the house and many cockroaches. The dogs go freely in and out, and the cats use the piles of old newspapers as litter boxes. The smell is horrible. John and Mary are extremely dirty at all times. They seem to eat junk food a lot. They have no toys and play with various odds and ends. However, aside from runny noses, they appear to be healthy and developing normally.

   • The massage parlor case: Sharleen, age 7, lives with her mother, Barbara, in a small apartment over the men-only massage parlor where Barbara works from 4:00 p.m. until midnight. Drinks are served in the waiting room of the massage parlor, and it is possible that there is some drug use on the premises as well. There are pornographic magazines available and soft-porn programs on the television sets. Some of the videotapes may have been made on the premises. Sharleen spends her after-school time at the massage parlor, sometimes coloring or playing with her own toys, sometimes helping to straighten up the waiting room, and sometimes just going around talking to people. She stays there until Barbara takes her up and puts her to bed, usually around nine o'clock at night.

- The truant case: Bobby, age 8, skipped school several times. A neighbor told his father about it, but when his father confronted the boy, Bobby lied, saying he had gone to school every day. The father viewed these as serious offenses on Bobby's part and he punished Bobby by beating him with a leather strap hard enough to leave marks on the back of Bobby's legs.

- The suicidal child: Margaret, age 14, took a large overdose of medication and then called the hospital. Due to prompt action, she survived. The hospital requested that she have a psychiatric evaluation before her discharge. Margaret's parents refused initially, but when they were threatened with court action, they capitulated. Margaret's evaluation indicated that she was of normal intelligence but showed signs of "depression, hostility, and impulsiveness." A foster home placement and individual therapy were recommended. Margaret's parents refused to follow the recommendations. (Hypothetical cases taken from material used at the MCLE/NELI Child Abuse and Neglect Program, Boston College Seminar, October 25, 1984.)

2. A woman went to the physician with severe stomach pains. She was examined by a surgeon who, she stated, told her that her spleen was "hanging by a thread" from her collarbone. The surgeon recommended surgery to "build up ligaments" in her spleen. Following the operation, the surgeon informed her husband that it had been necessary to remove the spleen. The pathology report revealed no evidence of any disease in the spleen. The woman and her husband brought a cause of action against the surgeon for fraud. Should the court rule in their favor?

3. Charles Venner swallowed 24 or 25 balloons of hashish oil in Morocco, flew to New York, passed 5 balloons, went on to Baltimore, and was brought by friends to the emergency room of Sinai Hospital "euphoric, disoriented, and lethargic, but responding to verbal orders." While under observation, he passed in bedpans the remainder of the balloons, one broken. The hospital staff saved the balloons and turned them over to the Baltimore police without a warrant. Should the police require a search warrant to use the balloons as evidence in a cause of action for possession of an illegal substance with the intent to distribute?

4. A patient went to a plastic surgeon to have repairs made on his nose. The surgeon took pictures before and after the operation. These were published without the patient's consent in a medical journal article titled "The Saddlenose." The patient sued the plastic surgeon, stating that the pictures were being used to advertise the surgeon's work. Should the patient win?

5. Parents took their 13-year-old daughter to the family physician for treatment of a foot infection. He advised the parents that she should stay at home in bed and that they should ask the school for a home teacher. The form the physician signed that went to the superintendent of the school incorrectly stated that the girl was pregnant. The child's parents requested that the physician change the report, but he told them that he had checked his files and found nothing that would indicate that he had made such a report. He also told them that if they brought the report to his office, he would do what he could to correct any error if he had made one. The school would not release the report. The parents continually called the physician. The office told the parents to stop bothering the physician about the matter and that he would not call the school. The father brought charges against the physician for libel. Do you think the physician had a defense that would convince a jury?

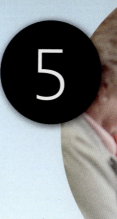

What Makes a Contract

> If the maintenance of public credit, then, be truly so important, the next enquiry which suggests itself is, by what means it is to be effected? The ready answer to which question is, by good faith, by a punctual performance of contracts. States, like individuals, who observe their engagements, are respected and trusted: while the reverse is the fate of those, who pursue an opposite conduct.
>
> *Alexander Hamilton*

OBJECTIVES

Contracts are a fundamental part of any medical practice. After reading this chapter, you should be able to:

1. Explain the elements necessary to make a contract.
2. Recognize how oral contracts can be formed.
3. Explain the difference between express and implied contracts.
4. Identify who can and who cannot be a party to a contract.
5. Describe the law of agency.
6. Identify the various ways to terminate a contract.
7. Recognize patient-related contracts that you will encounter.

BUILDING YOUR LEGAL VOCABULARY

Abandon	Agent
Acceptance	Age of majority
Advance directives	Breach

(continues)

Conservator
Consideration
Contract
Duress
Emancipated minors
Express contract
Guardian
Implied contract
Incompetent persons
Injunctive relief
Legal capacity
Legal disability

Mature minor
Memorialize
Mental incompetence
Minors
Mutual agreement
Offer
Principal
Remedies
Specific performance
Undue influence
Warranty

offer a proposal to perform or refrain from a certain action

acceptance an agreement to the terms of an offer

consideration something promised that results in making an agreement a lawful, enforceable contract

contract a voluntary agreement, written or unwritten, between two parties that creates an obligation to do or not do something

express contract a clear, definitive agreement between two or more parties

implied contract an agreement not indicated by direct words but evident from the conduct of the parties

legal capacity legal ability to enter into contracts because no legal disabilities exist

breach breaking a law, promise, or agreement

remedies legal ways to make someone whole

specific performance the remedy of requiring someone to perform a contract as specified

injunctive relief remedy preventing or requiring someone to perform or to refrain from performing a particular action

CONTRACTS, IN GENERAL

The patient–physician relationship is the foundation of medical practice. That relationship is contractual and can be illustrated in its simplest form as follows: The patient seeks medical care (the **offer**) and the physician agrees to provide the medical care (the **acceptance**). The promises made to the other party (the patient's promise to pay a fee and the physician's promise to provide health care) are the **consideration** needed to form a legally binding contract.

A **contract** is a voluntary agreement between two or more parties that establishes a legally enforceable obligation. A contract can be written or oral, and it can be **express contract** or **implied contract**. The parties must have the **legal capacity** to form a contract. Either party to a contract can appoint an agent to form the contract or to perform some or all of the contractual obligations.

A **breach** of contract occurs when either party fails to perform one or more terms of the agreement. Contracts are enforceable by the courts, and there are **remedies** for damages that occur as a result of a breach, including money, **specific performance**, and **injunctive relief**.

Contracts are an essential and pervasive part of any health care facility. If there is more than one physician in the practice, the entire practice is considered to have formed a contract with a patient. Medical practices, insurance companies, hospitals, nursing homes, and other health care facilities are held together through contract law. Health care personnel may have employment contracts that state that they are employed, at what rate, what the job consists of, and whatever other terms are necessary to define the framework of employment. If there is no employment contract, the employee is deemed to be an employee-at-will, which means that the employer can dismiss the employee at any time, without warning, and for any nondis-criminatory reason.

In addition to contracts related directly to the patient–physician relationship, contracts encountered in any health care facility can include:

- contracts with insurance companies.
- contracts for office or medical supplies.
- contracts to lease office space.
- contracts for employment.
- contracts with other health care facilities.
- contracts for clinical laboratories services, medical record software, or medical equipment lease or purchase.

ELEMENTS OF A CONTRACT

A contract comes into being when one party makes an offer, the other party accepts, and some form of consideration passes between them. Parties enter into a contractual relationship by mutual agreement, also referred to as assent or "meeting of the minds." By entering into a relationship with a health care provider, the patient makes the offer of his or her person for treatment. By opening the office doors or scheduling a patient's appointment, the health care facility accepts the patient's offer. The consideration is that the patient promises to pay the fee and that the physician promises to treat the patient. Once an offer, an acceptance, and consideration exist, the parties have formed a contract.

Consideration

In any contract, each party promises something in exchange for what is received. These promises are referred to as consideration. The promise made must be something that the party is not already obligated to do or to refrain from doing. In a patient–physician contract, the patient promises to pay a fee for the medical care received and the physician promises to provide the agreed-upon treatment. In a contract for leased medical office space, the health care facility promises to pay the rent and abide by the terms of the lease, and the landlord promises to make the leased space available as described in the lease. In a contract for medical supplies, the medical supply company promises to supply its products at certain prices, and the health care facility promises to pay for the products it orders. All contracts have some form of consideration. Without consideration, a contract is not enforceable.

Mutual Agreement

To form a contract, there must be a clear understanding between the parties, known as **mutual agreement**, assent, or meeting of the minds. Both the party who makes the offer and the party who accepts must be

mutual agreement common agreement of both parties

thinking and saying the same thing. In a health care facility, the patient seeks medical treatment for a fee and the physician must be offering to treat the patient for a fee. Whether there was mutual agreement, and, therefore, a patient–physician relationship, is often implied by the parties' actions. The courts have found that a variety of acts by physicians can create mutual agreement. Legal duties and obligations exist once a patient–physician relationship exists, so it is important to understand when the relationship begins and ends.

The cases that have decided the issue of whether a patient–physician relationship exists are heavily fact specific and rely upon state law. Generally, the relationship does not exist until the physician affirmatively undertakes to diagnose and treat the patient or participates in some manner of the patient's diagnosis and treatment.

The circumstances that create a patient–physician relationship can be simple and clear. For example, a new patient arrives for her first appointment. Often, however, the situation presents additional facts that require consideration to determine when the relationship began. Courts have held that a physician need not interact directly with a patient to establish a patient–physician relationship. As a result, the start of the patient–physician relationship can be unclear in situations involving on-call specialists, informal consultations with a colleague (sometimes referred to as "curbside consultations"), or physicians who are covering for others on vacation, among others.

> ⚖️
>
> The patient presented at the emergency room with a three-day headache. After examination and observation, the emergency room physician Dr. Boyle decided that the patient should be admitted to the hospital, which based upon the patient's health care plan, required approval from Dr. Tavera. Dr. Boyle briefed Dr. Tavera and recommended hospitalization. Dr. Tavera did not approve the admission and directed that the patient be treated on an outpatient basis. The patient was sent home and suffered a stroke a few hours later. The patient sued and alleged, in part, that his heath care plan created a patient–physician relationship by contract. The court agreed, in part, because the health care plan obligated its contracted doctors to treat the health care plan members as they would treat their other patients and the patient had essentially pre-paid for the medical care of Dr. Tavera, the health care plan's doctor on duty that night.
>
> *Hand v. Tavera*, 864 S.W.2d 678 (Tex.App.-San Antonio, 1993)

Courts have differed on whether indirect contact between the physician and patient, such as telephone communication between a hospital emergency room physician and an on-call physician regarding the treatment of an emergency room patient, can create a patient–physician relationship.

⚖️

The patient arrived at the emergency room with back pain, fever, and a history of a recent back surgery. Dr. Suarez, the emergency room physician, examined the patient and telephoned Dr. St. John, the hospital's on-call internist that night. Because Dr. St. John was not a neurologist or neurosurgeon, and the hospital was not able to handle such cases, Dr. St. John recommended that the patient be referred to a hospital with the requisite neurosurgeon or to the physician who had performed the surgery. The patient's wife requested the patient be transferred to a specific hospital closer to their home. The requested hospital refused the transfer. The patient's wife took the patient home. Subsequent complications due to meningitis caused permanent damage to the patient. The patient sued Dr. St. John. The court found that Dr. St. John had not formed a patient–physician relationship by recommending that the patient be transferred to another hospital after hearing the patient's history. Dr. St. John listened to the patient's history, symptoms, and condition to decide if he should accept the case, not to diagnose the condition or offer treatment.

St. John v. Pope, 901 S.W.2d 420, 38 Tex.Sup.Ct.J. 723 (Tex., 1995)

A physician, who is covering for another physician, does not automatically establish a patient–physician relationship with every patient of the physician who requested the coverage.

⚖️

The patient had been admitted to the hospital and assigned to Dr. Verm. The next evening, Dr. Johnson was the on-call physician for the patients of Dr. Verm, who was taking time off. As was standard practice, and unless advised otherwise, Dr. Johnson would first see Dr. Verm's patients during rounds the next morning. Dr. Johnson would have gone to the hospital had a nurse called with concerns or had Dr. Verm suggested an earlier visit. Test results that the patient claimed would have changed her outcome were completed at 7:24 a.m., but not available on the hospital computer until after 10 a.m. The first time Dr. Johnson was aware of the patient at all was in the morning when he saw her name on his list of patients. The court held that there was no patient–physician relationship until Dr. Johnson saw the patient during his rounds sometime after 10 a.m. that morning. Consequently, the patient's claim for damages attributable to the delay in reading the test results had to fail against Dr. Johnson, as there was no patient–physician relationship at the time of the alleged delay.

Wax v. Johnson, 42 S.W.3d 168 (Tex.App.-Hous., 1 Dist., 2001)

Physicians can refuse to establish a patient–physician relationship. Historically, the rule has been that a physician has no duty to accept a patient, regardless of the patient's illness. Mutual agreement allows physicians to limit or to avoid contracts with patients.

A physician can refuse:

- to treat patients outside of a particular specialty.
- to make house calls.
- to treat patients via video appointments.
- to have extended office hours or to not take vacation.
- a patient if the practice is not accepting new patients.
- a patient if the physician does not have a relationship with the patient's health insurance company.
- a patient if the patient cannot pay for the costs of treatment.
- a patient if the patient or immediate family member is a medical malpractice attorney.

A physician's right to refuse to treat a patient is broad provided the refusal is not based upon a discriminatory reason, such as race, gender, sexual orientation, national origin, or religion.

> ## 1.1.2 – Prospective Patients
>
> As professionals dedicated to protecting the well-being of patients, physicians have an ethical obligation to provide care in cases of medical emergency. Physicians must also uphold ethical responsibilities not to discriminate against a prospective patient on the basis of race, gender, sexual orientation or gender identity, or other personal or social characteristics that are not clinically relevant to the individual's care. Nor may physicians decline a patient based solely on the individual's infectious disease status. Physicians should not decline patients for whom they have accepted a contractual obligation to provide care.
>
> *AMA Code of Ethics: Opinions on Patient–Physician Relationships (June 2016)*

TYPES OF CONTRACTS

A contract can either be express or implied. An express contract is an actual agreement between the parties, the terms of which are openly stated in distinct and explicit language, either orally or in writing. In medicine, it is generally recognized that without an express contract, a physician or surgeon does not **warranty** the results of his or her work or contract to achieve a particular result.

warranty a promise that specifically named results will occur

An implied contract gives rise to contractual obligations by some action or inaction without specifically stating the terms orally or in writing. For example, if an individual is taken to an emergency room unconscious, it is implied that the patient will accept treatment and that responsibility for payment of the treatment will be assumed by the patient. If a nurse prepares an injection, and the patient rolls up his or her shirtsleeve to receive the injection, it is implied that the patient consents to the treatment.

CAPACITY OF THE PARTIES

Any person or legal entity (such as a corporation) can contract provided that the contracting party does not have a **legal disability** and is authorized to act as represented in the contract. A person with a legal disability cannot form a contract because a contract cannot be made by or enforced against a person who does not have the legal capacity for mutual agreement. **Minors**, **incompetent persons**, and individuals under the undue influence of a drug that alters their mental state are considered legally disabled for the purpose of forming a contract. The capacity to contract is also affected when individuals are under **duress** or required to make an agreement while under the undue influence of another person. In some circumstances, an exception to the requirement that both parties have the legal capacity to contract for health care services can be made when the contract is for emergency treatment that is reasonably needed to continue life.

legal disability lack of legal capacity for mutual agreement

minors persons who are under the age of majority as set forth by state law

incompetent persons those who lack the necessary qualifications to perform a duty

duress being influenced by threat to do something one would not ordinarily do

Minors

The general, common law rule in the treatment of minors is that a minor cannot give effective consent for the administration of medical treatment. Therefore, without the consent of the parents or **guardian**, medical practitioners can be held liable for assault and battery (a criminal charge) or medical malpractice (a civil matter). A minor is any person under the **age of majority**. In most states, the age of majority is 18 years. There are a few states where the age of majority is 19 years or 21 years. Exceptions to this rule are made in medical emergencies and for mature and **emancipated minors**. Other exceptions include states that allow minors to obtain birth control, prenatal, and sexually transmitted disease services without parental involvement. Where parents are also minors, most states allow the minor parent to make medical decisions regarding their own children. The majority of states require that one or more parents be advised of or consent to a minor's abortion.

guardian a person entrusted to take care of the person, property, and rights of someone too young or otherwise incapable of managing his or her own affairs

age of majority the age, as determined by state law, at which a person becomes legally able to contract

emancipated minor a person under the age of majority who is completely self-supporting and able to contract

State law determines a minor's ability to consent, and these laws have been changing in recent years.

In most, but not all, instances, a minor's emancipation is governed by state law and requires a court order. Common reasons for emancipation are the minor's marriage, enlistment in the military, abandonment by the minor's parent or legal guardian, or express agreement by the minor's parents. Many state statutes set forth the circumstances under which the court will order emancipation either entirely or for a limited purpose (health care, residential leases, insurance, banking, etc.).

A 17-year-old minor lived away from home with a woman who gave her free room and board in exchange for household chores. The girl made her own financial decisions and "managed her own affairs." Even though the minor's parents provided part of her income by paying for her private schooling and certain medical care, [she is] considered...[emancipated.]

Carter v. Cangello, 164 Cal. Rptr. 361 (1980)

Generally, neither a minor nor a minor's parents may consent to sterilization, transplants, experimental medical care, or refusal or withholding of treatment without a court order. Yet, in the following action for damages from a vasectomy performed without the consent of parents, the court held that the minor could make his own decision:

A minor and his wife decided to limit their family, and at 18 years of age, a physician performed a vasectomy on the husband. The minor was married, completed high school, the head of his own family, earned his own living, and maintained his own home. Because he was afflicted with a progressive and incurable disease that could affect his future earning capacity and ability to support his family, the court held that the minor could make the decision without involving his parents.

Smith v. Sibley, 431 P.2d 719 (Wash. 1967)

mature minor a person under the age of majority who has the mental capacity to make certain medical decisions without parental consent

A **mature minor** is a nonemancipated minor in mid- to late-teens who has the intelligence and emotional maturity to be able to grasp the information necessary to make an informed decision. The complexity of the medical treatment can affect whether the minor is sufficiently mature to give informed consent. The standards determining a minor's maturity and an individual's capacity to give informed consent are closely related and are often governed by state law.

Constitutional Rights and Minors   American citizens, including minors, enjoy Constitutional rights. The Constitutional right of privacy is fundamental but not absolute for minors in matters of abortion. While the Supreme Court has established that abortion is legal, it has also upheld state laws that require some form of parental involvement in a minor's decision to have an abortion. The majority of states now have laws requiring some form of parental consent or notification for minors who seek an abortion.

Mental Incompetence

Mental incompetence exists when a person does not have the mental capacity to understand the nature and consequences of his or her actions. Some individuals are adjudged incompetent by the courts and have an appointed legal guardian. Generally, the guardian will be appointed by the court to make decisions and enter into contracts on behalf of the incompetent. Many of the contract rules that apply to minors also apply to people adjudicated as mentally incompetent.

mental incompetence lack of reasoning faculties needed to enable someone to contract

   Incompetence is not necessarily adjudicated just for severe mental illness or developmental disability only. In some situations, an individual can be competent to care for himself or herself but unable to attend to personal finances. For such individuals, a **conservator** can be appointed to oversee financial matters. A conservator differs from a legal guardian in that a legal guardian is responsible for both the person and the person's financial matters.

conservator a court-appointed person given authority to manage the financial affairs of an incompetent person

Undue Influence

Undue influence occurs when one party to a contract improperly uses personal influence over the other to cause actions not in the second party's best interests. In the patient–physician relationship, physicians are in a position to influence their patients' decisions. When the physician uses the influential position to form an agreement that is more beneficial to the physician than to the patient, the physician is using undue influence.

undue influence any improper persuasion to make someone act differently from his or her own will

An elderly woman saw a psychoanalyst for many years before she died. During the period of treatment she gave him $116,050, and left him a large sum of money in her will. Part of the money was for professional fees, part was for a loan that he had never repaid, and $30,000 was a gift. After her death her heirs attempted to recover all the money except legitimate fees on the grounds of undue influence. The court ordered a hearing. The psychoanalyst had to prove that the transfers were "fair, open, voluntary, and well understood."

Estate of Reiner, 383 N.Y.S. 2d 504 (1976)

AGENCY

principal the employer, or source of authority, of the agent or employee

agent someone who acts on another's behalf

When a person agrees to work for and under the direction or control of another, a principal–agent relationship is created. The **principal** is the employer, and the **agent** is the employee. In a health care facility, the principal is usually the physician or the medical practice itself, and the agent can be a medical assistant, a nurse, a receptionist, or other employee. Special rules, called the law of agency, govern this relationship. When acting within the scope of their employment, agents are performing tasks on behalf of their employers. Business owners, physicians, hospitals, and other employers—who generally have greater financial resources than employees and for whose benefit the agent is acting—are required to compensate third parties who suffer damages caused by the employers' agents.

The employee answering a physician's phone or making the appointment acts as the physician's agent in forming an oral contract, as depicted in the telephone conversation below.

> Medical Assistant: "Good morning. Doctor's office."
> Patient: "Hello, this is Mrs. West I would like to make an appointment with the doctor for a flu shot."
> Medical Assistant: "I can schedule you for Thursday morning at 10:00 a.m."
> Patient: "That's fine; I'll see you on Thursday at 10."

A middle-aged man was worried after a consultation with a surgeon. "Looks like I'll have to have a heart bypass," the patient remarked to the assistant at the front desk.

"Don't worry," she assured him, "the doctor is very good at that procedure. You won't have any trouble. I can promise you that."

The operation was prolonged by unexpected complications, and the patient died several weeks later. His family successfully sued the surgeon on the grounds that his assistant had made a promise that amounted to a warranty.

Belli, Melvin M., *Belli for Your Malpractice Defense* (1986)

TERMINATION OF CONTRACTS

A contract between a physician and a patient can be terminated in several ways. The most satisfactory outcome is that the physician treats the patient, the patient pays the physician the required fee or copayment, both parties are satisfied, and the contract concludes.

Just as the patient–physician relationship requires mutual agreement by the parties to form a contract, the parties can mutually agree to terminate the relationship. When a physician enters into a patient–physician relationship, the physician is obliged to attend the case as long as it requires attention, unless the patient is given reasonable notice of the physician's intention to withdraw or the patient informs the physician that the services are no longer desired.

If the physician desires to withdraw from the case, the reasonableness of notice becomes an issue that depends on the patient's condition, the availability of other competent physicians, the manner of notice, and, indirectly, the patient's educational and economic status. If a patient discharges a physician and the patient is in need of further medical attention, the responsibility lies with the physician for protection from a charge of abandonment by confirming discharge by the patient. A letter to the patient confirming discharge using certified mail will usually protect the physician. Some physicians follow this procedure when a patient does not keep an appointment or fails to follow the physician's medical advice.

A physician's termination of a patient should be with a written notice sent by certified mail, return receipt requested and filed in the patient's chart, and it should explain the patient's medical problems. The terminating physician must allow time for the patient to receive medical care. The amount of time should be stated, as well as the projected termination date. If a patient relationship is not properly terminated, the physician can be sued for a breach of contract, abandonment, or medical malpractice.

BREACH OF CONTRACT

A breach of contract occurs when one of the parties does not keep a promise—by not performing, not paying for services, not keeping to schedule, or not doing the procedure as had been agreed. Breach of contract also occurs when one party prevents the other party from performing.

Examples of breach of contract can occur in the practice of medicine when the patient does not pay the physician's bill or when a physician makes a warranty that the physician will cure the patient but fails to do so.

When the promised cure does not take place, the physician becomes liable for breach of contract regardless of whether there was negligence.

When the court determines there is a breach of contract, the objective of the court becomes making the nonbreaching party whole. The most common means for accomplishing this is to award the nonbreaching party monetary damages in an amount sufficient to offset the losses incurred. The amount of damages varies greatly based upon the facts and the relevant state law.

Abandonment

abandon to give up or cease doing

To **abandon** a patient means that the physician gives up completely—deserts the patient—and implicitly indicates that the physician intends to terminate the contractual relationship before the contract's obligations are complete. A physician is free to withdraw from a case for nonpayment of fees but is liable for abandonment if proper termination procedures are not carried out or if the patient continues to need services.

Statute of Limitations

The statute of limitations is the length of time a person has to file a lawsuit after injury. Included in the statute of limitations is usually a "discovery rule," which maintains that the statute of limitations does not begin to run until the injured party knew, or should have known, that there was injury.

A minor does not have the capacity to sue in court and is dependent on the parent to file lawsuits before the age of majority. For one reason or another, a parent or legal guardian can decide not to pursue a cause of action. To cover this possibility and safeguard the minor's best interest, many states have maintained a statute of limitations extending two or more years beyond the age of majority. If a state has this provision, health care providers must keep the records of pediatric patients longer than the time that is legally required for adults or at least until the required number of years after the patient reaches the age of majority.

WHO PAYS?

Even though managed care has changed some of the relationship between physician and patient, the relationship between physician and patient still remains contractual in nature. The physician provides the service, and the patient pays the fee, usually a copayment or deductible. The reliability of this arrangement is essential to the fundamental principles of contract law and necessary to continuing commerce. As illustrated in the quotation at the beginning of this chapter, the U.S. economic system is built on the expectation that parties will honor their contracts.

Generally, the patient who receives treatment is responsible for payment even if someone else requests the services. In certain circumstances—for example, in the care of minor children and incompetent persons—others are responsible for payment. In a situation involving minor children or those who are mentally incompetent, the parent or legal guardian is responsible for payment.

Minors lack the legal capacity to contract without a parent or guardian's permission. The interest of the state in this matter is to protect minors from the consequences of their unknowing acts. If a minor contracts for basic necessities, such as food, shelter, and certain life-saving medical services, the policy of protection from unknowing acts is not urgent. When medical care is considered a necessity, however, the court will generally conclude that a fair trade was made and an implied contract will be upheld. The minor, or the person legally responsible for the minor, must pay.

When a minor contracts for plastic surgery for cosmetic purposes, the issue of necessity can be questioned, and the need to protect the minor becomes more urgent. In this situation, the minor may or may not be obligated for the cost. It is reasonably certain that an emancipated or mature minor would be responsible for the fee.

A minor who arranges for medical care can, by statute, invoke the parent's responsibility because parents are responsible for children's necessities. Yet, under certain circumstances, even if a child is living with a parent or guardian, the liability for medical services can rest entirely on the minor if the services were rendered entirely on the credit of the minor. For example, when the expense of treatment was a material and substantial consideration in a judgment recovered by a minor as the result of litigation or settlement, the minor was liable for the medical bills.

When an individual, who is not legally obligated to pay the physician's fee, agrees to pay the physician's fee, a legal principle called "the statute of frauds" requires that the agreement be in writing. An agreement to pay made by an individual, who is not legally obligated to pay the physician's fee, is not legally enforceable unless it is in writing.

Divorce, Minors, and the Single-Parent Family

Today's society offers particular challenges to the collection of bills for minors due to the number of divorces and "yours, mine, and ours" families. Often the parent who brings the child to the physician is not the parent who pays the bill. The party carrying the children's health insurance can be the noncustodial parent. In addition, there might be special arrangements for uninsured medical expenses.

In some cases, the divorced parties have resolved their differences, and the payment of children's medical expenses is not the battleground for further argument. In other situations, this might be the one place where an unhappy ex-spouse can still make a statement of anger by delaying or refusing payment. Sometimes medical insurance is deliberately allowed to expire. In any of these instances, the parents remain responsible for the payment of the minor's medical necessities.

HEALTH CARE ADVANCE DIRECTIVES

The Patient Self-Determination Act, enacted in 1990, requires health care facilities to provide written information to each adult admission regarding patient rights under state law to make **advance directives** involving the acceptance or refusal of medical or surgical treatment. It also requires documentation of the patient's receipt of this information in the medical record as well as whether a patient has executed an advance directive. Institutions cannot condition care on the provision that the patient execute an advance directive or agree to accept treatment. This act does not apply to individual physicians or to private medical offices.

advance directives
written instructions about a person's future medical care

Examples of advance directives, discussed in more detail in Chapter 12, are the living will and health care power of attorney (also referred to as a "health care proxy" or a "medical power of attorney"). It is common for these two directives above to be merged into one comprehensive health care advance directive. In addition, a health care advance directive can include choices regarding organ and tissue donation, as well as other instructions. Contact your state bar association or department of elder affairs for information appropriate to your jurisdiction.

A living will is a written, legal document that identifies treatments you want or don't want if you cannot speak for yourself due to terminal illness or a persistent vegetative state. A living will usually applies only to end-of-life decisions and the instructions tend to be general.

A health care power of attorney is a written, legal document that gives someone the authority to act on another's behalf with regard to specific health care decisions. A health care power of attorney is typically related only to health care decisions, while a durable power of attorney can relate to just about any matter. The document itself will identify the duration and the subject matter it covers.

A "comprehensive health care advance directive" includes the terms of a living will, a health care power of attorney, as well as any other directives, such as location of treatment or organ donation. The comprehensive health care advance directive is the favored form of advance directive because it is inclusive.

☑ SUMMARY

- A contract is a voluntary agreement between two or more parties that creates, modifies, or destroys a legal relationship.
- To have a contract, there must be an offer, acceptance, and consideration.
- An offer is a written or oral statement or other conduct by one party that invites acceptance by a second party.
- The offer can be accepted in an express or implied manner.
- Consideration is the promise or other item of value that is transacted for service or goods.
- To have a legal contract, there must be mutual agreement between parties who have the legal capacity to contract.
- Minors, incompetent persons, and those under undue influence are able to engage in contracts only on a limited basis. In these situations, the court must weigh the rights of the individual with rules of contract law, balancing private and public interests.
- Employees are the agents of their employers and, under the law of agency, able to contract for the principal.
- Contracts made by an authorized agent are valid and enforceable. The principal is usually held responsible for any damages.
- Contracts terminate upon completion of the terms or by agreement of the parties.
- In the contract between physician and patient, the patient may desire to change physicians before treatment has been completed or the physician may desire to refuse further treatment. The discharged physician should **memorialize** the circumstances and conditions of the discharge in a certified letter sent to the patient.

memorialize to put something into writing

- If a physician terminates the relationship, further provisions must be made for the care of the patient or the physician can be found to have abandoned the patient.
- Contracts not performed according to agreement are termed breached.
- A party who sustains a breach of contract is entitled to be made whole by the award of damages. In the medical field, the most common remedy for a breach is monetary damages.
- A comprehensive health care advance directive includes the provisions of a living will and a health care power of attorney, among others.

SUGGESTED ACTIVITIES

1. Consider what the quotation at the beginning of this chapter tells you about why contracts are valuable.

2. What is the age of majority in your state?

3. Find an advance health care directive on the Internet that is applicable to your state. How would you complete it?

4. Identify the various contracts you encounter in your personal life. What was the last contract you signed? What was the last contract you signed on behalf of someone else (an employer, a child, a disabled relative, etc.)?

5. Go to your favorite website and find the "terms and conditions" page, which is sometimes referred to as "legal policy." On that page, find the warranty terms and conditions, which are usually in all capital letters and entitled "Disclaimer, Limitation of Liability and Indemnity." What type of warranty does this company provide?

STUDY QUESTIONS

1. Review the Alexander Hamilton quotation at the beginning of this chapter. Based upon the material you have just read, list the questions that come to mind regarding the phrase "punctual performance of contracts."

2. Give examples of implied and express consent to medical treatment in a hospital emergency room situation.

3. A patient has just been informed by the physician that she must have a hysterectomy and that there is a question of malignancy. As she leaves the office and you schedule her for hospital admission, she comments: "The doctor makes me feel so good about this. She says that I will be out of the hospital in four days and on my own within a week. Isn't she a wonderful person? She says that I will be completely cured following my surgery." How would you handle this situation?

4. A 16-year-old male comes to the office without an appointment and asks to see the physician because he thinks that he has AIDS. He does not wish to give you his name, parents' names, or address. You have seen him around town and know that he is a local resident. The physician is not available, but you expect her within an hour. As the agent of the physician, what is your responsibility in this situation?

5. A 15-year-old girl comes to the office with a diagnosis of first-trimester pregnancy. A year ago, she visited the physician twice, and then miscarried. There is an outstanding fee to be collected from the patient. Her parents are also patients of the physician but do not

know that their daughter is pregnant. It is your job to collect the fees from patients. What would you do as an agent of the physician in this situation?

6. A woman and a 15-year-old minor present at your office for medical care. The woman declares she is the minor's conservator, and she shows you a court document that confirms this. Can she consent to medical treatment on behalf of the minor? How would you handle this situation?

CASES FOR DISCUSSION

1. A 16-year-old female was pregnant and wished to get married to give the child legitimacy. Her mother objected strenuously and took her daughter to a gynecologist to have an abortion. The gynecologist refused to enter into a contract to perform the abortion without a court order. Should the court allow the abortion?

2. A teenage boy suffered from a massive deformity of the face and neck. His appearance was so grotesque he was excused from attendance at school and therefore was illiterate. The condition could be corrected by surgery, but the mother objected to blood transfusions on religious grounds and would not consent to the surgery. (a) Did the minor have the right to surgery? (b) Did the mother have the right to refuse to enter into a contractual relationship with the physician?

3. The director of a drug treatment center called a physician friend and requested that he admit one of the center's patients to the hospital. The physician friend had been seriously ill and was at home recovering when he received the telephone call. He was in no condition to visit the patient in the hospital and conveyed that information to the director but did allow the patient to be admitted to the hospital under his name. The patient never saw the physician before she died of an undiagnosed brain abscess within a few days after admission. Her father sued the physician, claiming that there was a patient–physician relationship between his daughter and the physician. Should the court agree with the physician or the father?

4. A woman was hit by a car and complained of injuries to her leg, knee, hip, and thigh. She was taken to the nearest hospital, where, on the orders of a physician, she received X-rays of her arm and pelvis. No X-ray was taken of her leg, and she was released from the hospital on crutches. The pain in her leg increased, and she went to another hospital some hours later, where an X-ray was taken and revealed that her leg was fractured. She was admitted to the second hospital and remained an inpatient for a month. Ten days after admission to the second hospital, she received a letter from the first hospital

telling her to return for a leg X-ray. She sued the first hospital and the radiologist. Does the radiologist, who never saw her, have a contractual relationship with the patient?

5. A clinic patient was operated on by a hospital resident for removal of his gallbladder. It was later determined that a piece of gauze was left in the patient's abdomen. The defendant in this case was a consultant physician who saw the patient before and after the operation but who was not present at all times during surgery. He was not paid a fee for his services and did not expect payment. Was the consultant physician liable for the gauze in the patient's abdomen?

6. A man had a vasectomy. He and his wife were the parents of two developmentally disabled children, and the vasectomy was desired to prevent the birth of another disabled child. After the vasectomy, another child was born who was developmentally and physically disabled. Should the surgeon who performed the vasectomy be liable for breach of contract?

7. A woman went to a plastic surgeon for an operation to improve the appearance of her nose. Before the operation, the woman's nose had been straight but long and prominent. The surgeon undertook, with two operations, to reduce its prominence and shorten it, thus making it more pleasing in relation to the woman's features. Actually, the patient was obliged to undergo three operations, and her appearance worsened. Her nose now had a concave line to about the midpoint, at which it became bulbous; viewed frontally, the nose from bridge to midpoint was flattened and broadened, and the two sides of the tip had lost symmetry. This configuration could not be improved by further surgery. Should the surgeon be liable for breach of contract?

8. An 18-year-old girl, one of 10 children whose mother was a welfare recipient, was allegedly told by a county social worker that if she refused to be sterilized, her mother would lose her welfare payments. Although the state had an involuntary sterilization statute for mental incompetents residing in state institutions, there was no allegation that the plaintiff was developmentally disabled or incompetent. To the knowledge of the court, there had not been any intelligence tests administered. There was no court order. After her mother's death and upon reaching legal age, the plaintiff filed suit against the social worker who had required sterilization, the county welfare department, the physician who performed the procedure, and the hospital in which the operation was performed. Was the plaintiff unduly influenced, causing her to consent to a sterilization procedure?

9. The plaintiffs engaged a physician to perform a sterilization operation on the wife. Some 17 months later, the wife became pregnant, and nine months later, she was delivered of a child by cesarean section. At the time of this birth, one of her fallopian tubes was found to

be intact. This is alleged to have resulted from the negligent manner in which the physician performed the sterilization. The plaintiffs alleged a breach of warranty. Should the court allow them to recover damages under a breach of warranty action?

10. A patient was hospitalized for mental illness and as part of the treatment received electroshock therapy. When the psychiatrist realized that the patient could not pay his hospital bill, the physician sent the patient home immediately following electroshock treatment. The patient was prescribed a heavy sedative. The patient, confused from the combination of the drug and the effects of the treatment, fell asleep and ignited himself with a cigarette. He suffered nearly fatal third-degree burns over a wide area of his body. Did the physician have the right to discharge the patient from the hospital because he could not pay his bill?

11. The plaintiff, a blind person, accompanied by her four-year-old son and her guide dog, arrived at the defendant's "medical office" on a Saturday to keep an appointment "for treatment of a vaginal infection." She was told that the physician would not treat her unless the dog was removed from the waiting room. She insisted that the dog remain because she "was not informed of any steps which would be taken to assure the safety of the guide dog, its care, or availability to her after treatment." The physician "evicted" the patient, her son, and her dog; refused to treat her condition; and failed to assist her in finding other medical attention. Because of this conduct on the part of the physician, the patient was "humiliated" in the presence of other patients and her young son, and "for another two days while she sought medical assistance from other sources," her infection became "aggravated" and she endured "great pain and suffering." The plaintiff demanded damages resulting from "breach of the physician's duty to treat." Should she be awarded damages?

6

Medical Malpractice and Other Lawsuits

> " The physician must be able to tell the antecedents, know the present, and foretell the future—must mediate these things, and have two special objects in view with regard to disease, namely, to do good or to do no harm. "
>
> *Hippocratic Collection, Of the Epidemics,* book I, sect. II (2)

OBJECTIVES

After reading this chapter, you should be able to:

1. Distinguish between a cause of action for negligence and one for malpractice.
2. List the elements of a medical malpractice lawsuit.
3. Identify when there has been a breach of duty to a patient based on an inappropriate standard of care.
4. Analyze the legal cause of a patient's injury and assess accountability of the employee.
5. Give examples of the defenses available to the defendant.
6. Identify the legal, moral, and ethical aspects of informed consent.
7. Recognize the need for malpractice insurance.
8. Analyze emergency situations and determine whether a situation is covered by a Good Samaritan statute.
9. Distinguish between invitees, licensees, or trespassers and the duty of care owed to them for maintenance of equipment and premises.
10. Define strict liability in tort.
11. Identify a product liability cause of action.

BUILDING YOUR LEGAL VOCABULARY

Adversary	Nonverbal communication
Affirmative duty	Peer review
Assumption of risk	Pharmacopoeia
Burnout	Product liability
Comparative negligence	Proximate cause
Consumer	Reasonable care
Contributory negligence	Res ipsa loquitur
Ethical	Sanctioned
Expert witness	Sociological
Grossly negligent	Statute of limitations
Insurance	Statutory guidelines
Invitee	Suit-prone
Licensee	Trespasser

PRACTICING MEDICINE

The practice of medicine is generally held to mean diagnosis, treatment, and/or prescription for prevention or cure of any human disease, ailment, injury, deformity, or physical or mental condition. To practice medicine, one must have a license. Traditionally, only physicians could practice medicine. With the emergence of new health care providers such as nurse-practitioners, physician's assistants, and medical assistants there has been a trend toward allowing professionals other than medical doctors to engage in limited forms of medical practice.

State legislatures enact laws that govern what duties health care providers can perform based on the kind of license they have. Each individual who practices medicine is held to professional and/or **statutory guidelines** and accepted standards of care. A physician's assistant, a nurse practitioner (or advanced practice registered nurse), and others are permitted to engage in a variety of diagnosis and treatment activities. The precise limitations vary from state to state. The following is an example of a medical assistant practicing medicine without a license:

statutory guidelines
legislative enactments defining legal rights and responsibilities

The husband of a woman who died after undergoing a procedure to destroy a thin layer of her uterus lining through freezing brought a medical malpractice lawsuit against the doctors involved in the treatment. After the surgery, the patient experienced increasing pain, which radiated along the side of her torso to her back. She called the doctor's office and spoke to Lauren Gephart, an unlicensed medical assistant. Gephart thought that the patient might have a urinary tract infection, and she asked the patient about her symptoms. Gephart did not discuss the patient's symptoms with any doctor, nurse, or physician's assistant. Gephart told the patient that her symptoms could be normal and advised her to take 800 milligrams of Ibuprofen. Gephart, however, was not authorized to make medical diagnoses or to give medical advice. Because some of Gephart's actions amounted to the unlicensed practice of medicine, the trial court erroneously failed to explain to the jury that they should consider whether the medical assistant was engaged in the unauthorized practice of medicine.

Wong v. Chappell, 773 S.E.2d 496 (Ga. App. 2015)

A medical assistant is neither licensed nor certified to practice medicine and cannot decide the course of treatment for a patient on behalf of a physician. It is best for the assistant not to discuss the patient's symptoms with the patient but to listen only, making a memorandum for the physician of the complaints listed. If a patient makes the statement "I'm not happy with my care," the medical assistant should not hide the information from the physician or attempt to handle the complaint alone. If the patient is not cooperating with the treatment prescribed by the physician, the medical assistant should make a note informing the physician and attach it to the front of the record. Medical assistants are the first contact with a patient, and often the last, and are therefore in a key position to positively influence the patient–physician relationship.

Because it is unlawful for the medical assistant to practice medicine, it is also unlawful to diagnose over the telephone or during an office visit. Even though the assistant knows that a particular illness is prevalent and that the physician will prescribe an over-the-counter drug, to decide the course of treatment for a patient is practicing medicine. It is similarly illegal to take or order an X-ray of an obviously broken arm without a physician's directive.

NEGLIGENCE OR MALPRACTICE?

"Negligence" is generally defined as "conduct that falls short of a standard; the most commonly used standard in tort law is that of a so-called 'reasonable person'" (Bal, 2009). Medical malpractice is a specific type of negligence. It is defined as "any act or omission by a physician during treatment of a patient that deviates from accepted norms of practice in the medical community and causes an injury to the patient" (Bal, 2009). Malpractice differs from negligence in that malpractice is the negligence of a professional, such as a doctor, educator, pharmacist, or lawyer.

A negligence lawsuit alleges that the defendant did not act in accordance with what a "reasonable person" would have done. A lawsuit that alleges malpractice involves the misconduct of professionals and implies a greater duty of care to the injured person than the reasonable person standard because of the professional's specialized expertise. The term implies that a physician, nurse, or other licensed health care professional has special knowledge that raises society's expectations.

For example, a surgeon performing an appendectomy is held to a higher standard of care than a general practitioner performing the same operation. The surgeon has special knowledge, education, training, and experience, which indicates to society that he or she is better qualified to perform an appendectomy.

In a medical malpractice case, each party must have an **expert witness** to testify as to the particular standard of care and whether it was met. Expert witnesses have experience in the field in which they are testifying. Attorneys will try to find the best qualified expert to testify, with the hope that the jury will receive the expert's testimony as credible. Because medical assistants are not always licensed or certified, the standard of care for medical assistants can be difficult to predict.

The American Association of Medical Assistants (AAMA) and the American Medical Technologists (AMT) maintain national certifying and registration programs; therefore, they are certifying organizations. Difficulties arise, however, because the medical assistant works under the supervision of a physician or other health care professional and performs delegated tasks. The variety of procedures performed, the varying educational levels of medical assistants, and the differences in state statutory requirements make it difficult to establish a national professional standard for the medical assistant. In addition, medical assistants are emerging health care professionals working to carve out professional recognition in the health care delivery system. They are hybrid professionals performing tasks of nurses, secretaries, and technicians. When performing the work of a secretary or receptionist, the medical assistant may be regarded as a reasonable person (rather than a professional); however, when performing clinical procedures, such as giving an injection or doing blood tests, the medical assistant may be regarded as a professional. These same guidelines may be used in establishing the standard of care for all cross-trained professionals.

> **expert witness** a person whose education, profession, or specialized experience qualifies him or her with superior knowledge of a subject

ELEMENTS OF A MEDICAL MALPRACTICE LAWSUIT

To have a medical malpractice lawsuit, the patient must show the following:

1. There was a physician–patient relationship.
2. This relationship established duty by the physician to the patient.
3. The duty had been upheld at a professional standard of care.
4. The physician breached the duty to the patient.

5. The patient had a resulting injury.

6. The physician's breach was the **proximate cause** of the patient's injury.

proximate cause an event from which an injury results as a direct consequence and without which the injury would not have happened

Not only must all these elements be present, but they must be sequential. For example, a physician does not have a duty to a patient before there is a patient–physician relationship.

The elements of a medical malpractice case are the same whether the defendant is the physician, as in the preceding cases, or a nurse, therapist, technician, medical assistant, or other defendant. For the plaintiff to win, each element must be met by a preponderance of the evidence. This means that the fact finder (the jury or judge) must find that evidence supporting the plaintiff's allegations is more likely than not to be true.

Relationship

The relationship between the physician and the patient is established by contract law, which is covered in Chapter 5. If there is no professional relationship between the physician and the patient—for example, if the physician is at a cocktail party and, during a social conversation with the patient, discusses an illness or some symptoms that the patient reveals—there is no malpractice, even if the patient suffers injury from something that was said during the conversation.

The patient–physician relationship establishes duty of the physician to the patient when it can be shown that the patient consulted the physician for medical advice and the elements of a contract were met: offer, acceptance, consideration, and mutual agreement. The specific profession and/or society's expectations establish the duty (also called the "standard of care") required of the physician. When a contract is made between a physician and a patient for medical care, the physician has a duty to the patient that must meet a professional standard of care. Breach of the duty by the physician, by action or inaction, is measured against the standard of care. For example:

A patient visited his physician because of chest pains. While in the office an electrocardiogram was taken. The physician did not tell the patient about the results nor did he prescribe rest or other treatment. A week later the chest pains recurred and were more severe, and the patient called the doctor. The physician told him to go to the hospital. The physician did not tell him to go in an ambulance. The patient walked down several flights of stairs and drove to the hospital in his own car. Examination revealed that he had had a heart attack several days before and open heart surgery was necessary to repair the heart damage. The patient sued and recovered damages from the physician. The court held that a duly careful, reasonably prudent physician would have told his patient about the electrocardiogram results and would have hospitalized the patient immediately.

Armstrong v. Svoboda, 49 Cal. Rptr. 701 (1966)

Duty

In the above example, the first breach of the physician's duty occurred when he did not inform the patient of the irregularities in the electrocardiogram (ECG) and of the possibility that he had or was at risk of having a heart attack. The second breach of duty occurred when the physician did not advise the patient to go to the hospital in an ambulance. A majority of physicians would have explained the ECG irregularities and sent the patient to the hospital via an ambulance. Therefore, the physician performed below an acceptable standard of care. In addition, society expects that a physician will tell a patient of a life-threatening situation, especially when simple modification of the patient's behavior could be lifesaving.

Standard of Care

Standard of care is undergoing many changes. In the past, physicians were held to a local standard of care because of inequities in education and funding for the latest technology between urban and rural localities. Subsequently, the trend in the court was a shift toward a national standard due in part to advances in communications technology allowing for physicians at any place in the United States to access training experiences. More recently, standards of care appear to be reverting back to a local standard of care due to health maintenance organization and other managed care organization guidelines used as the basis. Theoretically, physicians should be protected from malpractice actions by following these recognized practice guidelines because the law sets the standard of care according to accepted medical practices. The guidelines usually set ideal levels of competency, and the law recognizes different medical practices as long as they are generally accepted. There have not been enough cases tried in the courts to accurately assess this trend, but as the managed care networks grow larger and encompass broader areas of the country, the standard of care may again focus on national acceptance.

Injury

To sue for malpractice, the patient must have an injury. Without an injury, there is no case, as described in the following:

A child had Perthes disease in one leg. The physician, by mistake, placed a cast on the other leg. No harm was proven to have occurred as a result of the error; therefore, no damages were awarded.

Redder v. Hanson, 338 F.2d 244 (1964)

Causation

The physician's breach of duty must be the cause of the injury. There are two definitions of the legal cause of injury. The first is "but-for" causation. This means that but for the action of the physician, the injury would not have occurred. In addition to but-for causation, proximate cause must be established. Proximate cause differs in that it takes into consideration any incidents that may have occurred between the original negligent act and the outcome that is the basis for the lawsuit. For example:

> The plaintiff was involved in an automobile accident and fractured a cervical vertebra. The fracture was not discovered for two months and it was determined that a bone graft was necessary. The patient sued the physician for failure to discover the fracture immediately. A witness for the defense, at the trial, testified that the treatment would have been the same regardless of whether the fracture had been discovered immediately and that it would have been necessary to perform a bone graft. The court held that no proximate cause existed because a graft would have been necessary even if the fracture had been discovered immediately. The period of time between the accident and treatment did not cause further injury.
>
> *Rudick v. Prineville Memorial Hospital*, 319 F.2d 764 (1963)

In the case *Holtzclaw v. Ochsner Clinic* (831 So. 2nd 495, La. App. 5th Cir. October 30, 2002), the Court of Appeal of Louisiana found a clinic guilty of malpractice when a nurse answered a phone call after the physicians had left for the day, prescribed aspirin with directions for the patient to "call back in the morning," and did not relay information on the patient's distress to the admitting physician in a timely fashion. The patient had undergone an outpatient colonoscopy and the next day felt intense abdominal pain.

The attending physician rationalized that even if the patient had come to the hospital on the night he began experiencing abdominal pain, the "treatment plan" would not have been different. The court found that an 18-hour delay in administering antibiotics foreseeably caused the patient's injuries. "Since time is critical in arresting any infections the jury could have found that this delay, caused by the nurse's malpractice, denied the plaintiff the opportunity to avoid the [surgical procedure and the hospitalization] by receiving timely treatment."

The courts—recognizing that, in certain cases, evidence of what occurred is not available to the injured person—developed the doctrine of **res ipsa loquitur**. Translated res ipsa loquitur means "the thing speaks for itself." The following is a classic example of res ipsa loquitur:

res ipsa loquitur evidence showing that negligence by the defendant may be reasonably inferred from the nature of the injury occurring to the plaintiff

The physician performed an emergency cesarean section on the plaintiff. At the conclusion of the surgery, two operating room nurses stated that the sponge count was accurate. A sponge was, however, left in plaintiff's abdomen, which required another surgery to remove it. Plaintiff sued and, among other evidence presented, alleged that the doctrine of res ipsa loquitor supported an inference that the physician was negligent. The jury agreed and found in favor of the plaintiff patient. The defendant physician appealed the judgment and argued, in part, that the trial court should not have instructed the jury on the doctrine of res ipsa loquitor.

The trial court properly instructed the jury that the evidence must show "(1) the occurrence of a harmful event ordinarily not occurring in the absence of someone's negligence, (2) caused by an agency or instrumentality within the exclusive control of the defendant, (3) without any voluntary contribution by the plaintiff, and (4) under circumstances such that evidence explaining the event causing the harm is more accessible to the defendant than to the plaintiff." In the instant case, the plaintiff in no way contributed to the sponge being left in her abdomen during the surgery when she was anesthetized and under the control of the physician.

Ochoa v. Vered, 186 P.3d 107 (Colo. App. 2008)

INFORMED CONSENT

Informed consent is an important part of medical practice today. Physicians are often sued for malpractice because of failure to adequately inform patients of drug reactions, possible adverse surgical results, or alternative forms of treatment. Many times, the office staff is actively involved in the consent process. In the next case, the physician was sued because he did not adequately inform the patient of alternative procedures once her condition changed.

Plaintiff sued her obstetrician and alleged medical malpractice and lack of informed consent after her son was born with cerebral palsy. Plaintiff argued that the defendant failed to inform her of risks and available alternative treatments related to material changes in her pregnancy. A jury found in favor of the plaintiff, and the defendant made a motion to set aside the verdict because "it is well established in Maryland that the doctrine of informed consent pertains only to affirmative violations of the patient's physical integrity." On appeal, the court held that an informed consent claim is viable even in cases where there was no "affirmative violation of the patient's physical integrity, because it is the duty of a health care provider to inform a patient of material information, or information that a practitioner knows or ought to know would be significant to a reasonable person in the patient's position in deciding whether or not to submit to a particular medical treatment or procedure."

McQuitty v. Spangler, 976 A.2d 1020 (Md. App. 2009)

Analysis of the elements of this case results in the following:

1. *Relationship*: The relationship between the physician and patient is established. The physician offered services, the patient accepted, consideration was implied, and the fact that hospitalization and delivery took place indicates there was mutual assent.

2. *Duty*: The patient–physician relationship establishes a duty of the physician to inform the patient about the procedures to be performed, the associated risks, alternative methods, and the prognosis.

3. *Breach of duty*: The physician did not communicate to the patient the alternative methods of treatment once her condition changed, and therefore, the patient could not choose or consent to treatment.

4. *Injury*: The patient's child suffered severe cerebral palsy.

5. *The breach was the cause of the injury*: The cause of action is that the physician was negligent for not telling the patient about alternative course of treatment once the conditions of her pregnancy changed. There was no informed consent; therefore, because the patient would likely have chosen a course of action that would have delivered her baby earlier and without complications, the breach was the cause of the injury.

Informed consent is a legal tightrope on which physicians must walk. On one side is the physician's medical judgment about what information the patient must have to make a decision, and on the other side is the patient's right to know every possible outcome. Traditionally, the physician made the decision about how much information was given to the patient. Today, the patient and society exercise the patient's right to know, often requiring the physician to reveal more information than was thought necessary in the past.

Informed consent enters medical practice in many instances. Patients carrying the breast cancer gene have the opportunity to have their own vulnerability to the disease exposed. In a study by the New England

Medical Center, 50 percent of patients who had a history of breast cancer in their family refused the test. Of the remaining 50 percent, 47 percent made the decision to receive the results of the testing. The others did not wish to be informed. In addition, under certain circumstances, physicians may make the judgment that for "therapeutic" reasons, a patient should not be informed about his or her condition.

Another aspect of informed consent occurs when a physician has an "impairment" and has to decide whether to inform the patient. For example, the physician may have an infectious disease, or several malpractice actions may have been brought against the physician for whatever reason.

There are ethical and moral implications in informed consent, especially when a drug or procedure is in the research phase and physicians are experimenting on patients. Physicians' comments and studies reveal that some patients do not want to hear bad news from the physician. In addition, when the risks of a procedure or medication are communicated to a patient, the patient often does not remember what is said. In some situations, a patient may selectively remember comments by the physician and selectively forget other important statements. The sicker the patient, the less accurate the memory is for details of pending treatment; the less educated the patient, the less accurate the recall of information. Lawyers develop forms for patients to sign indicating that they have been informed of possible adverse reactions, but these are commonly not understood by the patient.

"Are patients who sign informed consent paperwork really informed about the treatment they're about to undergo? Of course not. The fine print on such forms is for lawyers, not sick people. But should patients understand the risks and tradeoffs of different options they face? Of course."

Mahar, M. (2007, Fall). Making choice an option. *Dartmouth Medicine*, 1, 39.

The Medical Assistant and Informed Consent

Medical assistants cannot be delegated the responsibility of receiving informed consent from a patient. However, the medical office staff is in a position to protect, or at least warn, the physician of potential malpractice actions when there is doubt whether the physician adequately informed the patient. Keeping accurate records, providing adequate documentation, and relaying patient misunderstanding to the physician can help prevent such actions.

Physicians are legally responsible for obtaining informed consent from a patient. The primary responsibility of the medical office staff is to be certain that copies of informed consent forms are available to the physician, properly dated and signed, and accurately and promptly filed in the patients' medical records. Following discussion with the patient, the physician should document the fact that the patient has been informed and the patient's reactions.

In addition, many times a member of the office staff knows the patient well enough to function as a sounding board for the physician. Patients often express confusion and ask questions of the staff that they will not ask of the physician. **Nonverbal communication** can cue the staff that something is amiss. Medical assistants should communicate with the physician and document personal observations on a sheet attached to the medical record but not part of the record. This information is for the physician only and gives the physician an opportunity to follow-up on the first discussion and correct a patient's inaccurate perceptions and misunderstandings.

nonverbal communication communicating with someone using body language

A patient may decide to withdraw consent. This is the patient's right even after the authorized treatment has begun. The presence of a third person offers assurance to the patient that his or her preferences will be honored.

IMPACT OF MEDICAL MALPRACTICE SUITS

It is a devastating experience for physicians to be sued by patients for whom they have done their best. Physicians may feel that everyone is pointing a finger; they may feel disgraced in the community. They may be afraid that one claim of poor treatment will negate all the good performed in a lifetime.

Researchers surveyed more than 7,000 surgeons and found that nearly one in four were in the midst of litigation. Surgeons involved in a recent lawsuit were more likely to suffer from depression and burnout, including feelings of emotional exhaustion and detachment, a low sense of accomplishment and even thoughts of suicide.

Chen, P. (2011, December 15). When the doctor faces a lawsuit. *The New York Times.* Retrieved from http://well.blogs.nytimes.com/2011/12/15/when-the-doctor-gets-sued-2/?_r=0

Families are affected by a medical malpractice suit. Emotional tension increases in the home as a result of stresses, such as children defending a parent to other children. The fact that the physician can be **ethical**, honest, and competent and still be sued is seldom remembered as the

ethical conforming to professionally proper behavior

defendant proceeds through the lawsuit. Nurses, pharmacists, therapists, and other professionals voice the same disbelief when informed that their actions and professional behavior are in dispute.

Emotions of a defendant may fester and potentially poison relations with patients. Embittered physicians can also have an impact on their colleagues. Physicians and patients can begin viewing each other as an **adversary** rather than as a partner. The ultimate result is that medical care becomes a business—an impersonal, cold, monetary transaction—rather than a trusting relationship between the patient and the physician.

adversary opponent

A defendant loses regardless of the outcome of a malpractice case. The substantial amount of time used to prepare for litigation, the stained reputation, the diversion of society's resources, and the emotional harm to the community can never be recovered or undone.

Defensive Medicine

Physicians, concerned that they might be sued for malpractice, may order every known test in search of a definitive diagnosis when presented with specific symptoms. Following the old adage—the best defense is a good offense—they may request more and more laboratory tests, X-rays, assorted diagnostic procedures, hospitalizations, consultations, and referrals. Many hospitals and most experienced physicians, when confronted with an accident victim, cynically "X-ray 'em wherever they hurt."

Advances in medical science and technology have led to increased specialization: general practitioners were no longer willing to deliver babies, and fewer general surgeons were willing to repair broken bones. The increased use of specialists, the development of managed care, and the threat of malpractice allegations all served to increase the psychological distance between physician and patient. The gap between the patient and the physician began to widen. Each viewed the other as a potential enemy. By continually guarding against litigation, patient hostility—of which physicians constantly complain—became a self-fulfilling prophecy. The trusting relationship the patient wanted was met with a screen of suspicion and wariness. The warm, intimate family physician relationship changed as the physician looked at every patient as a potential malpractice suit. Entrepreneurs published lists of patients who were known to have been involved in malpractice actions against physicians. Medical magazines published articles describing **suit-prone** patient behavior in an attempt to alert physicians that particular kinds of patients should be avoided. In addition, patients have become more knowledgeable and demanding consumers. The Internet has contributed to an increased patients' awareness of medicine. Some of the information patients retrieve in this way may be perfectly good; some may be harmful. Once armed with this "knowledge," however, patients may become more assertive over their care. Likewise, the advent of advertising prescription drugs on television has increased patient demand for certain medications, regardless of whether a patient fully understands the drug's purpose.

suit-prone likely to sue someone or be sued

A recent survey published in the Archives of Internal Medicine revealed that 91 percent of doctors said that their fear of medical malpractice lawsuits impels them to order more tests and procedures for their patients. According to the Associated Press, the survey polled 1,231 ER doctors, surgeons, primary care doctors and other specialists... The survey also revealed that male doctors are more likely to over treat patients than their female counterparts. Overall, 93 percent of male doctors versus 87 percent of female doctors said their fear of medical malpractice changes the way they treat patients... A 2003 study by the US Department of Health and Human Services estimated the cost of defensive medicine at $60 billion a year, but the American Medical Association pegs it at $200 billion. A 2008 study by PricewaterhouseCoopers' Health Research Institute calculated the cost of defensive medicine at $210 billion per year, or 10 percent of all healthcare spending.

Crane, M. (2010, June 28). New study finds 91% of physicians practice defensive medicine. *Medscape Medical News.* Retrieved from http://www.medscape.com/viewarticle/724254

Although it is not known whether the practice of defensive medicine aids in preventing professional liability suits, physicians are caught between protecting themselves by ordering tests and being **sanctioned** for ordering unnecessary procedures by professional **peer reviews** in a society that is extremely interested in containing medical costs.

sanctioned penalized for violating a law or accepted procedure

peer review assessment of academic, professional, or scientific work by others who are experts in the same field

The economics of medicine has also changed behavior. When physicians were getting paid by fee for service, there may have been an incentive to do more than clinically necessary. With the proliferation of capitation, in which a physician is paid a set fee per month for each patient covered by an insurance company, there may be an incentive to do too little.

In any event, the atmosphere surrounding medical errors, the source of malpractice, may be changing. More and more frequently, errors are being attributable to the failure of the system of care rather than blaming an individual. More commonly now, a physician may actually engage in apologizing to a patient; a hospital may work with a patient's family to improve systems of care to benefit individuals beyond the potential malpractice plaintiff.

Economics of Medical Malpractice

Practicing defensive medicine, in short, transformed the malpractice crisis into a vicious circle. Not only did it contribute to the deterioration in the patient–physician relationship, but it contributed to the increased cost of medical care. Physicians formerly had a stake in selling a lot of health care because they got paid on a fee-for-service basis.

An example of the widespread trend of defensive medicine was shown in an article in the *Journal of the American Medical Association (JAMA)*. Reporting on the results of a 2005 survey in Pennsylvania, *JAMA* reported:

Nearly all (93%) reported practicing defensive medicine. "Assurance behavior" such as ordering tests, performing diagnostic procedures, and referring patients for consultation, was very common (92%). Among practitioners of defensive medicine who detailed their most recent defensive act, 43% reported using imaging technology in clinically unnecessary circumstances. Avoidance of procedures and patients that were perceived to elevate the probability of litigation was also widespread. Forty-two percent of respondents reported that they had taken steps to restrict their practice in the previous 3 years, including eliminating procedures prone to complications, such as trauma surgery, and avoiding patients who had complex medical problems or were perceived as litigious.

Studdert, D. M., Mello, M. M., Sage W. M., DesRoches, C. M., Peugh, J. (2005). Defensive medicine among high-risk specialist physicians in a volatile malpractice environment. *Journal of the American Medical Association, 293,* 2609–2617.

The excessive number of tests ordered by physicians to ensure accurate diagnosis is passed on to the patient in the form of dollar cost and lost time and to the American public as a major cause of medical inflation. Physicians, employers, patients, and insurance companies become paper shufflers, adding to the fixed costs of the medical industry. As inflation spirals upward, the American public succumbs to stress-produced illnesses, anxiety, and despair, which hurts the economy by reducing the nation's productivity.

For the physician, one of the immediate effects of the increase in malpractice litigation is seen in higher malpractice insurance premiums and the decline in the number of carriers willing to assume the risk. As the size of awards and number of suits increase, insurance companies suffer losses. Small insurance companies have dropped out of the medical malpractice insurance coverage arena altogether or are selective about who they insure. It is common knowledge that insurance companies are in business to make money and that physicians are also. Since physicians cannot absorb the burden of additional insurance premiums, the public again picks up the tab.

Malpractice continues to be a significant concern. Although the issue seems to have a cyclical nature—the "crisis" reappears every 20 years or so—there is also a geographic component to it. In areas of the country where jury verdicts for "punitive damages" are extraordinarily high relative to the rest of the country, malpractice coverage premiums become a significant barrier to many physicians continuing in the practice. Some leave and go to another jurisdiction, some retire, and some find new careers in administration with either a provider or a payer organization.

Negative Defensive Medicine

When the penalty for unsuccessfully performing a procedure becomes too high, the thinking person avoids the act. Some physicians today are shying away from the treatment of difficult cases with a potentially poor result. Many physicians have refused to take emergency room duty, which has created another specialty in medicine. Fear of malpractice action may prevent a physician from attempting new procedures or employing new drugs. Physicians have protested the hike of medical malpractice insurance premiums by refusing to treat certain classes of patients, primarily obstetric and orthopedic.

An example of this behavior serves to demonstrate how this limits access to care and contributes to physician shortages in certain areas and subspecialties. It is common, for example, for primary care physicians in urban areas to no longer perform ECGs, but rather to refer the patient—even one who has no symptoms—to a cardiologist. The cardiologist is then seeing a relatively healthy patient who may have risk factors but no symptoms or history of heart disease. As this volume of patients increases, those who do have heart disease may find it difficult to get in to see the cardiologist. This underscores a perceived shortage of cardiologists, provides a measure of protection against malpractice to the primary care physician, and contributes to the rising costs of health care through what may be overutilization of specialty care.

ANALYSIS OF THE PROBLEM

A malpractice lawsuit usually arises from two factors: the objective, which is the patient's injury, and the subjective, which is the patient's alienation, anxiety, frustration, and potential anger. Although medical malpractice as a legal concept requires both injury and negligence, the injury alone does not usually bring about the intense hostility that a lawsuit expresses. Many malpractice suits are brought because of poor communication.

Something dawned on attorney Richard Boothman when he defended his first client, a Detroit surgeon, against a malpractice claim in 1981: Sometimes patients just want to be heard. The plaintiff, a woman who'd suffered a major infection after abdominal surgery, hadn't spoken with her doctor in

(Continues)

(Continued)

the six years between the surgery and the trial. While listening to her doctors' testimony in court, however, the woman realized he'd done his best. She won the case, but as the jury filed out, she turned to the surgeon and said, "If I'd known everything I know now, I would never have sued you."

Sanghavi, D. (2013, January 27). Medical malpractice: Why is it so hard for doctors to apologize? *The Boston Globe.* Retrieved from https://www.bostonglobe.com /magazine/2013/01/27/medical-malpractice-why-hard-for-doctors-apologize /c65KIUZraXekMZ8SHIMsQM/story.html

In the preceding example, the role of the physician in addressing the error to the patient has become a form of risk management to avoid litigation while serving as a major factor in improving the safety of medical care.

The Suit-Prone Physician

The working habits and personality of a physician can make the difference between a dangerous, unhappy patient and a friendly, satisfied one. The Richardson Commission warned that there is a suit-prone physician. They portrayed the physician as follows:

One who cannot admit his own limitations… When such a doctor is confronted by a dissatisfied patient, he dismisses the complaint as being trivial instead of making the patient feel less angry, afraid or depressed by showing understanding and explaining matters.

Wilson, P. T. (1975). Anesthesiology and malpractice lawsuits. *Medical Trial Technique Quarterly, 76,* 73.

An attorney who specializes in defending physicians in malpractice suits describes the typical physician who gets sued for malpractice as follows:

… the surgeon who will read the *Wall Street Journal* while the jury is out. He's got the businessman's personality and it shows in the way he runs his practice. He's usually the one who has eight patients in six rooms, with half a dozen

more in the waiting room, and with a flock of nurses checking Blue Shield cards. He is also arrogant, egotistical, condescending, and aloof.

... The doctor who wants to get in trouble after an incident of actual malpractice can do so easily. All he has to do is avoid the patient, blame the patient for the bad result, refuse to talk to the family, refuse to apologize, refuse to listen in humility to patient castigation, and then to send his bill as usual.

Landers, L. (1978, July). Why some people seek revenge against doctors. *Psychology Today*, 94.

The Patient Litigator

Can a physician spot the patient who will sue? An unnamed general practitioner commented in a poll taken by *Medical Economics*, "I have a list above the phone of suit-prone patients who are not to be given appointments." In trying to recognize the patient who is a potential troublemaker, a well-known anesthesiologist has found that patients in the lower middle-class tend to be more demanding about medical activities before and after surgery. Likewise, when a patient's family situation may be emotionally disturbing, there is a greater tendency or predisposition to initiate a lawsuit.

Being sick is uncomfortable, often painful, often embarrassing, and frequently terrifying and involves one's self-image. If there is a malignancy involved, the emotions of the patient, as well as those of the family, are highly charged.

Insults in the Medical Office

It has been said that a malpractice suit is a sort of reverse class action suit—one individual suing the entire medical profession to revenge all the insults of long delays in crowded waiting rooms and physicians with too little time to give each patient. John A. Appleman, attorney for the plaintiff in *Darling v. Charleston Community Hospital*, has summarized several factors he believes contribute to the problem. First on his list: the physician guilty of overbooking the number of patients that can be seen in a day. Many schedule all patients for a given hour. Patients who are depressed may have to wait two hours or more while being exposed to other patients who are coughing or sneezing.

Lack of Empathy

Empathy is a form of communication that is one level deeper than understanding. Empathy requires vicariously experiencing the feelings or thoughts of another person. Health care professionals cannot identify with each patient but can communicate, through nonverbal cues and listening skills, their recognition of the patient's situation.

Often the physician's casual attitude indicates a lack of empathy for his or her patients. Because members of the office staff pick up their cues from the physician for acceptable behavior toward patients, too much casualness may lead to a situation that implies contempt for the patient and the patient's complaints. In contrast, too formal an atmosphere may inhibit the staff's freedom to share their observations about the patient with the physician, as well as give the office a snobbish, uncaring, cold environment.

Today's practice involves a group of physicians, with a primary care physician assuming the role of the family physician. The rules of managed care schedule a certain number of minutes for each patient visit with little flexibility to allow for lengthy conversation in any area. Some patients can express their concerns about their health in this time frame, but others require a few minutes to establish or reestablish a trusting relationship in which to reveal troubling problems. It is difficult to exhibit empathy for a patient's situation when the subject causing distress is never broached.

The Effect of a Prescription

pharmacopoeia a book officially listing medical drugs along with information about their preparation and use; a stock of drugs in a pharmacy

Today's physician has at hand a **pharmacopoeia** that dazzles the imagination. One need only spend a weekend with an elderly grandparent to see an array of pills that will match a flower garden in full bloom for color, and a precious gem display for variety in size and shape.

Nearly 3 in 5 American adults take a prescription drug, up markedly since 2000 because of much higher use of almost every type of medication, including antidepressants and treatments for high cholesterol and diabetes.

In a study published Tuesday in the Journal of the American Medical Association, researchers found that the prevalence of prescription drug use among people 20 and older had risen to 59 percent in 2012 from 51 percent just a dozen years earlier. During the same period, the percentage of people taking five or more prescription drugs nearly doubled, to 15 percent from 8 percent.

Dennis, B. (2015, November 3). Nearly 60 percent of Americans—the highest ever—are taking prescription drugs. *The Washington Post*. Retrieved from https://www.washingtonpost.com/news/to-your-health/wp/2015/11/03/more-americans-than-ever-are-taking-prescription-drugs/

The American public is impatient, sees serious illnesses "cured" in 30 minutes on television soaps, and anticipates being back in the swing of things the next day if the proper pill is prescribed. If the prescribed drug does not work against a particular illness, the patient becomes angry at the physician. Even worse, if the prescribed drug causes an allergic reaction, it is the physician's fault for prescribing the medication. In certain segments of the population, the physician is viewed as a dispensing technician and trust is placed in the drug, not the physician. One of the challenges of the Internet is the inclination of patients to self-diagnose. The patient's "diagnosis" may be right or wrong, but ultimately the physician not only has to deal with the real malady but may need to reeducate the patient as well.

One of the most serious outcomes of the American prescription-conditioned society is that patients do not properly take prescribed medication. Again, the physician is battling the time problem. Physicians do not take, or do not have, the time to explain to patients the importance of properly taking medication and continuing to do so even when they feel better.

Problems arise when more than one physician is involved in prescribing and incompatible drugs are ingested or complications result from a double dosage of the same drug. Many elderly have blind loyalty to the physician, little understanding of the purpose of a particular medication, and fear of asking questions that might brand them as "stupid." When trouble comes, angry relatives enter the picture and view the physician as negligent.

The changes that have taken place in the delivery of health care have affected pharmacies and the dispensing of medications. Where there used to be a small pharmacy on Main Street in every town, there are businesses, such as CVS, Walgreens, and so on, dispensing pharmaceuticals from megastores strategically situated to draw customers from a defined geographic area. Competition also emerges in the form of discount stores such as Walmart and Target utilizing generic list discounting. A national drug chain has its advantages when the customer is away from home and forgets a prescription, but it also has affected the personal relationship that pharmacist and customer enjoyed in the past. Large pharmaceutical stores coach their personnel to be friendly and helpful and to interact with customers as part of the health care team, but often this is a bit much and becomes offensive rather than helpful.

RISK MANAGEMENT ISSUES IN THE MEDICAL OFFICE

Anger is a thread running through the entire medical malpractice saga. The patient is angry, the physician is angry, relatives of both are angry, and the American public is angry about the spiraling medical costs, illness, and the inevitability of old age and dependence. And, physicians are angry because they generally feel as if they are wrongly accused.

Within the past 20 years much has been done to prevent injuries, but attention is just beginning to be drawn to the skills and systems necessary to prevent patients from becoming angry and hostile in their relationships with health care professionals. Legally, the first element of the malpractice case that must be proven is that the patient–physician relationship exists. The case, at this point, turns on the physician's assertion that the relationship exists or does not exist. Psychologically and **sociologically**, the first element of the malpractice case again involves the patient–physician relationship. Here, the question is not whether a relationship exists but what kind of relationship exists. Again, the onus is on the physician.

sociological pertaining to human social behavior

As can be seen from the preceding analysis of the medical malpractice problem, no amount of defensive medicine will aid in reducing the irritants that interfere with a friendly relationship between physician and patient. Without a good patient–physician relationship, the patient's inclination to sue skyrockets, and the resulting malpractice situation becomes increasingly destructive to physician and patient alike. In an effort to eliminate or reduce the threat of a malpractice lawsuit, physicians practice assertive preventive medicine.

Fortunately, physicians are becoming aware of the need for a friendly, professional office environment. A professional office staff can complement the physician in all areas. The physician's staff stands in the physician's corner. Most are working in the health care field because they see themselves as caregivers. Just as patients prefer to stay with one physician, stability in the office staff adds to the sense of security and continuity. A medical assistant or office nurse who knows the patients can alleviate some of the anxiety associated with a visit to the physician and fill gaps caused by the physician's schedule. Training in the art of making immediate contact with patients and basic skills in good human relations will help the assistant meet the patient's needs, avoid confrontations, and contribute to a cheerful office environment.

burnout exhaustion from overwork

Burnout is both a result and a cause of many problems between people working with the public and the public they are serving. A burned-out health care worker only adds fuel to the fire if a patient is incubating a malpractice action. Burnout can be addressed in an office by staff meetings and training sessions to help the employees support each other. They can work together rather than drain personal resources coping with interoffice interpersonal insensitivity. Without dwelling further on the intricacies of informed consent, a well-trained office staff can minimize the difficulties in educating patients.

And so, poor communication still remains the norm. A short while ago, the Annals of Emergency Medicine published a study that examined patient-physician communication in the emergency room on the management of acute coronary syndrome, which is chest pain caused by decreased blood flow to the heart, as with a heart attack or angina. About two-thirds of patients left conversations thinking they were having a heart attack, while physicians believed this to be the case less than half the time. The median estimate of whether a patient might die at home of a heart attack was 80 percent in patients and 10 percent in physicians. Doctors and patients were reasonably close in their estimates of danger only 36 percent of the time. They clearly weren't hearing each other.

Carroll, A. E. (2015, June 1). To be sued less, doctors should consider talking to patients more. *The New York Times.* Retrieved from http://www.nytimes.com/2015/06/02 /upshot/to-be-sued-less-doctors-should-talk-to-patients-more.html?_r=1

A well-educated office staff can either assist the physician in informing a patient or refer the patient to an educational center for instruction. They can tactfully question the patient after the physician's explanation to assess the patient's comprehension and state of acceptance. Many times a patient feels more comfortable asking a nurse or other assistant questions. Hospitals are educating personnel and developing quality assurance systems to improve the quality of care and reduce malpractice claims. Medical societies are educating physicians in the "art" of practicing medicine. It seems logical to extend this educational process to those office personnel who are at every patient's entrance into the maze of modern medical care.

Melvin Belli, an internationally known attorney who has practiced extensively in medical malpractice, wrote a chapter in his book for physicians, *For Your Malpractice Defense*, on the medical office staff and titled it "Is Your Staff Leading You into Legal Hot Water?" Following is the beginning of that chapter:

A woman once came to me with a complaint that she'd been incorrectly treated by a "dumb doctor."

"How do you know he's dumb?" I asked her.

"Because everybody who works for him is dumb."

It's common for patients to relate a doctor to his or her staff. Therefore, quite often, patient dissatisfaction with an office assistant will put the doctor on a malpractice spot.

Belli, M. M. (1986, December). *Belli for your malpractice defense* (1st ed.). Advanstar Medical Economics (p. 47).

This is just another example of how important it is for health care professionals to conduct themselves in a professional manner. What you do and say matters.

DEFENSES TO A MEDICAL MALPRACTICE CAUSE OF ACTION

Common defenses available to a defendant in a medical malpractice cause of action include **statute of limitations**, **contributory negligence**, **comparative negligence**, **assumption of risk**, and emergency.

Statute of Limitations

The statute of limitations sets forth a particular number of years within which one person can sue another. Attorneys representing physicians who have been sued for malpractice will typically first determine whether the statute of limitations has run out by determining how much time has passed since the time the patient knew or should have known there was an injury and the time the lawsuit was filed. Different causes of action have different statutes of limitations. In medical malpractice actions, the statute of limitations is specified in each state's medical malpractice law. Statutes of limitations are necessary because as the years go by, evidence vanishes, witnesses' memories dim, and witnesses die. By setting a time frame within which a lawsuit may be initiated, there is assurance that relevant evidence is available for the fact finders and the parties.

The statutes of limitations of medical malpractice lawsuits usually give the patient two years to sue for damages but can be as long as 10 years depending on the state and the injury. This does not necessarily mean that the medical practitioner is free from concern about malpractice as soon as the statute of limitations expires. In most states, the statute of limitations begins to run when the injured patient becomes aware of the injury. In the case of minors, the statute may not begin to run until the minor reaches the age of majority; therefore, if a child is injured at the age of 1 year, and 18 years is the age of majority, it may be 19 or 20 years before the statute of limitations has expired. If a surgeon leaves a sponge inside a patient, and the patient has no symptoms and does not know the sponge is there, the statute of limitations will likely not start to run until the patient knew or should have known of the surgeon's error.

In some states, the statute of limitations for negligence is longer than that for malpractice. This may be an issue for medical assistants, depending on whether the medical assistant is viewed as a layperson or professional. If the medical assistant is held to be a layperson, the negligence statute of limitations determines the length of time between the

statute of limitations the law setting a time limit within which one person can sue another

contributory negligence conduct by a plaintiff that is below the standard to which he or she is legally required to conform for his or her own protection

comparative negligence negligence measured by percentage, with the determined damages lessened according to the extent of injury or damage committed by the party proven guilty

assumption of risk voluntary acceptance of a known danger

injury and the filing of a cause of action. If the medical assistant is held to be a professional, the malpractice time frame will rule. Following is a case that demonstrates how the statute of limitations defense works:

> A patient had pain in her leg, which began immediately following surgery on her kidney. For several years following surgery she knew that she had phlebitis. She went to another surgeon, who informed her that a vein in her leg had been severed at the time of her first operation. She filed a malpractice action against the first surgeon. The court determined that the pain in her leg and other symptoms put her on notice that something was wrong and that she should have filed an action immediately. Her failure to do so within the statutory period eliminated her right to sue.
>
> *Crawford v. McDonald*, 187 S.E.2d 542 (Ga. 1972)

Contributory Negligence

Contributory negligence is a term used to describe any unreasonable behavior on the part of the patient that contributed, in part, to the cause of injury. In other words, if a patient does anything that contributes to his or her suffering and constitutes behavior that is non-self-preserving, the patient is contributorily negligent. For example:

> Two men, following arrest, were taken to the emergency room following their declaration that they were heroin addicts. The physician on duty observed one of the men writhing, twitching, and moaning, and behaving in a manner that gave the appearance of a person suffering withdrawal symptoms. The physician administered methadone to both men. An hour later one patient stated that he was still having difficulty and the physician gave him an additional dose. The police returned both men to jail. The next morning one of the men was found dead in his cell of an overdose of methadone.
>
> Investigation revealed that one of the men was a drug addict but that the one who died was intoxicated from the combination of Librium, beer, and methadone. The dead man's family brought an action against the emergency room physician. The court held that a patient has a duty to be truthful to a physician, and that failure to do so, in this case, was the sole cause of the death. The dead man had stated he was an addict when he was not an addict. The patient's negligence, or more accurately, his intentional misconduct, barred a malpractice action.
>
> *Rochester v. Katalan*, 320 A.2d 704 (Del. 1974)

The preceding case gives an example of a patient contributing to his own suffering by giving a physician false information. What follows is an example of a patient unwilling to follow the physician's directions and, as a result, contributing to the injury:

The patient arrived at the hospital complaining of pain in his lower abdomen, nausea, and vomiting blood for two weeks. Several blood tests were ordered, and the patient's vital signs were recorded as slightly elevated. The doctor ordered a nasogastric tube to be used to check for blood in the patient's stomach. This test required a painful process wherein the tube is inserted through the nose and down the patient's esophagus into his stomach. One nurse tried to insert this tube, but the patient complained that the procedure was painful. A second nurse explained the procedure and why it was necessary. Nevertheless the patient continued to refuse to have the tube inserted. The nurse then had the patient sign a form indicating that he was refusing medical treatment against medical advice. The nurse then advised the patient that signing out against medical advice could result in dire consequences. The patient died three days later, and the administrator of his estate brought a medical malpractice lawsuit. Because the patient had left the hospital against medical advice, the defense of contributory negligence was appropriate.

Lyons v. Walker Regional Medical Center, 868 So.2d 1071 (Ala. 2003)

Comparative Negligence

In states that allow the defense of contributory negligence, the plaintiff is unable to recover any damages for injury if he or she has contributed in any manner to the injury. Under comparative negligence, the plaintiff is allowed to recover damages proportionate to the defendant's fault, at least in a situation in which the plaintiff's negligence is less than that of the defendant.

Assumption of Risk

Assumption of risk is defined as voluntarily accepting a known danger. The consent to assume risk may be express or implied. This is a defense similar to the doctrine of informed consent in that the only way a patient may assume the risk of a procedure is if the patient is informed of it by the physician.

Emergency

Both common law and the Good Samaritan acts protect health care professionals when they respond to an emergency situation. Under common law, the elements of a medical malpractice action are applied to the emergency situation. For example, if a medical assistant witnesses an automobile accident and no one else is available, is the medical assistant liable for what happens to the victim?

1. *Relationship*: No contractual relationship exists between the medical assistant and the victim as long as the medical assistant does not stop to give help. As soon as help is offered—merely stopping a car may prevent someone else from coming to the aid of the victim—a relationship is established with the victim.

2. *Duty*: As long as the medical assistant passes the accident, he or she has no legal duty to assist the victim. After a medical assistant stops, the victim cannot be abandoned unless care is being provided by someone with comparable or better training, or until the first responders arrive on the scene and assume responsibility for the victim. This reasonable person duty applies whether the Good Samaritan is a health care professional or a layperson.

3. *Standard of care*: In an emergency situation, to encourage trained people to stop and assist, states have enacted Good Samaritan statutes to protect the rescuer from liability. The level of training of the Good Samaritan and the standard of care are important to the person being rescued, but the rescuer will only be held liable for reckless behavior.

4. *Breach of duty*: If a person passes an accident, no breach of duty exists because no relationship with the victim from which a duty arises has been established. If a helper stops and assists, he or she will be held to a standard of care appropriate to the individual's training and experience. If the procedures are performed below standard, the usual question of the court is whether the actions increased the victim's injury.

5. *Injury*: The victim is already injured. The Good Samaritan has a responsibility to help the victim, but for the helper to be held liable for the injury, the helper's acts must cause a considerable amount of additional harm.

6. *The breach was the cause of the injury*: Under negligence law, the victim must prove by a preponderance of the evidence that the help offered caused injury. Since the victim is already injured, the helper's behavior would have to be **grossly negligent** to increase the victim's injuries.

grossly negligent failing intentionally to perform a necessary duty in extraordinary disregard of the consequences to the person neglected, particularly if it can be proven that there is more than a 50 percent chance the negligence caused an injury

As can be seen from the preceding analyses, there is only a slim chance of being charged with malpractice under common law for aiding an accident victim. The reason courts are reluctant to find those who help accident victims guilty is that the public has an interest in encouraging people to stop and aid someone who is injured. Pursuing this reasoning one step further, the states have enacted Good Samaritan laws to encourage trained professionals to provide services at accident scenes.

Good Samaritan statutes provide immunity to volunteers at the scene of an accident as long as they do not intentionally or recklessly cause the patient further injury. It is important to remember that the basis of negligence law is that everyone is responsible for the consequences of his or her own acts.

Office emergencies usually do not fall under the protection of Good Samaritan laws. For example, someone walks into a medical office off the street, obviously ill, and requests medical help. Add to this scene the facts that the potential patient is dirty and has no money, and the physician has asked the medical assistant to get rid of this person. It will probably not go well for the physician in court if the patient sues for not receiving emergency medical care. It is the public's expectation that emergency care will be provided; therefore, the patient should be treated prior to arranging for transportation to the closest emergency room.

MALPRACTICE INSURANCE

insurance a contract binding a company to compensate someone for proven damages or injury caused by the party who has paid premiums in the contract

Malpractice **insurance** is a subject that frequently makes headlines because of rising costs to health care providers. In a society in which many are willing to litigate situations that they believe violate their rights and there is the opportunity to do so, it is understandable that the premiums for coverage increase. The subject is complex. Litigation is expensive, and the damages that are awarded to successful plaintiffs are rising. This is an issue that changes over time; sometimes (and in some places) costs become so excessive that malpractice coverage is either prohibitively expensive or simply unavailable.

Most, but not all, states require that physicians have malpractice insurance. Hospitals, health care facilities, physicians, nurses, and other health care employees may also have malpractice insurance. Because a medical assistant works under the direct supervision of the physician and is not licensed to practice, the physician's insurance usually covers the assistant. This is part of the employment benefits package. If the physician's office does not offer this as a benefit, the medical assistant may need to acquire his or her own malpractice insurance coverage. The reasoning behind this is that a medical assistant extends the effectiveness of the physician. Problems arise when an assistant is named a codefendant in a lawsuit and the physician's insurance will not represent the assistant, or the positions of the assistant and the physician conflict.

PRODUCT LIABILITY

A product liability case is negligence against a manufacturer, a distributor, or some other supplier of goods. Product liability becomes of concern in the medical office when equipment malfunctions, proper instructions are not given for medication, or supplies used in a procedure are defective. The basic theories of recovery are negligence and breach of warranty. In some states, an action filed under strict liability is allowed. Examples of product liability in a health care setting include the following:

A pediatric nurse checks on a patient, then leaves the room. She returns later to discover that the child has been crushed to death by the automatic lowering device on his electric bed. Several children at other hospitals have been killed by activating such bed-lowering buttons.

A nurse in the post-anesthesia care unit breaks a left-atrial catheter while trying to remove it from a patient's chest after open heart surgery. A piece of it remains permanently embedded.

An ICU patient dies when nurses fail to hear a ventilator disconnect alarm through the plate glass doors. Respiratory therapists rig a remote alarm system. Four more patients die before it's debugged.

A nurse's aid manages to keep a patient from falling when the caster drops off a shower chair, but sustains a disabling injury herself.

Tammelleo, A. D. (1990, October). Who's to blame for faulty equipment? *RN*, 67.

Product liability cases have surfaced in court when patients have been injured by tampons, pacemakers, wrinkle cream, implant prosthetics, and so on. In the past, common products have become the object of these suits: blood transfusions, Tylenol, silicone breast implants, infant car seats, heart pacemakers, and tobacco. Those who have standing to sue include persons injured by the product, their relatives in certain circumstances, and employees, among others.

product liability a tort making a manufacturer liable for compensation to anyone using its product if damages or injuries occur from defects in that product

Product liability actions that will be faced by workers in medical offices most often include those classified as "failure to warn" suits. Medical office personnel are often responsible for educating patients about the medications that the physician has prescribed. *The Wall Street Journal* reported as a result of its research:

A new study found that 11% of the statements that drug industry sales representatives made in pitches to doctors falsely described the benefits of their products. The report, based on 13 lunchtime sales presentations sponsored by drug companies at the University of San Diego School of Medicine, said

(Continues)

(Continued)

the inaccurate statements contradicted information in federally approved labeling for the drugs in the companies' own brochures.

In one case, a sales representative said an anti-inflammatory drug had a low incidence of "gastro-intestinal upset," when the product's own package insert said that minor problems "are common" and that fatal bleeding is possible. [Another] was an assertion that monitoring a patient for potentially dangerous blood-count changes should be at a doctor's discretion, when the insert actually advised taking daily blood counts and included a boxed warning to draw attention to the side effect.

The findings offer a new glimpse of the pharmaceutical industry's controversial and enormously effective marketing practices, particularly the thousands of sales people known as drug detailers who visit doctors' offices, hospitals and medical meetings to tout the industry's products.

Winslow, R. (1995, April 26). Drug-industry sales pitches to doctors are inaccurate 11% of the time, study says. *The Wall Street Journal*, B6.

The plaintiff in a product liability suit may include a passenger in an automobile accident if a physician fails to warn the driver about mixing drugs with drinking and driving.

The driver, a hospital patient, was given the drugs by two psychiatrists the day he was discharged from the hospital. He then had an alcoholic drink and drove his car into a tree, permanently injuring his passenger.

The court held that the drug manufacturers, the doctors, and the hospital had a duty to warn the patient of the drugs' adverse effects. What happened was "within the realm of reasonable foreseeability absent a pertinent warning." The burden of preventing injuries to the general public is not undue in light of the great risks to the public, it continued, declaring that "the fast pace at which new drugs are presently being introduced and utilized demands that the public be protected from their varying adverse effects."

Kirk v. Michael Reese Hospital, No. 81-2408 (Ill. App. Ct., August 28, 1985)

Duty to Provide Adequate Warnings and Directions for Use

A manufacturer is obligated to provide adequate directions for use of a product. The extensive written material that accompanies a prescription drug is an example of the manufacturer's duty to give directions for use and to warn of any untoward results. Directions are primarily to secure the efficient use of a product. When a departure from the directions may create a serious problem, a separate duty to warn arises. The following is a case in point:

Heat blocks are used to help revive injured persons. Instructions to wrap the blocks in insulating material before using were given, but there was no statement that if used without insulation, the blocks would cause serious burns. The plaintiff was seriously burned by the blocks. The court, in dictum as to the need for warning, observed that "instructions, not particularly stressed, do not amount to a warning of the risk at all…" and found against the defendant.

McLaughlin v. Mine Safety Appliances Co.,
11 N.Y.2d 62, 226 N.Y.S.2d 407, 181 N.E.2d 430 (1962)

STRICT LIABILITY

Strict liability is used in product liability cases in which the seller is liable for any and all defective or hazardous products that unduly threaten a **consumer**'s personal safety. Strict liability may arise when the product is defective and unreasonably dangerous. To prevent the product from being unreasonably dangerous, the seller may be required to give directions or warning, on the container, as to its use. For the most part, actions in strict liability are not applied to physicians and hospitals because of the requirement that there be a sale of goods. Health care is primarily a sale of services. However, there have been a few exceptions. For example:

consumer one who buys products and services

In Texas, a patient was injured when his hospital gown caught fire after the patient dropped a lighted match on it. The court held that where a hospital supplies a product unrelated to the essential professional relationship with the patient, the hospital may be considered the entity to have introduced the harmful product into the stream of commerce for purposes of a strict liability cause of action.

Thomas v. St. Joseph Hospital, 618 S.W.2d 791 (Tex. Civ. App. 1981)

Problems of strict liability arise in medicine with use of drugs. For the most part, physicians and health care facilities are not liable under strict liability but drug manufacturing companies are. The courts must balance the risk of taking the drug versus the risk without it, and whether the physician and patient were warned. If the drug has known side effects and the physician warns the patient of these, the patient *assumes the risk* of the treatment.

PREMISES LIABILITY

Hospitals, clinics, and individual practitioners are responsible to the public for their offices, laboratories, buildings, and equipment, as shown in the following:

Plaintiff was rendered a quadriplegic when he fell on a mat while waiting for an elevator in defendant hospital. Plaintiff contended that the fall was caused by a fold or buckle in the mat and that the hospital was negligent in using and failing to secure the mat. There was a triable issue of fact as to whether the hospital breached its duty of care to plaintiff.

Caburnay v. Norwegian American Hosp., 2011 IL App (1st) 101740 (Ill. App., 2011)

Property owners must observe certain standards of care for the protection of others, regardless of whether they come onto the property legally. Persons coming on property are classified as **invitees**, **licensees**, or **trespassers**.

invitee a person who enters property for business as a result of express or implied invitation

licensee a person who enters property with implied permission of the owner

trespasser someone who enters a property illegally

reasonable care the amount of care a rational person would use in similar circumstances

Trespassers   Someone who enters property illegally is a trespasser. Despite the fact that such a person is not invited and probably not wanted, the owner and the occupier have obligations for the safety of this person. There is a duty to warn of dangers and a duty to reduce and eliminate dangers existing on the property. This duty should be carried out with **reasonable care**. The care necessary to fulfill the duty required, in most cases, is merely giving warning of the activity or condition. There is a stricter responsibility to trespassing children because they are often unable to recognize danger. The law limits the extent to which property may be protected against trespassers, as shown in the following:

The house was inherited from the defendants' grandparents and had been unoccupied for some time. There had been a series of intrusions, and the defendants had boarded up the windows and the doors in an attempt to protect the property. They had posted "no trespass" signs on the land, the nearest one being 35 feet from the house. On June 11, 1967, the defendants set a "shotgun trap" in the north bedroom. After Mr. Briney cleaned and oiled his 20-gauge shotgun, defendants took it to the old house, where they secured it to an iron bed with the barrel pointed at the bedroom door. It was rigged with wire from the doorknob to the gun's trigger so it would fire when the door was opened. Briney first pointed the gun so an intruder would be hit in the stomach, but at Mrs. Briney's suggestion it was lowered to hit the legs. He admitted he did so "because I was mad and tired of being tormented," but he did not intend to injure anyone. He gave no explanation of why he used a loaded shell and set it to hit a person already in the house.

The plaintiff entered the old house by removing a board from a porch window which was without glass … As he started to open the north bedroom door, the shotgun went off, striking him in the right leg above the ankle bone. Much of his leg, including part of the tibia, was blown away. Only by…assistance was the plaintiff able to get out of the house and then to a hospital. He remained in the hospital 40 days.

The trial court held that an owner may not protect personal property in an unoccupied boarded up farmhouse against trespass by use of deadly force. This decision was affirmed by the appeals court.

Katko v. Briney, 183 N.W.2d 657 (Iowa 1971)

Licensees   A licensee differs from a trespasser in that a licensee enters property with implied permission. Examples of licensees include public servants, such as the police and firefighters, those who may cross property to take a shortcut, social guests, those who come into the office to get out of the rain, traveling salespersons, and charitable solicitors. There is a duty to warn these people about any dangerous conditions that they would not anticipate or easily see.

Invitees   Invitees are persons who enter property for business as a result of express or implied invitation. Store customers; patrons of restaurants, banks, and places of amusement; delivery persons and plumbers; and electricians and carpenters doing work at an owner's request are all invitees. The duty owed to invitees is higher than that owed to trespassers or licensees. Generally, it is to make the premises safe by exercising reasonable care to warn the invitee of known defects in the property, or of those which could be discovered with reasonable care. This includes an **affirmative duty** to protect the invitee. Reasonable care may include inspection of the premises to discover possible defects, an example of which is seen in the following:

affirmative duty responding to an incident in a predetermined manner

> ⚖️
>
> A mother took her 5-year-old son to the pediatrician's office. After the visit she left by the back door, stepped into a hole and hurt her ankle. The hole was hidden by some very high grass and neither she nor the pediatrician had noticed it on prior trips through the door. The court found that she was an invitee, even though she was not herself a patient, but held that there was no evidence that the physician had known of the hole.
>
> *Goldman v. Kossove*, 117 S.E.2d 35 (N.C. 1960)

Premises owners are increasingly being held liable for injuries intentionally inflicted by third parties unrelated to the victim or the premises owner. For example:

> ⚖️
>
> Plaintiffs who were injured or killed by a fellow patron at a movie theater complex in Aurora, Colorado brought a premises liability claim. The defendant Cinemark sought to have the premises liability claims dismissed and argued that plaintiffs could not show that Cinemark knew or should have known of the danger resulting from the theater's layout and operation. The gunman was able to cause such a tragedy, in part, because he was able to exit the theater via a side door, make at least one trip to his car, and return to the theater through the same side door with assault rifles, handguns, tear gas canisters, body armor, and tear gas canisters. There was no system to survey or monitor the parking areas behind or to the sides of the theaters, and the gunman was undetected by Cinemark personnel. In addition, the side doors to the theaters did not have alarm systems or any other security or alarm features that would alert theater personnel that someone had used the side door. The court held that the plaintiffs had sufficiently stated a claim to survive a motion to dismiss.
>
> *Traynom v. Cinemark USA, Inc.*, 940 F.Supp.2d 1339 (D. Colo. 2013)

While the *Traynom v. Cinemark USA, Inc.* case is an extreme example of premises liability, there are potential premises liability situations you will encounter while at work where you can make a difference. If you see a piece of paper on the floor, pick it up; if you notice a spill on the floor, ensure it is cleaned as soon as possible and prevent others from getting near the spill until it is cleaned; if you see a frayed electrical cord, bring it to the attention of the appropriate person in your office. The saying "if you see something, say something" applies here, as you are on the frontline and can prevent lawsuits.

☑ SUMMARY

- When one person hurts another without intent, the legal cause of action is negligence. Negligence by a professional is known as malpractice. The difference between negligence and malpractice is the standard of care required of the injuring party.

- If the defendant is a layperson who is held to the reasonable person standard, the act (or failure to act) is considered "negligence." If the inflicting party is a professional who is held to the standard of a profession with prescribed education, training, and experience, the act (or failure to act) is considered "malpractice."

- An expert witness provides evidence for the jury to the standard for the profession with testimony in court.

- Medical assistants are hybrid health care professionals. Receptionist and secretarial duties are categorized under a layperson standard, and clinical tasks may be labeled professional. In either case, the responsibilities extend the effectiveness of a physician and are delegated by the employer.

- The AAMA and the AMT are the national certifying bodies, and membership would be recognized in the qualifications of an expert witness.

- The elements of a civil medical malpractice cause of action include the following:

  1. There was a relationship between the physician and the patient.
  2. This relationship established duty by the physician to the patient.
  3. The duty had been upheld at a professional standard of care.
  4. The physician breached the duty to the patient.
  5. The patient had a resulting injury.
  6. The physician's breach was the proximate cause of the patient's injury.

- Informed consent requires that a physician communicate information to a patient regarding the treatment he or she is about to receive. The patient has a right to refuse treatment; therefore, the physician must provide enough information to allow the patient to make an informed decision. Only a physician can accept consent from a patient.

- The medical assistant performs the duties of preparing and filing the consent forms, as well as listening and observing to determine whether the patient understood and accepted the proposed treatment plan.

- Some malpractice lawsuits can be avoided simply with better communication.

- Five defenses are available to a defendant in a medical malpractice cause of action: tolling of the statute of limitations, contributory negligence, comparative negligence, assumption of risk, and emergency.

- Medical malpractice insurance is available to cover monetary awards against a defendant. Medical assistants may or may not be covered under a physician's insurance. Insurance is available for the protection of a medical assistant.

- Hospitals, clinics, and individual practitioners are responsible to the public for their offices, laboratories, buildings, and equipment.

- Different standards of responsibility are required for trespassers, licensees, and invitees. The standard of property maintenance for a trespasser is reasonable care. The standard of maintenance increases for licensees. The highest standard of maintenance is due to invitees and requires affirmative behavior on the part of the landlord or occupier to warn the invitee about dangerous conditions or activities that are known or could be discovered with reasonable effort.

SUGGESTED ACTIVITIES

1. Play the childhood game of rumors. Begin by giving directions for taking medication. As the rumor travels around the circle, document the changes. After 15 minutes, try to remember the directions first given. This will give each player an opportunity to learn about some of the confusion a patient experiences in the informed consent process.

2. Role play. Show empathy to a patient who has just learned that he has cancer of the larynx.

STUDY QUESTIONS

1. Describe a situation that might place a medical assistant in the position of being negligent.

2. Describe a situation that might cause a medical assistant to be charged with medical malpractice.

3. List the qualifications for an expert witness in a legal action involving a medical assistant who works in a pediatrician's office.

4. What is meant by the following: "Even if a doctor wins, he or she loses in a medical malpractice lawsuit"?

5. What relationship is necessary between a physician and patient to establish duty of care for the physician?

6. List the elements of a medical malpractice cause of action.

7. A newly diagnosed cancer patient comes to your desk after being informed of two alternatives for treatment, one involving surgery and the second involving chemotherapy. He asks your advice. How do you handle the situation?

8. List, define, and give examples of the five defenses available to a defendant in a medical malpractice suit.

9. An automobile accident occurs in front of your office. You hear the crash and go to the door to see what has happened. One of the passengers in the car is walking around the street in a daze with blood dripping from a facial laceration. What do you do?

10. Prepare a question for your employer to determine whether his or her malpractice insurance covers a medical assistant working in the office.

11. An individual comes onto property owned by the medical office, is drunk, has been told to leave, but remains in the building. There is a floor board in the front hallway that everyone knew needed to be fixed, but nothing has been done about it. The individual falls when the board gives way and breaks his leg. What is the responsibility of the medical office?

12. While sitting in the waiting room of a medical office, a patient falls when the chair gives way under him. The man is a very heavy person and chose to sit on a regular chair. There was a large chair available for him. The patient ends up in the hospital for observation and later for pneumonia related to his inactivity. Who is responsible for the pneumonia?

13. List equipment one might find in a medical office that could injure a patient and give rise to a product liability claim.

CASES FOR DISCUSSION

1. A negligence action was brought by a mother on behalf of her minor daughter against a hospital. It alleged that when the mother was 13 years of age, the hospital negligently transfused her with Rh-positive blood. The mother's Rh-negative blood was incompatible with and sensitized by the Rh-positive blood. The mother discovered her condition eight years later during a routine blood screening ordered by her physician in the course of prenatal care. The resulting sensitization of the mother's blood allegedly caused damage to the fetus, resulting in physical defects and premature birth. Did a patient relationship with the transfusing hospital exist?

2. The patient was admitted to the hospital for dilation and curettage. The defendant was an anesthesiologist who injected sodium pentothal into the patient. The patient developed a laryngospasm, which prevented oxygen from entering the lungs and bloodstream. Attempts were made to break and relax the spasm but were unsuccessful. The plaintiff suffered severe and disabling brain damage. Conflicting evidence was submitted with regard to whether the defendant left the operating room to attend another patient before or after an equally qualified physician arrived to provide patient care. Was the physician at liberty to withdraw from the patient?

3. A woman was in labor. The nurse on duty refused to call the obstetrician. Instead, the nurse sat and read a magazine, ignoring repeated requests from the patient and her husband to call a physician. The husband informed the nurse when his wife was about to deliver, and the nurse told him to sit down. The woman delivered before the obstetrician arrived, and she was injured. Was the hospital liable for the nurse's negligence?

4. A 16-year-old boy was hit by an automobile while riding his bicycle. He was taken to the emergency room by a parent; the physician on call looked him over and sent him home. The boy died a few hours later. Autopsy revealed that he had a massive skull fracture. Was the physician's lack of a thorough examination the cause of the patient's death?

5. A male patient was admitted to the hospital with pneumonitis. He was ill with a high fever and in his confusion walked out on the balcony outside his room and told construction workers below that he was going to jump. They notified the nurse on the patient's floor, who called his physician. The physician told her to watch and restrain the patient. The nurse called the patient's wife and told her what was happening. The wife explained that she had to get a babysitter before she could get to the hospital but that the patient's mother could be there in five minutes. The wife asked the nurse to stay with the

patient until a family member could get there, but the nurse stated that they were too busy. The man jumped or fell from the balcony. Was the nurse guilty of malpractice?

6. The plaintiff was a 21-year-old student who severely injured his right index finger while working in a bakery. He is left-handed. The defendant, a board-certified orthopedist who specializes in hand surgery, testified that the value of the hand had been reduced by some 40 percent. At the plaintiff's request, the defendant took over the case. There were two operations. The first went well, but after the second, circulation could not be restored to the finger and it had to be amputated at the base. With the amputated finger, the plaintiff had 80 percent use of the hand, which was more than prior to surgery. The plaintiff sued, alleging that the defendant did not inform him of the risks of the operations and that he might lose his finger. Should the court find the defendant guilty of malpractice?

7. The plaintiff, Bonner, was a 16-year-old Washington resident who had a severely burned cousin. The cousin was brought to the defendant, a plastic surgeon, for treatment. The physician advised a skin graft. After many unsuccessful attempts to find a donor, Bonner's aunt asked him to go to the hospital for a test to see if his blood would match with that of his cousin. He went to the hospital, had the test, and his blood matched. The defendant performed the first operation on Bonner's side. Bonner's mother, with whom he lived, was ill and knew nothing of the operation. Bonner later returned to the hospital for a second operation. He told his mother that he was going to have his side "fixed up." Instead, Bonner remained in the hospital, where an unsuccessful graft was attempted. In the course of the operation, Bonner lost a lot of blood and skin and had to remain hospitalized for two months. There was sufficient evidence for the jury to believe that Bonner's mother never knew the exact nature of the operations or consented to them. When his mother did learn of the operations, she made no attempt to prevent them but instead allowed Bonner to return to complete them. Bonner was a minor. Must the parents of a minor give consent before an operation for the benefit of another may be performed?

8. Kennedy, the plaintiff, consulted the defendant, a surgeon. The surgeon diagnosed appendicitis and recommended an operation, to which the plaintiff agreed. During the operation, the defendant discovered some enlarged cysts on the plaintiff's left ovary, which he punctured. After the operation, the plaintiff developed phlebitis in her leg, which caused her considerable pain and suffering. The plaintiff alleged that the puncturing of the cysts on her ovary was unauthorized, and she brought an action for damages. Can a surgeon extend an operation without consent?

9. The plaintiff, Anderson, was undergoing a back operation. During surgery, the tip of a forceps-like instrument broke off in Anderson's spinal canal. The surgeon was unable to retrieve the metal, and the patient suffered significant and permanent physical injury caused by the fragment, which lodged in his spine. The plaintiff-patient sued the defendant-surgeon for medical malpractice, the hospital for furnishing a defective instrument, the medical supply distributor for furnishing the defective instrument to the hospital on a warranty theory, and the manufacturer on a strict liability theory for making a defective product. The trial court held that there was no cause to the surgeon and the other defendants. Did the appeals court support the trial court's decision?

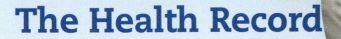

7

The Health Record

> **"** Electronic health records are, in a lot of ways, I think the aspect of technology that is going to revolutionize the way we deliver care. And it's not just that we will be able to collect information, it's that everyone involved in the healthcare enterprise will be able to use that information more effectively.
>
> *Risa Lavizzo-Mourey, M.D., M.B.A.* **"**

OBJECTIVES

After reading this chapter, you should be able to:

1. Define the characteristics and benefits of an EHR.
2. List different types of health records.
3. Identify the owner of a health record.
4. Recognize new dimensions of confidentiality with the use of computers for health records.
5. Identify the procedures necessary for release of information from the health record.
6. Determine who has access to a health record.
7. Identify the concerns associated with faxing medical information.
8. Define the importance of health record credibility.
9. Follow an acceptable method for making corrections to a health record.

BUILDING YOUR LEGAL VOCABULARY

Data
Premises
Property right

Subpoena
Subpoena duces tecum

INTRODUCTION

Despite the changes in the way a health record is kept, the foundational elements remain intact, including privacy, accuracy, timeliness, and reliance. The medical assistant is one of many care providers who manage patient health records.

A medical record, also referred to as a health record, is a recorded collection of **data** on a patient. It includes past history, a statement of the current problem and diagnosis, and the treatment procedures used to solve the problem. Health records are created for many reasons, including the following: Records are often required by licensing authorities; records may contain information required by patient's insurance companies to pay claims; records are essential for communicating important data to all those who participate in a patient's care; records create a legal document to record and substantiate a standard of care; and specific records and pieces of data may be required by physicians' liability insurance.

The move from paper charts to electronic health records (EHRs) has been one of the most significant changes in health care. Federal legislation that penalizes Medicare providers who continue to use paper charts has accelerated the transition to EHRs. The Health Information Technology for Economic and Clinical Health (HITECH) Act has created incentives for using EHRs, as well as penalties for not using them.

Largely due to the data available from EHR, the health record is increasingly being used to determine the necessity for and the quality of health care. This is reflected in the greater use of the health record by health maintenance organization (HMO) peer review teams and insurance company audits. In addition to the fact that insurer reimbursement may depend on adequate documentation of services provided, the quality of a health care provider's health records often tells a lot about the quality of the practice.

data pieces of information

ELECTRONIC HEALTH RECORDS

The HITECH Act was enacted as part of the American Recovery and Reinvestment Act of 2009 economic stimulus bill. According to the U.S. Department of Health and Human Services, HITECH Act provides the "authority to establish programs to improve health care quality, safety, and efficiency through the promotion of health IT [information technology], including electronic health records and private and secure electronic health information exchange." Among other changes to the use of information technology in health care, HITECH Act has provided incentives for the "meaningful use" of EHR, and it assesses penalties for noncompliance. Complying with the meaningful use requirement relies on accomplishing specific objectives related to the use of information technology.

> **" "**
>
> HITECH proposes the meaningful use of interoperable electronic health records throughout the United States health care delivery system as a critical national goal. Meaningful Use is defined by the use of certified EHR technology in a meaningful manner (for example electronic prescribing); ensuring that the certified EHR technology is connected in a manner that provides for the electronic exchange of health information to improve the quality of care; and that in using certified EHR technology the provider must submit to the Secretary of Health & Human Services (HHS) information on quality of care and other measures.
>
> The concept of meaningful use rested on the "5 pillars" of health outcomes policy priorities, namely:
>
> 1. Improving quality, safety, efficiency, and reducing health disparities
> 2. Engage patients and families in their health
> 3. Improve care coordination
> 4. Improve population and public health
> 5. Ensure adequate privacy and security protection for personal health information
>
> Centers for Disease Control and Prevention. (n.d.). *Meaningful uses.*
> Retrieved from http://www.cdc.gov/ehrmeaningfuluse/introduction.html

Objectives that support a provider's meaningful use of health technology include computerized provider order entry; prescribing prescriptions electronically; providing patients with an electronic copy of their health information; providing clinical summaries for patients for each office visit; recording patient demographics; maintaining an up-to-date problem list of current and active diagnoses; protecting electronic health information; generating lists of patients by specific conditions; sending reminders to patients per patient preference for preventive/follow-up care; providing electronic syndromic surveillance data to public health agencies; recording electronic notes in patient records; identifying and report specific cases to a specialized registry; and providing structured electronic lab results to ambulatory providers, among many others.

EHR technology includes both computer hardware and software systems that store patient information. Many times, physicians and hospitals will have similar or identical systems, allowing shared access to the patient's record. Despite the adoption of EHR, there remain several challenges to the universal adoption of EHR systems that can all "talk" to one another. Although there is general agreement that these very expensive systems will help to improve the quality of care, and perhaps the efficiency with which it is provided, the question of "Who pays for it?" looms large. Second, not all forms of EHR "talk" to each other. So the patient who resides in a community and has a physician and hospital that use a particular system may not be able to easily access her record if she becomes ill in another location. Interestingly, this was underscored in the aftermath of Hurricane Katrina. Patients of the Veterans Administration (VA) hospital found that, because the VA has fully integrated all of its patient record keeping, their records could be accessed from anywhere in the United States.

While the majority of health care providers have transitioned to EHR, there are still some who have not. Typically, they are (1) smaller practices who have decided the penalty is less daunting than purchasing, installing, and learning an EHR system or (2) physicians who just do not want to integrate computers into the way they practice medicine. Some physicians have even chosen retirement over using EHR. Association of Physicians and Surgeons' President Melinda Woofter, M.D., says, "The number of physicians practicing medicine has been decreasing. The environment to practice medicine has become unbearable and too toxic. Many have chosen early retirement, while others have changed career paths. The number of physicians choosing to opt out of Medicare has been increasing as well."

TYPES OF HEALTH RECORDS

The typical form of the health record has morphed from a collection of handwritten notes and hard copy test results to an electronic file stored on a computer. As with a paper chart, EHR technology is typically tailored toward the health care provider's type of practice.

In large outpatient clinics associated with teaching hospitals, the integrated health record is common. With an integrated health record, the patient is represented by a single record that includes all outpatient and inpatient activity. Hospitals, HMOs, or private physicians' offices are completely separate and distinct organizational and legal entities. Cross-indexing of the hospital and outside office records is very limited and usually represented by a copy of the discharge summary from the hospital chart in the office record of the attending physician. The hospital record seldom carries any direct report of medical office visits unless the medical office is part of the hospital. And, even then, the technologies of a hospital and one of its practices may not be compatible.

The health record of the nonhospital situation, identified as a record of medical care given in a facility that does not retain the patient overnight, has unique qualities, depending on the specialty of the physicians and the requirements of the state. The more the outpatient facility resembles a hospital, the more the record resembles a hospital record. The medical assistant's care of the health record requires the same attention to detail and confidentiality regardless of whether it is in a hospital setting or a specialist's private office or whether it is a paper chart or an EHR.

For most Olympic athletes, the biggest fear is not failing to win a gold medal but falling victim to a last-minute injury that destroys years of hard work and endless hours of practice. But doctors working with big data and cloud-based software are competing to make those heart-breaking injuries less likely.

The 2016 Olympic Games in Rio de Janeiro, for example, is using a cloud-based version of GE Healthcare's Centricity Practice Solutions (CPS) as the official electronic medical records (EMR) keeper. Moving these records into the cloud eliminates the need to ship pallets of paper around the globe in order to monitor athletes' health. The technology is available at all medical posts throughout the games and at the central clinic in the Olympic Village where doctors can deliver more complex care.

"To win the Olympics you have to be the best in the world on a particular day, at a particular time, in your sport," says Bill Moreau, the U.S. Olympic Committee's managing director of sports medicine. "To achieve that is extremely difficult. But, can you imagine training for 20 years and showing up sick or hurt when it could have been prevented? Our goal with electronic medical records is helping to ensure that athletes can deliver their best performance at the right time."

...

By drawing on the massive amounts of data, the system also helps the medical team develop new ways to improve the health and performance of all athletes by preventing injuries. Team USA tracks 1,000 data points on each athlete and runs retrospective and forward-looking analytics to spot trends and offer solutions. Using EMR, for example, doctors helped reduce incidence of anemia among women athletes. Using blood tests, doctors can track hemoglobin levels and other lab results and then watch how various nutritional approaches impact stores of hemoglobin in the body, says Dr. Moreau.

Egan, M. (2016, August 9). A winning idea: How the cloud helps Olympic athletes avoid injury. *GE Reports*. Retrieved from http://www.gereports .com/a-winning-idea-how-the-cloud-helps-olympic-athletes-avoid-injury/

PRIVACY AND PRIVILEGED COMMUNICATION

Professional confidentiality dates back to the time of Hippocrates:

> **❝ ❞**
>
> Whatever in connection with my professional practice, or not in connection with it, I see or hear in the life of men, which ought not to be spoken abroad, I will not divulge as recommending that all should be kept secret.
>
> *Hippocrates*

Privacy, in the medical setting, involves at least two different kinds of interests. One is individual interest in avoiding disclosure of personal matters; the second is interest in independent decision making. The federal government, in the form of the Health Insurance Portability and Accountability Act (HIPAA), has weighed in on the issue of patient privacy. See Chapters 2 and 9 for detailed treatment of this important federal law.

In this context, the challenge is to maintain that patient privacy in an era in which electronic storage of records has become commonplace. That method of storage makes access to that data easier—and more easily subject to violation.

OWNERSHIP OF THE HEALTH RECORD

State law determines who owns a patient's health record. In the majority of states, the health care provider owns the health record. In at least one state, the patient owns the health record. And, in several other states, there is no express statute that indicates who owns the health record. Although the physician and others as owners have a **property right** to the record and can restrict its removal from the **premises**, the patient's interest in the information is protected by law.

property right a right of ownership to a certain thing

premises physical location, such as an office or building

Ownership usually carries with it the exclusive right and power to exercise authority and control over the use of the property. In the case of the health record, the owner cannot control the record exclusively. The fact that a hospital or physician owns the piece of paper on which the record is written does not prevent other individuals, professionals, corporations, and courts from claiming a right to see and copy the information. There are competing interests in and claims on the contents of a health record. For example, a physician is ethically obligated to furnish office records to another physician who assumes responsibility for the care of a patient. The following case involves ownership of a health record.

A dispute occurred between a physician who was employed by a clinic and the estate of a deceased physician, owner of a medical clinic. Following the death of the owner, the employee removed from the clinic the Daily Reference Book, which disclosed the identity of all the persons treated…, the receipt book which contained a statement of funds, and all current patient records. The estate accused the physician employee of wrongfully removing the records from the clinic.

The court held that the employee had wrongfully removed the records from the clinic but the importance of the rights and the interests of the patients who elected to receive [the physician employee's] professional services required that he be allowed to retain such of the health records of these patients as might be found necessary to enable him to render them proper care and treatment.

Jones v. Fakehany, 67 Cal. Rptr. 810 (1968)

Another example of the physician's inability to absolutely control health records occurs in the disbursement of property at death. Following the death of a physician, the records, which are owned by the physician, cannot be dispensed with or distributed in the same manner as other property. For example:

The doctor's will directed his executor to burn and destroy all of his office records and files without opening them. The court held that this was against public policy and ordered the executor to make available records and notes pertaining to patients to succeeding physicians upon authorized request.

In re Culbertson's Will, 292 N.Y.S.2d 806 (1968)

Consequently, a physician who sought to destroy patient medical records rather than provide patients with an opportunity to transfer their records to new providers would not be acting in accord with the American Medical Association standards:

3.3.1 Management of Medical Records

Medical records serve important patient interests for present health care and future needs, as well as insurance, employment, and other purposes.

(Continues)

(Continued)

In keeping with the professional responsibility to safeguard the confidentiality of patients' personal information, physicians have an ethical obligation to manage medical records appropriately.

This obligation encompasses not only managing the records of current patients, but also retaining old records against possible future need, and providing copies or transferring records to a third party as requested by the patient or the patient's authorized representative when the physician leaves a practice, sells his or her practice, sells his or her practice, retires, or dies.

American Medical Association. (2016, June). *Opinions on privacy, confidentiality, and medical records, 3.3.1. Management of medical records.*

X-rays, magnetic resonance imaging, electrocardiograms, and the results of other diagnostic tests are a form of health record and belong to the physician or the hospital where they are taken. Access to x-rays depends on the policy of the owner. Policy is affected by statutes that may require the owner to give the films to another physician selected by the patient but may not require the owner to give them to a patient for personal viewing. When a physician refers a patient to a radiologist for x-ray studies, the films usually belong to the radiologist and not to the referring physician who receives the radiologist's report.

ACCESS TO THE HEALTH RECORD

Hospitals and physicians should have a written policy on file detailing the procedures for releasing patient information. The policy must reflect federal law, and, if applicable, state law as well. In certain states, legislators have given the patient, the patient's physician, and/or the authorized agent the right to examine or copy the health record. In other states, judicial precedence has been set for those who base the right to examine the record on the patient's rights.

There is general authorization for the physician or hospital to release information to insurance companies about patients submitting third-party payment claims. In addition, office records, as well as hospital records, are subject to inspection by an attorney authorized by the patient to examine them for use in possible litigation against either the physician or a third party. When a patient submits a claim to litigation, the authorization is not clear-cut and must be determined on an individual basis, but a patient cannot use the privilege as a sword and a shield.

Patients are often required to submit to a physical examination before receiving benefits such as life insurance or welfare, participating in school athletics, obtaining a marriage license, or employment. In these situations, the patient consents implicitly or expressly to the sending of a truthful record to the third party. For example:

Following a physical examination, the physician disclosed to a patient's employer that the patient had a long-standing nervous condition, despite the patient's express orders not to release such information. The disclosure caused the patient's dismissal. The court found that the duty for the physician to maintain confidentiality was qualified and depended on the context of the patient-physician relations. The physician was authorized to release the information.

Horne v. Patton, 287 So.2d 824 (1973)

Health Insurance Portability and Accountability Act of 1996

To improve efficiency in transferring information about patients within the health care system, the HIPAA directs Health and Human Services to adopt standard "data elements" and "code sets" for electronic coding throughout the entire health care industry. All providers of health care are required to participate in these provisions. In addition, HIPAA sets standardized guidelines for the protection of a patient's privacy related to health records.

Facsimile (Fax) Transmission of Medical Information

Society is increasingly dependent on the use of the fax to transmit information. However, there are times when a faxed message goes astray, either because of error on the part of the sender or imprecise handling by the receiver. In the health care industry, this may cause a breach in the confidential relationship between physician and patient. Because of the importance of the timely receipt of information about patients in emergency circumstances, a fax may be an appropriate mode for the delivery of medical information. Under other circumstances, either because of the content of the information or the lack of urgency, another method of transferring sensitive information may be more appropriate.

> A physician should be sure, however, to comply with the Privacy Rules' requirements for disclosures generally. For example, the physician should check whether the "minimum necessary" rule applies and, if it does, limit the information in the fax to the minimum necessary information.
>
> Also, a physician should be sure to have appropriate security safeguards in place that are administrative, technical, and physical in nature. For example, the physician should use policies and procedures that require office staff to verify the recipient's fax number and use a cover sheet that does not include protected health information.
>
> American Medical Association. (n.d.). *Frequently asked questions about HIPAA.*

Patient Access to Health Record

An issue of chronic aggravation between the public, their representatives (lawyers), and the medical establishment is gaining access to health records. HIPAA protects the privacy of patient's medical information, and it also gives patients the right to access much of the information contained in their health records.

> "Based on recent studies and our own enforcement experience, far too often individuals face obstacles to accessing their health information," said Jocelyn Samuels, the director of the Office for Civil Rights at the Department of Health and Human Services, which enforces federal health privacy standards. "This must change."
>
> When patients can see their medical records, the administration said, it is easier for them to participate in their health care. They can, for example, review what they were told by their doctors and, perhaps, consider other options for care.
>
> Pear, R. (2016, January 16). New guidelines nudge doctors to give patients access to medical records. *New York Times.* Retrieved from http://www.nytimes.com/2016/01/17/us/new-guidelines-nudge-doctors-on-giving-patients-access-to-medical-records.html

Physicians disagree about whether patients should have access to their own records. Some believe that there is the possibility of misinterpretation by the patient; others are of the opinion that a little knowledge can be more dangerous than no knowledge at all. Legal commentators view patients' access to their own records cynically, observing that almost everyone except the subject of the records can know what is in them. HIPAA requires that patients have the right to see their records, to obtain copies, and to make corrections in them.

Physicians who do not support a patient's direct access to health records comment that there may be information in the records that the patient or members of the family should not see; for example, confidential information on past pregnancies, abortions, sexually transmitted diseases, or mental illness. Artificial insemination presents ethical dilemmas in that the availability of the record to the family affects the woman's privacy regarding conception; on the other side of the issue, there is the responsibility of the physician to maintain an accurate record as well as to preserve information for the future benefit of the child. HIPAA requires, however, that certain health information be provided regardless of the provider's wishes. In very limited cases, a health care provider may refuse to provide a patient with certain information.

> 66 99
>
> Under certain limited circumstances, a covered entity may deny an individual's request for access to all or a portion of the PHI requested. In some of these circumstances, an individual has a right to have the denial reviewed by a licensed health care professional designated by the covered entity who did not participate in the original decision to deny.
>
> *Unreviewable* grounds for denial (45 CFR 164.524(a)(2)):
>
> - The request is for psychotherapy notes, or information compiled in reasonable anticipation of, or for use in, a legal proceeding.
> - An inmate requests a copy of her PHI held by a covered entity that is a correctional institution, or health care provider acting under the direction of the institution, and providing the copy would jeopardize the health, safety, security, custody, or rehabilitation of the inmate or other inmates, or the safety of correctional officers, employees, or other person at the institution or responsible for the transporting of the inmate. However, in these cases, an inmate retains the right to inspect her PHI.
> - The requested PHI is in a designated record set that is part of a research study that includes treatment (e.g., clinical trial) and is still in progress, provided the individual agreed to the temporary suspension of access when consenting to participate in the research. The individual's right of access is reinstated upon completion of the research.
> - The requested PHI is in Privacy Act protected records (i.e., certain records under the control of a federal agency, which may be maintained by a federal agency or a contractor to a federal agency), if the denial of access is consistent with the requirements of the Act.
> - The requested PHI was obtained by someone other than a health care provider (e.g., a family member of the individual) under a promise of
>
> *(Continues)*

(Continued)

confidentiality, and providing access to the information would be reasonably likely to reveal the source of the information.

Reviewable grounds for denial (45 CFR 164.524(a)(3)). A licensed health care professional has determined in the exercise of professional judgment that:

- The access requested is <u>reasonably likely</u> to endanger the life or physical safety of the individual or another person. This ground for denial does not extend to concerns about psychological or emotional harm (e.g., concerns that the individual will not be able to understand the information or may be upset by it).
- The access requested is <u>reasonably likely</u> to cause substantial harm to a person (other than a health care provider) referenced in the PHI.
- The provision of access to a personal representative of the individual that requests such access is <u>reasonably likely</u> to cause substantial harm to the individual or another person.

Department of Health and Human Services. (n.d.). *Individuals' right under HIPAA to access their health information 45 CFR § 164.524*. U.S. Retrieved from http://www.hhs.gov/hipaa/for-professionals/privacy/guidance/access/index.html

HIPAA also provides guidelines on what healthcare providers can charge patients for copies of their records. And, while states may pass laws that include costs that are less than those set forth in HIPAA, a state may not pass a law that allows for higher charges for patient records than HIPAA allows.

Innocent Party in the Health Record

In the case of the mentally ill patient, health records may contain sensitive and private information regarding the patient's family, friends, employers, and associates. A therapist frequently will record intimate aspects of relatives' and associates' lives. This information may contain falsehoods and inaccuracies based on the patient's delusions and misconceptions. The patient's record may also contain the therapist's assessment of the patient's interaction with family members and other patients.

Release of information involving other persons contained in the patient's health record is potentially harmful to all parties involved. Disclosure may damage reputations within the community, affect employment opportunities, cause severe emotional distress, and infringe on the individual privacy of others. If the patient obtains access to the health record and learns about others' opinions, an adverse clinical reaction may occur, and family and social relationships may be severely and permanently disrupted. Information in the health record may be used against persons other than the patient in legal proceedings—for example, divorce, child custody, and competency hearings.

At least three courts have held that when family members participate in counseling sessions along with the patient, the health records of the patient may not be disclosed without the consent of the patient and family members. Another potentially troublesome area is the maintenance of confidentiality in group psychotherapy settings.

Release of Information

When working in a physician's office, the best rule to follow, unless instructed otherwise, is to refuse to disclose information—even to the point of acknowledging whether the individual is a patient. It is always possible that an enterprising sleuth could figure out the nature of a patient's illness from the specialty of the physician.

Six basic principles are suggested for preventing unauthorized disclosure of information:

66 99

1. When in doubt, err by not disclosing rather than by disclosing. There are exceptions to this principle, but a mistaken refusal to disclose confidential data is, at least, reversible.
2. Remember that the owner of the privilege to keep information confidential is the patient, not the physician. If the patient is willing to release the data, the physician may not ethically decide to withhold it even "for the patient's own good."
3. Apply the concept of confidentiality equally to all patients despite the physician's assessment of their goals, mores, and lifestyles. A physician cannot ethically inform an insurer of suspicions that a patient is trying to defraud an insurer or that a young man is trying to use a medical excuse to evade the draft.
4. Be familiar with the local statutes including federal, state, and local law plus ordinances, rules, regulations, and administrative decrees of various agencies such as public health departments.
5. When required to divulge a confidence, discuss the situation with the patient. When obligations to society conflict with those of the patient, the physician should discuss the conflict with the patient. When legal guidelines are absent or vague, the criteria of decision are the immediacy and degree of danger to either the patient or society.
6. Get written authorization from the patient before divulging information. To meet standard situations such as requests from third parties, have the patient sign a blanket authorization in advance to release pertinent data to specific third parties.

Beck, L. C. (1972, April 15). Patient information—when and when not to divulge. *Patient Care, 72,* 60.

Information should not be released unless the request is specific. The request should have time limits, identify the purposes for which the records will be used, and identify the particular information requested. It is important to check and confirm the credentials of the person and/or organization requesting information from the record. Your office should have a protocol that describes the steps necessary when you have a request for a copy of a health record, and it is highly advisable to follow the protocol.

Capacity to Consent to Release of Information

Any patient who has reached the age of majority can consent to the release of health records. If a former patient is dead, the executor, administrator, or personal representative may release the record. If an adult patient is temporarily unable to consent, a court-appointed guardian has authorization. If an attorney is authorized by a patient to view a record, the patient need not be of sound mind at the time the decision to consent is made. In an emergency, a record may be released to the extent necessary without consent, because the emergency creates the power to act.

Minors have particular problems with regard to the release of medical information. In a drug abuse or sexually transmitted disease diagnosis, only the minor involved can release the record, even to his or her parents or guardians. Normally, a parent or guardian can release the minor's records until the minor reaches majority. If one parent has been awarded custody of the minor, it is preferable to get that parent to release the medical information. The mature minor doctrine allows minors to release their records under certain circumstances such as when they are living away from home, self-supporting, or married. Under certain conditions, when a minor knows the nature, quality, and consequences of his or her actions, a minor can authorize the release of a health record.

Release of Information to Attorneys

Attorneys need information from health records under many circumstances. If there is likelihood that medical malpractice charges will be brought against a physician, an attorney will usually ask to examine the records before going to court. By responding indifferently to a lawyer's request for records, a physician frequently causes problems. The attorney may find that it is more efficient to file the lawsuit and engage in formal discovery than to fight with a doctor for the records. This attitude hardens feelings between attorneys and physicians. Health records cannot be withheld pending payment of the patient's bill to a physician or a hospital.

Release Forms

A patient's in-person oral request or telephone call is insufficient to properly authorize the release of health records. The request must be in writing. And, when the information requested is disclosed, it must be accompanied by a instructions that forbid its re-disclosure to others who are not authorized to receive it.

To compel, or force, the production of health records, a **subpoena** is necessary. A subpoena is a command to appear at a certain time and place to give testimony on a certain matter. The particular type of subpoena used for documents or objects is called a **subpoena duces tecum**. It identifies the records that are requested in court. Legal subpoenas do not automatically require the release of all requested health information. When sensitive information about patients and other persons has been requested without consent of the parties, the issues can be discussed with the judge and attorneys. The judge may then make the decision to review the material privately to determine whether it should be allowed into evidence.

subpoena a written order to appear at a specified time and place to testify

subpoena duces tecum a written order to produce documents or things

CREDIBILITY OF THE HEALTH RECORD

Credibility of a health record refers to whether the information recorded in the record is believable. An article written for lawyers informing them how to recognize a good medical malpractice case (one they can win) stated the following:

> If you take on a case where the doctor or the hospital changes something in the records, you will need less than the usual quantum of fault to prevail before a jury. The same is true if a record or x-ray is missing. Even a change that the doctor argues was made for a good faith reason or a record lost with the explanation, "fire," "flood" or "robbery," will suggest to the jury that there was a guilty motive afoot-and there probably was.
>
> Gage, S. M. (1981, Spring). Alteration, falsification and fabrication of medical records in medical malpractice actions. *Medical Trial Quarterly, 27,* 476.

Even though the above article was written before the widespread use of EHR, the premise remains valid and true today: If a health record has corrections, amendments, modifications, changes, or even misspelled words, it will raise suspicions. The credibility of the health record is crucial in the defense of a physician, medical facility, or employee.

Health information is needed to try cases in nearly every area of law. When a lawyer meets with a client who has a complaint about medical care, the first step is to obtain all health records available and have them reviewed by an independent physician. The second physician's evaluation may prompt the attorney to further investigate the potential malpractice claim or to explain to the client why there is no evidence of malpractice. Sometimes attorneys find that they can settle with a potential defendant or the insurance company before filing a malpractice suit. This prelawsuit settlement usually happens when the health record has credibility issues.

The credibility of the record-keeping procedure is subject to question when investigation reveals delayed filing of laboratory test results, incomplete files, illegible records, altered or fabricated records, or the loss or concealment of information. The following sections describe conduct that has caused problems for defendant–physicians.

Delayed Filing of Laboratory Tests

Sixty-seven closed claims with a diagnosis of melanoma were reviewed by the Aetna Life and Casualty Company. Failure to diagnose was the most common allegation in the claims, and the physician's office was the setting most often identified as the site of the alleged malpractice. The study suggested that the flow of medical reports, such as x-ray readings, may be a factor in malpractice suits involving malignancy. In four cases, the physician who ordered an x-ray study did not see the final positive radiology report—the one that probably would have led to earlier diagnosis and treatment. For example:

A 78-year-old woman was evaluated by an internist for recurrent indigestion. The radiologist's report suggested the presence of a small soft tissue mass below the left diaphragm, but the patient did not call the physician's office to ask about the result as she had been told to. The physician did not see the results until approximately eight weeks later. An upper G.I. series confirmed the diagnosis. Surgical exploration and biopsy disclosed the unresectable reticulum cell sarcoma of the stomach. The patient died within six weeks. The original report may have been placed in the patient's file during the physician's vacation.

Mittleman, M. (1980, February). What are the chances when malignancy leads to a malpractice suit? *Legal Aspects of Medical Practice*, 42.

Incomplete and Error-Filled Records

Health records must be accurate, complete, and correct. In the worst case scenarios, these types of mistakes in health records can have fatal results. In less severe cases, health record mistakes can damage a health care provider's reputation. Consider how you would feel if you were the patient in the following real-life example:

Marilyn Mullins, 62, said she was shocked when she received a note from a chaplain at Sentara Martha Jefferson Hospital that said she had died…

A hospital chaplain called Mullins with an apology and explained that a technical error caused the mistake. The hospital said a secretary accidentally checked the box for deceased patient instead of checking discharge to home.

Woman leaves hospital, finds out she died. (2016, June 11). Retrieved from http://www.nbcwashington.com/news/local /Woman-Leaves-Hospital-Finds-Out-She-Died-382568031.html

Altered Health Records

If a record is damaging to a physician, he or she may be strongly tempted to change it. The use of EHR has, however, changed the way someone might alter a health record. With EHR, any changes to a record will be reflected as an amendment and be marked with the user's identification and time and date of the amendment.

For any alteration to be plausible, all other people involved—physicians, nurses, administrators—must go along with it. Somewhere along the line the chain is almost bound to snap. Altered records demonstrate the defendant's consciousness of wrongdoing and strongly establish liability. If a jury learns that a physician has intentionally altered a record for improper reasons, they will award much larger damages. Insurance companies are well aware of this. It is no coincidence that when a medical malpractice case involves altered records, defense lawyers will advise their clients to settle the case.

A 23-year-old woman was admitted for delivery of her first child and was administered a spinal anesthetic by the obstetrician. Her chart indicated that her blood pressure was normal when the anesthesia was given and no change was indicated until the "moment her infant delivered." At that time a "heart

(Continues)

(Continued)

stat" emergency was called, and artificial respiration and other resuscitative efforts were promptly instituted to restore breathing and heart rhythm.

Photocopies of the mother's hospital record showed close monitoring of the patient-consistent with the defendant's claim of no malpractice. As the litigation continued, plaintiff's counsel sent out a photocopy service to obtain the baby's chart. The record contained a carbon copy of the delivery room record from the mother's chart. Although these records were duplicates of the originals, comparing the two revealed that significant alterations had been made in the mother's chart. The carbon copy revealed these alterations and demonstrated that the defendants were guilty of malpractice.

Gage, S. M. (1981, Spring). Alteration, falsification and fabrication of medical records in medical malpractice actions. *Medical Trial Quarterly, 27*, 476.

Fabricating Health Records

Altering health records modifies the content of the record, and fabricating records means inventing facts. The motive is typically to cover up an error or wrongdoing.

The court upheld the denial of unemployment benefits where the employer terminated the employee for fabricating a patient's medical record. The court found that credible testimony proved that a patient's complaint that the employee had never visited the patient despite making a health record entry to the contrary.

Zeo v. Unemployment Comp. Bd. of Review (Pa. Commw. Ct., 2015)

Loss or Concealment of Records

Related to the alteration of health records is the destruction, unavailability, or loss of relevant x-rays, laboratory test results, and other physical evidence. Health records may also be summoned in fraud situations in which a physician claims excessive amounts from insurance companies or welfare agencies, as in the following:

Dr. Emanuel Stolman, a diplomate of the Academy of Family Physicians, had practiced for over twenty-five years when he was indicted in 1976 on twenty-three felony counts of illegally receiving state funds from the

Medi-Cal program. Dr. Stolman's method of treatment was a folksy sort of approach, and did not match the rigid bookkeeping methods required by the state. The main question was whether or not Dr. Stolman was present in hospitals and nursing homes on the dates he claimed he had examined patients. At issue was whether Dr. Stolman altered his records when he discovered the state was investigating him.

Dr. Stolman followed the motto, "Patients, not Paper," and had been writing pulse counts and blood pressure measurements from memory as long as a week later. He stated that he had a good memory, and would write prescriptions for patients from memory within a week's time after a visit. Dr. Stolman's memory became difficult for nurses, ward clerks and medical records clerks to verify during the ten-week trial. The entire medical community went on trial with Dr. Stolman as discrepancies surfaced in records in nursing homes, extended care facilities, hospitals and within the doctor's office.

Poulos, C. J. (1987, May/June). A case of fraud.
The Professional Medical Assistant, 14.

Acceptable Method of Making Changes in Health Records

Although maintaining the record perfectly should always be the goal, it is important to recognize that incorrect entries may happen. Most EHR systems track each entry by user, date, and time. So, if a mistake is made and the record needs to be changed, the original error will remain but there will be an addendum with the correct information.

When an error occurs with a paper chart, cross out the mistake, initial and date it, and then write the correct information. It is highly inadvisable to use correction fluid or some other method to try to hide the mistake.

There are occasions when making a change in a patient's records is necessary. If the changes are made while the patient is under treatment, they may be accepted as rewritten or amended. But if the changes are made beyond a reasonable period of time following discharge, particularly after a physician or hospital is on notice of a potential lawsuit, changes in the health record are almost always serious and raise red flags.

It is the responsibility of individuals charged with keeping health records to be accurate. They must bring any error in record keeping to the attention of the physician at the time it is discovered, as well as any ambiguous section that may affect the reader's understanding. It is the physician's responsibility to correct his or her own error. Keeping good notes is as important to the physician as the diagnosis. If the record keeper is in dispute with a physician, the facts should be recorded and reviewed by a neutral third professional. The physician is ultimately responsible; the assistant is responsible only if negligent in the performance or omission of assigned duties, or if conspiring to defraud.

☑ SUMMARY

- EHRs are electronic health records, which are required by federal law for all health care providers who treat Medicare patients. A provider's failure to use EHR will result in a monetary penalty.

- Health records and information regarding patients are subject to privacy laws.

- The patient–physician relationship is one protected from disclosure by privileged communication, which extends to the office personnel and other delegated employees.

- The owner of a health record is usually the facility that generates the record: A hospital record is owned by a hospital, and an office record by the physician or corporation that owns the medical practice. Each facility has a health record that is adequate to meet its own needs.

- Patients often wish to see their records. HIPAA allows patients to see their records and make corrections in them. Physicians are required to transfer medical information to other physicians engaged by their patients and to allow attorneys access to records of their clients.

- Contents of a health record should not be transferred or disclosed without the patient's authorization.

- Records are often required in court and can be ordered by the issuance of a subpoena duces tecum. The subpoena must be accompanied by a court order with the information required clearly spelled out.

- Health records must be credible. This means that there can be no alterations, fabrications, or concealments in a record.

- Corrections to a health record should be made with great care.

SUGGESTED ACTIVITIES

1. There are many HIPAA-compliant health record release forms on the Internet. Find one and complete it so you can obtain a copy of your health records from one of your health care providers.

2. Draft a letter for a fictitious patient who has requested a copy of her health records. Include a copy of the release form you found on the Internet.

STUDY QUESTIONS

1. List the type of information contained in a health record.

2. Discuss the difference between ownership of a health record and ownership of other property.

3. A patient requests his x-rays to take home and show to the family. Role-play how you would handle this matter.

4. Privacy means many different things in a medical setting. Distinguish between the patient's right to physical privacy and privacy of privileged communication.

5. As a medical assistant, privileged communication includes your knowledge of the patient. Your office has a famous celebrity as a patient. A well-known newspaper reporter calls and asks you to go to lunch with her. How will you handle this matter?

6. Your office has a strict policy with regard to release of information in health records, and despite a state statute allowing patients access to their records, the physicians you work for will not give patients their records. An obnoxious attorney storms into the office and demands access to your files. The patient has signed a release form. You are at the front desk and the office is full of patients. What do you do?

7. Your office has a relaxed policy with regard to the release of information in health records. A patient asks to see his record. You know that there is information in the record regarding telephone calls from the patient's relatives that would interfere with the family relationship. The physician is away for a week. How would you handle the matter?

8. A health record has been subpoenaed and a court order accompanies it. The physician has removed important parts of the record. You know that this information is missing. The office sends you to court as the keeper of the record. You must testify about the completeness of the record. What are you going to say?

9. There is an error in a health record that has been subpoenaed. This is a good-faith error and should be corrected. It has to do with the information the plaintiff is interested in and could be damaging to the defendant–physician if changed, but also damaging if unchanged. The physician asks you to blot out the error, write in the correct information and put the paper, with surrounding papers, through the copy machine. What do you do?

CASES FOR DISCUSSION

1. The plaintiff's physician received a release of information from the plaintiff to an insurance company following the plaintiff's application for major medical insurance. The physician released the following information: Enclosed is a summary of Mr. Millsaps's recent hospitalization. Physically the man has no notable problems; emotionally, the patient is quite mercurial in his moods. He is a strong-willed man obsessed with faults of others in his family, for which there has been no objective basis. He has completely resisted any constructive advice by his wife, family, minister, or myself. The man needs psychiatric help for his severe obsessions and depressions, some of which have suicidal overtones. He is an extremely poor insurance risk.

   The application for major medical insurance was rejected. Did the physician have a right to release this information to the insurance company?

2. The plaintiff was committed to the Hastings State Hospital by order of the Probate Court, which found him to be "mentally ill—inebriate." The commitment petition was brought by the plaintiff's mother, apparently to secure treatment for him for a developing drug and alcohol problem. Several attempts at voluntary treatment, prior to the commitment proceedings, had proven unsuccessful. Shortly after admission, the plaintiff allegedly attempted to strangle a member of the hospital staff and was transferred to the Security Hospital. Upon admission to the Security Hospital, the plaintiff was diagnosed with simple schizophrenia. He was treated with tranquilizing and antidepressant medications but apparently failed to improve. Consent was sought from the plaintiff's mother to administer electroshock treatment. Consent was not given, but the mother did request the consultation of a second psychiatrist, who concurred with the physicians at Security Hospital. Without the consent of the plaintiff or his mother, electroshock treatment was begun. Did this treatment without consent invade the patient's privacy?

3. The defendant was executive director of Planned Parenthood. A second defendant was the physician who served as medical director for Planned Parenthood. Both gave information, instruction, and medical advice to married persons about how to prevent conception. The defendants were arrested and found guilty of violating a statute that forbade the use of contraceptives. They then appealed, contending that the statute as applied violated the Fourteenth Amendment. Does a law forbidding the use of contraceptives invade the zone of privacy in violation of the due process clause of the Fourteenth Amendment?

4. The patient alleged that the defendant–physician fraudulently and negligently advised her that she had a brain tumor that required

immediate surgery, that the physician negligently performed an unneeded craniotomy on her at the hospital, and that the physician had held staff surgical privileges at the hospital on a continuing basis. The plaintiff–patient further alleged several theories against the hospital. Underlying these was the contention that the hospital had sufficient prior information to be put on notice that the defendant–physician was an incompetent, overaggressive neurosurgeon with a history of performing unnecessary operations, particularly elective craniotomies. The court ordered the hospital to produce copies of all preoperative consultations, operative notes, interpretations of preoperative x-rays, and brain tissue analyses obtained on 140 patients. Included in the order were provisions to ensure the privacy of the patients. The hospital refused the records on the grounds that consent had not been obtained from any of the 140 patients and the production order was in violation of the patient–physician privilege statute. Should the appeals court agree with the hospital?

5. Following a visit to a physician's office, the physician wrote the patient a letter informing her that she had a sexually transmitted disease. The patient showed the letter to two or three friends. When the physician came to her home to talk with her about it, a friend was visiting her, and the patient discussed the matter in the presence of the physician and the friend. The patient then sued the physician for breach of confidentiality. Did the physician breach her confidentiality?

6. The plaintiff was seen by a physician for a blocked tear duct. During the treatment, an instrument brushed her cornea with resulting abrasions. Following the incident, the plaintiff's daughter, who was a nurse, requested permission to review the physician's records. After seeing the records, the plaintiff filed against the physician. At the trial, the daughter testified that her mother's records, which she had seen in the physician's office, had been materially altered by the time they were admitted into evidence. It was also noted that a visit that the patient made after the accident was not documented in the record. Should the court presume from this testimony that there was negligence?

7. A patient came to the emergency room of the hospital complaining of nausea and chest pains. The nurse on duty refused to call a physician, determining that there was no need at that time. The patient died of a myocardial infarction minutes after leaving the hospital. The widow's attorney attempted to review the records during discovery but found that they had been destroyed. Could the court presume from this information that there was negligence?

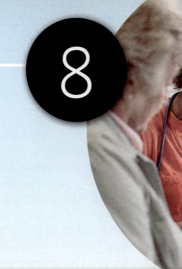

Introduction to Ethics

> 66 Ethics is the difference between knowing what you have a right to do and what is right to do.
>
> *Potter Stewart, Chief Justice of the U.S. Supreme Court* 99

OBJECTIVES

After reading this chapter, you should be able to:

1. Distinguish between law, morals, ethics, and etiquette.
2. Appraise the impact of economics in the making of ethical decisions.
3. Analyze conflict between personal and professional ethics.
4. Discuss the importance of studying ethics.
5. Develop a thought process for making ethical decisions.

BUILDING YOUR LEGAL VOCABULARY

Amoral
Bioethics
Ethics
Etiquette
Immoral

Philosophy
Political
Values
Virtue

ETHICS

Ethical dilemmas are found in every aspect of health care delivery. The study of law in the earlier chapters has introduced the process of thinking legally as well as applying legal doctrine to real-life situations in a health care setting. The study of **ethics** is related to, yet distinguished from, the study of law. For example, celebrity actress Sofia Vergara and her former boyfriend Nick Loeb created frozen embryos when they were dating. They prepared a written agreement that stated their mutual consent would be needed to bring the embryos to term, but the agreement did not specify what would happen to any remaining embryos if the couple broke up. The frozen embryos became the subject of a lawsuit when the couple broke up. Mr. Loeb believed that the destruction of the embryos or simply leaving the embryos frozen was the same as killing a life, and he sued for the right to obtain custody of the embryos. Ms. Vergara wanted the embryos to remain frozen and sought to prevent Mr. Loeb from implanting the embryos in a surrogate.

ethics the study of moral choices that conform to professional standards of conduct

---

NEWS

When we got engaged, in 2012, I began to push for children. As I said in my complaint, my fiancée insisted that we use a surrogate. With her eggs and my sperm we created two female embryos. I was so excited once the lives were created that I began to suggest names we could call our girls. The first embryo we implanted didn't take. The second time, the surrogate miscarried, and I felt crushed.

A year later, we tried again, creating two more embryos, both female. But as we began to discuss other potential surrogates, it became clear once more that parenthood was much less urgent for her than it was for me. We had been together for over four years. As I was coming on 40, I gave her an ultimatum. When she refused, we split up.

A few months later, I asked her to let me have the embryos, offering to pay for all expenses to carry our girls to term and raise them. If she did not wish to share custody, I would take on full parenting responsibilities and agree to have her declared an egg donor. She has refused. Her lawyer, Fred Silberberg, has told reporters that she wants to keep the embryos "frozen indefinitely." In my view, keeping them frozen forever is tantamount to killing them.

Loeb, N. (2015, April 29). Sofía Vergara's ex-fiancé: Our frozen embryos have a right to live. *New York Times.* Retrieved from http://www.nytimes.com/2015/04/30/opinion/sofiavergaras-ex-fiance-our-frozen-embryos-have-a-right-to-live.html?_r=0

Both parties have positions with which we can empathize. The legal issues embedded in this story include who has the legal right to decide what to do with an embryo. This story also illustrates ethical dilemmas: Are the embryos life that require protection via implantation in a surrogate? Is keeping the embryos frozen forever tantamount to the murder of a life? Whose rights are more important: the father who wants to implant the embryos in a surrogate and raise any resulting children as his own or the mother who does not want any children to be born from the embryos?

The study of ethics is grounded theoretically in **philosophy**, which can be defined broadly as the pursuit of wisdom. The word is derived from the Greek term *ethos*, meaning custom, usage, or character. Ethics referred traditionally to a custom of a particular community and evolved to include standards of good or bad and questions of moral duty and obligation.

philosophy a basic viewpoint of an individual's or a society's value system

The study of **bioethics** deals with ethical implications of biological research and applications, especially in medicine (medical ethics). Medical ethics applies to conflicts between theories and positions, to questions involving traditional ethical positions and threats posed by modern medical technology, and to the interaction between ethical constraints and the law.

bioethics refers to life and death ethical issues and the implications of the application of biological research

Distinguishing between legal and ethical issues can be difficult. Ethical dilemmas in medicine occur when the enforcement of law does not seem to bring about justice, when there is no obvious right or wrong behavior, when "right" behavior appears to have the wrong effect, or when personal sacrifice is the consequence of following ideals. Studying ethics involves examining emotions, reasoning, and constitutional issues of freedom and personal responsibility.

Some people may perceive being ill as a degrading and dehumanizing experience and may view themselves as being at the mercy of the physician. Because of the perceived unequal status of physician and patient, ethical constraints are necessary. In the United States, individual privacy and an individual's right to make decisions are highly valued. As a result, ethical codes restrain a physician's right to take action without informing and receiving consent from the patient. To touch a patient without permission changes the physician's action from ethical misbehavior to a legal claim of battery and/or negligence. Breaking ethical codes results in the disapproval of at least a segment of society, but breaking legal codes results in penalties enforced by the law.

MORALS

Morals are recognized as principles of "right" conduct. Right moral conduct is based on traditional religious teachings found in Judeo-Christian, Buddhist, Islamic, and other traditions and cannot be separated from these thought systems without distorting its meaning. The term *moral* is sometimes used as a word of praise, as in "she is a very

virtue goodness conforming to the standard of moral excellence

immoral not moral

amoral without any consideration of morals

moral person," but on other occasions it has a much broader meaning, taking into consideration the **virtues** of courage, wisdom, balance, or fairness. Morally bad actions are characterized by opposite qualities. Behavior that goes against morals is known as **immoral**; behavior that does not take moral principles into consideration is known as **amoral**.

In 1992, the Lakeberg twins, who shared a defective heart, were separated at the parents' request despite the fact that doing so would inevitably result in one child's death. The family followed Islamic religious traditions.

values principles of thought and conduct that are considered desirable

In an Islamic society, religious traditions and **values** guide such decisions. Although the desires of the parents and the advice of medical experts are considered, powerful cultural influences ultimately determine the course of events. In Saudi Arabia, sharia law, shaped by the Koran, governs everyday life. Making the unique decision about whether Nura and Sarah [the twins] should be separated required the opinions of religious leaders and scholars at various judicial levels in Saudi Arabia. They were asked to interpret and apply the precepts and guidance of the Koran to this case and make an appropriate judgment.

The twins' primary physician first contacted the Islamic Opinion Committee (IOC), a religious advisory group established to handle cases such as this one. The IOC instructed the doctor to complete all the feasibility studies on the separation and to form a medical committee that would make a final recommendation. If the medical findings indicated that the twins could be viably separated, the surgery could take place under Islamic law. But if the medical committee decided that one or both of the twins were likely to die as a result of separation, the IOC would review the case further in light of Islamic religious beliefs. It could well have ruled against surgery.

The Lakeberg Siamese twins: Were risks, costs of separation justified? (1992).
Medical Ethics Advisor, 9(10), 121.

Right conduct for a person practicing in the Islamic tradition follows Islamic law and is a matter requiring a moral decision. Determining whether an operation will be conducted to separate the twins, and which twin will live if a decision must be made to terminate the life of one of the two individuals, is moral in its substance. Unless the consequence of practicing within sharia law conflicts with the law of the U.S. Constitution or the state in which the situation occurs, it is moral to follow the practice advocated by those affected by the decision. It would be immoral for the parents to go against the tenets of their religion. It is difficult to make an argument for or against amorality in this matter because the morality of the clinical decision makers would have to be taken into consideration along with that of the parents. A situation like the separation of the Lakeberg Siamese twins might end up in court and be subject to the decision of the judge if the parties cannot agree on a course of action.

In U.S. society, which is a melting pot, ideas about right moral conduct may differ widely and cause the terms *moral* and *ethical* to have several different meanings. In general, ethics provides a framework within which right and wrong can be studied. When one group attempts to enforce its concept of right conduct on others, a **political** process occurs. In contrast, an ethical solution to moral differences occurs when the conscience, or that "still small voice within," activates a sense of moral obligation within an individual.

political administration of public affairs, particularly those of a government

ETIQUETTE

Etiquette is the socially accepted procedure for interacting in society and changes with the times and the community. It does not require moral understanding or ethical reasoning even though it is based on societal laws, morals, customs, and beliefs. Etiquette requires specific behavior in a given situation. For example, *Emily Post's Wedding Etiquette* spells out the etiquette for preparing a family wedding. Each military branch has highly developed customs and rituals requiring strict adherence to its code of etiquette.

etiquette the prescribed code of courteous social behavior

A less structured code of medical etiquette and protocol exists for those working in the health care community. Politeness, proper dress, and courtesy are at its core. Etiquette extends privileges to other medical professionals. For example, a physician will usually instruct staff to put through all calls immediately from other physicians. In addition, individual medical offices have their own etiquette for staff to follow.

Telephone etiquette is at the core of medical office management. One person's poor telephone etiquette can reflect negatively upon the entire office and can result in dissatisfied patients and families who express negative comments.

ETHICAL ENVIRONMENT OF HEALTH CARE

In the past, the U.S. economic system, based on supply and demand, has operated to regulate the health care system. When demand exceeded supply, the cost determined who could afford access to what services. In 1946, the Hill-Burton Act provided millions of dollars for the construction of hospitals. Hospitals built with Hill-Burton money were required to provide a "reasonable volume of services...to persons unable to pay." Although a universal health insurance bill was never passed, in 1965, Medicare and Medicaid amendments to the Social Security Act were enacted with the intent of ensuring access to health care for all the elderly and poor. The 1983 report of the President's Commission, "Securing Access to Health Care," concluded that society has a moral obligation to ensure equitable health care. Equitable health care implies that health care is a right. This requires adjustment in thinking and practice from treating the poor only in emergency situations to treating them as normal, fee-paying patients. It also leads to an overall increase in the cost of health care.

Managed care is synonymous with managing costs. To manage costs, managed care organizations must participate in making patient care decisions. Key to making decisions is the identification of what is to be decided.

Health Care versus Medical Care

Defining *health care* is a fundamental problem that affects decisions about financing health care. The World Health Organization (WHO) defines health as "a state of complete physical, mental, and social well-being, and not merely the absence of disease or infirmity." The WHO definition describes a utopia that may be an unrealistic goal and includes medical care within the broad definition of health care. Being healthy is a subjective state and means different things to different people. Being ill and requiring medical care to function is easier to objectively determine.

Preventive medicine straddles the dividing line between health care and medical care. Preventing illness with inoculations against communicable disease is important to the whole of society as well as the individual. It can easily be objectively classified as medical care. It makes sense to allow society to allocate funds and personnel to prevent communicable diseases. However, in matters of prevention of illness by controlling diet, smoking, exercise, driving habits, stress, and the like, there is too much subjective personal preference to allow a clearcut classification. In contrast, not caring for these aspects of health may cost society more in the long run because neglect may result in the development of an expensive disease. Also competing for a piece of the health care pie are alternative medical providers such as chiropractors, acupuncturists, herbal healers, massage therapists, and so on. The American public is interested in health. Newspapers, books, television, and politicians regularly comment on health and health care.

Private Choice versus Common Good

Increasing the number of individuals covered by medical insurance and ensuring coverage to a larger number of people can require certain restrictions, including limiting a patient's choice of medical providers. There may be a short time to choose a primary care physician when entering a plan and few opportunities to change a primary care physician if either the physician or the patient is unhappy with the arrangement. Choice of a specialist, if needed, must be from the confines of a plan's accepted list, with no opportunity provided for evaluation by physicians outside the plan unless prior provisions are written within the managed care contact. These conditions might result in the following scenario:

The doctors at Karin Smith's health maintenance organization kept telling her she was fine. She knew that wasn't true. She was sick and getting sicker. Frustrated and frightened, she went to an independent physician. The news couldn't have been worse. Ms. Smith had advanced cervical cancer. If she had been properly diagnosed when she first sought help, at age 22, her chances of survival would have been 95 percent or better. Now she is 28 and doctors say it is unlikely she will see 30.

"Even though my medical records were fully documented with the classic physical characteristics and symptoms of cervical cancer, no doctor or medical practitioner associated with my [health maintenance organization (HMO)] or its lab ever made the correct diagnosis." Three Pap smears and three biopsies were performed. "All but the fifth test were misread by the lab my HMO contracted with," Ms. Smith said.

"Unfortunately the one Pap smear they did read correctly was dismissed when they misread the biopsy they performed to confirm it. All six tests clearly indicated that I did, in fact, have cervical cancer." … Ms. Smith tried for three years to convince her HMO doctors that she was ill…

Herbert, J. (1994, September 11). Profits before patients. *The New York Times*, E19.

Ms. Smith is an example of a patient suffering because she required a referral to receive another opinion about her condition. This is an example of a missed diagnosis and the managed care process harming the patient. In the past, physicians' sole responsibility was to take care of the patient, but under managed care, physicians have evolved into "gatekeepers" who manage an HMO's purse strings as well as expenses for patient care and the course of treatment for the duration of the illness. Ms. Smith stayed with the HMO, but Carley Christie's family chose another route:

Carley Christie was eleven years old and lived in Woodside, California. She was diagnosed with Wilms' tumor, a rare childhood kidney cancer. Her parents, Harry and Katherine Christie, found a surgeon with expertise in removing this tumor. But the HMO refused to pay his bills, proposing a less experienced surgeon from its network. The Christies assumed the initial burden of paying their expert, and while nursing their daughter through chemotherapy they battled the bureaucracy for 15 months. The American Arbitration Association sided with the Christies' claim.

Chase, M. (1994, December 5). Can a doctor who's a gatekeeper give enough care?"
The New York Times, B1.

The American Medical Association Council on Ethical and Judicial Affairs reaffirms the priority of physicians' commitment to patient welfare within a managed care practice.

> The Council identifies two types of ethical conflict facing physicians: (1) balancing the interests of their patients with the interests of other patients; and (2) balancing the needs of patients with the financial interests of their physicians. ... When physicians are employed or reimbursed by managed care plans using financial incentives to limit care, a serious ethical conflict results. Financial incentives are permissible only if they promote cost effective delivery of quality care—not the withholding of necessary medical services.
>
> Ethical issues in managed care. (1995, January 25). *Journal of the American Medical Association, 273*(4), 330–335.

IMPORTANCE OF STUDYING ETHICS

Although medical assistants and other office personnel do not usually make life-and-death decisions for patients, they are involved with patients and the patients' families or significant others. Skilled health care practitioners know the patients, understand the risks involved in certain procedures, are sensitive to the mood swings and caring levels of other professional staff, and internally deal with their own personal questions of ultimate concern.

It is important that health care providers develop their own understanding of ethics. Without some basic recognition of the depth of thinking that goes into ethical decisions, a practitioner has few resources to deal with the conflict that may develop between personal value systems and daily occurrences within the profession of medicine.

These conflicts may potentially lead to either burnout or growth. Knowing that others are dealing and have dealt with many of the same issues encourages interdisciplinary support and understanding. Questioning conflicts may lead to further exploration, education, and the development of different perspectives about an issue. The resolution of conflict may lead to transfer to another job that is more in line with personal beliefs.

In addition, the medical employee's family members, friends, and the community may look to a health care provider for insight into troubling ethical issues facing society. Listening skills and knowledge gained from personal investigation may help others understand. Many ethical questions do not have "correct" answers, and acknowledging this also contributes to the education of the community.

The next four chapters address the ethical issues of confidentiality, allocation of resources, and autonomy versus paternalism under the following headings:

Chapter 9—Laws and Ethics of Patient Confidentiality

Chapter 10—Professional Ethics and the Living

Chapter 11—Birth and the Beginning of Life

Chapter 12—Death and Dying

As each of these sections is addressed, other ethical issues emerge.

After identifying the issues, the question becomes this: "Who owns them?" Is this a problem for the physician, other health care providers, a lawyer, or medical office personnel? Perhaps it is a problem for administration. Often we take on burdens that are not ours, and clearly identifying responsibility may shift the ethical perspective. In dealing with ethical solutions to health care problems, many individuals may have something to say about what is happening, but at some point, "the buck stops here." Where it stops is where the decision is "owned."

☑ SUMMARY

- Making an ethical decision may be quite simple or very difficult. Sometimes it is easy to get lost in a multitude of factual details or go off on a tangent without addressing the problem.

- When one is given a fact pattern that contains an ethical dilemma, resolution requires distinguishing between clinical (medical), legal, and ethical issues. After this analysis has been made, the next step is to further clarify the ethical issue(s).

- This chapter introduces the matter of medical ethics, sometimes identified as bioethics. The importance of distinguishing between clinical, legal, and ethical decisions is addressed.

- The distinctions between ethics, morals, and etiquette have been introduced; however, a process for making an ethical decision has not been offered because there is no one way to search for a solution to an ethical dilemma. Each individual approaches an ethical problem from his or her own perspective, which includes cultural values, moral upbringing, present circumstances, society's expectations, and a multitude of other variables.

SUGGESTED ACTIVITIES

1. Use your favorite Internet browser to find reports that deal with medical/legal/ethical issues. Review these stories and analyze the health, legal, and ethical components.

2. Use your favorite Internet browser to find "Letters to the Editor" columns and collect any letters relating to these matters. After doing this for a month or more, you will begin to sense the variety of ways the public views ethical issues. Document your reaction to the ethics of the article and review your documentation approximately three months later. If you have changed your mind about any matter, try to determine what personal or societal events caused this change.

3. Use your favorite Internet browser to find the latest transplant news and attempt to break down costs. Review the benefits of money being used for the transplant versus other places in society for the common good. Form personal opinions on these issues.

4. Within the past 24 hours, you probably performed an action out of a sense of etiquette. Remember what you did, how you did it, and why. Was this a satisfying experience for you?

5. Review your local hospital's bill of rights. Find out if it is given to the patient upon admission. Find out if it is explained to the patient. Determine who discusses this with the patient during the hospital stay. If possible, try to interview this person about the success or failure of the process.

6. Try the process for making an ethical decision. Identify something that happened in your life recently that required you to make an ethical decision. Attempt to divide it into its medical (if appropriate), legal, and ethical components. Identify your role and think of all the possible ways you could have handled the situation and their probable results. Weigh each alternative against your personal philosophy. Follow up on the situation and determine whether the outcome was what you expected.

STUDY QUESTIONS

1. List three situations that bring about ethical dilemmas in medicine.
2. Why are ethical constraints important in practicing medicine?
3. Define *morals* and give examples of medical moral dilemmas.
4. Describe one medical/ethical issue that was raised in your lifetime involving politics. How was political pressure brought on the public?

CASES FOR DISCUSSION

1. A premature infant was delivered at Woman's Hospital by the plaintiff. The child died shortly after birth, and the plaintiff was assured by the floor nurse that the hospital would take care of the infant's burial. When the mother went to the obstetrician for an examination six weeks later, she was given her folder to hold while waiting for the physician. She found in it a note from the pathologist about disposal of the baby's body. When the plaintiff asked the physician about the disposal of the body, he instructed his nurse to take her to the hospital across the street to see someone who would tell her what had been done with the baby. When the woman and the nurse found the person, the plaintiff was handed a large jar with the baby's body inside. As a result, the plaintiff suffered nightmares, could not sleep, was depressed when she was around children, had surgery for a pseudopregnancy, and required psychiatric treatment. Should a patient–physician relationship include the contract to dispose of a dead body?

2. The plaintiff's 18-year-old son died suddenly at home. His body was taken to the hospital, where the cause of death could not be found without an autopsy. The deputy medical examiner ordered a

postmortem examination. The plaintiff was a member of the Jewish Orthodox faith and refused the postmortem examination of his son on the basis that religious conviction prohibited any molestation of the body after death. Is freedom of religion curtailed by a law that has a compelling state interest?

3. The plaintiff was a 59-year-old woman who had been a practicing Christian Scientist for approximately 10 years. She was unmarried and on welfare. She was involuntarily admitted to Bellevue Hospital by the police when she would not leave her hotel room. Upon admission, she was examined by two psychiatrists and certified according to New York law for commitment for 60 days. The plaintiff informed the hospital staff of her religious preference and that, based on these beliefs, she was unwilling to receive medical treatment. Over her objections she was given tranquilizers. She was never adjudicated mentally ill or incompetent prior to the treatment. The plaintiff brought an action under federal civil rights statutes, claiming damages for violation of her right to freedom of religion under the First Amendment. Can an individual be determined mentally ill and treatment initiated without an adjudication of incompetence?

4. The plaintiff, a Jehovah's Witness, was injured in an automobile accident and was taken to the hospital, where it was determined that she would die without an operation. The operation required blood transfusions. A tenet of the Jehovah's Witness faith forbids blood transfusions. The plaintiff was accompanied by her mother. The plaintiff was in shock, and evidence was presented that she was incoherent. Her mother signed a release of the hospital for all liability, but the hospital went to the court for the appointment of a guardian who would consent to the transfusions. A guardian was appointed, and the operation, with transfusions, was successfully performed. Does a state have the right to authorize the use of force to prevent an individual's death?

5. The plaintiff was injured when a tree fell on him. At the hospital, he refused to consent to blood transfusions because of religious beliefs. The plaintiff's wife agreed that he should not be transfused. The hospital petitioned the court for the appointment of a guardian for the plaintiff. The court decided that the plaintiff understood the consequences of refusing the transfusion and that the plaintiff's wife and children would be taken care of, and refused to grant the petition. Should a patient refuse treatment?

6. The physician was licensed to practice medicine in Maine and, as a licensed physician, was a member of the Maine Medical Association. Following an informal meeting with the physician, the association's ethics and discipline committee, in a report, charged him with submitting invoices to the Maine Department of Health and Welfare that showed "gross overutilization, malpractice, and unethical practice." The physician was not informed of the charges against him before the

meeting. The committee placed into evidence confidential documents used against the physician without his consent. In charging the physician, the association went against procedures established in its own bylaws, which required that ethical complaints be disposed of at the county level. Should this report be withheld from disclosure?

7. The New York Legislature passed the New York State Controlled Substances Act of 1971 because of concern about the illegal use of drugs in the state. The act requires that records involving the use of certain prescription drugs be filed by physicians with the New York State Department of Health. These records are kept on computers and include the name and address of patients using the drugs. The concern of the physicians and patients who were plaintiffs was that patients in need of treatment with these drugs would decline treatment for fear of being labeled drug addicts. Was the collection of these records by the state a violation of the patients' Fourteenth Amendment rights?

8. The plaintiff was arrested in Denver and charged with solicitation and prostitution and held in the city jail. She had the choice of remaining in jail for 48 hours for examination and treatment for sexually transmitted disease or of taking penicillin without examination and being released from jail immediately. She chose to take the penicillin. In Denver, any person arrested for vagrancy, prostitution, rape, or any other sexual offense must be examined and treated for sexually transmitted disease. The plaintiff brought suit against the city and county of Denver, claiming that her civil rights under the Fourth and Fourteenth Amendments had been violated. Are the arrest, involuntary detention, and treatment of individuals suspected to have sexually transmitted disease a valid exercise of the state's police power?

9. The defendants, Griswold and Buxton, were arrested for violating a statute that forbade the use of contraceptives. Griswold, executive director of Planned Parenthood, and Buxton, a licensed physician and medical director for Planned Parenthood, gave information, instruction, and medical advice to married persons regarding the prevention of conception. Griswold and Buxton charged that the statute violated the due process clause of the Fourteenth Amendment. Did the U.S. Supreme Court find that the statute violated the due process clause?

10. An unmarried female, Jane Roe, brought an action against the District Attorney in Texas, charging that the Texas criminal abortion statutes were unconstitutional. The plaintiff stated that she was unmarried and pregnant, that she wished to end the pregnancy in safe clinical conditions, but that she was unable to get a legal abortion in Texas because she was not in a life-threatening situation. She claimed that the statutes abridged her right of personal privacy protected by the First, Fourth, Fifth, Ninth, and Fourteenth Amendments. Should her right of personal privacy include the right to have an abortion?

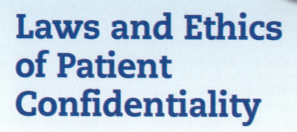

9

Laws and Ethics of Patient Confidentiality

 A secret spoken finds wings.

Robert Jordan, *The Path of Daggers*

OBJECTIVES

After reading this chapter, you should be able to:

1. Distinguish between privacy, confidentiality, and privileged communication.
2. Recognize the role that every member of the health care community plays in maintaining confidentiality.
3. Identify the challenge that the media presents to maintaining confidentiality.
4. Discuss the importance of confidentiality of the medical record.
5. Begin to develop a personal philosophy for dealing with confidentiality dilemmas within an ethical framework.

BUILDING YOUR LEGAL VOCABULARY

Egregious   Stringent
Patient–physician privilege   Waives
Privileged communication

INTRODUCTION

Matters tied to patient confidentiality, privacy, and **privileged communication** often raise both legal and ethical issues with conflicting interests. The public's need to know about a patient's medical condition may conflict with a patient's desire to keep the information private. A patient's interest in making an independent decision may also conflict with a predesignated outcome. The Health Insurance Portability and Accountability Act of 1996 (HIPAA) has everything to do with patient information confidentiality in health care. HIPAA is a foundational health care reference for contemporary patient confidentiality issues, including who can obtain a patient's medical information and under what circumstances.

DISCLOSURE OF PATIENT INFORMATION

Health Insurance Portability and Accountability Act of 1996 (HIPAA)

With the federal government's enactment of HIPAA in 1996 and the start of its enforcement in 2003, confidentiality has become a focal point in the practice of health care. HIPAA provides new, complex standards regarding health information security; the adoption of code sets for standard transactions; and the maintenance of the privacy and confidentiality of health records.

HIPAA's Privacy Rule ensures that patients' confidential health information is protected while also permitting sharing of health information to foster improved health care. The Privacy Rule pertains to protected health information (PHI), which is "individually identifiable health information" and, according to the U.S. Department of Health and Human Services:

[PHI] is information, including demographic information, which relates to:

- the individual's past, present, or future physical or mental health or condition,
- the provision of health care to the individual, or
- the past, present, or future payment for the provision of health care to the individual, and that identifies the individual or for which there is a reasonable basis to believe can be used to identify the individual. Protected health information includes many common identifiers (e.g., name, address, birth date, Social Security Number) when they can be associated with the health information listed above.

PHI includes all forms of health information, including electronic, written, or verbal.

You may have seen signs in hospitals and physician offices reminding staff members to keep patient conversations confidential. It is now routine procedure for a patient to receive a "HIPAA notification" once a year while checking in for an appointment. Some physician offices and urgent care facilities use pagers similar to those used in restaurants to avoid mentioning a patient's name when notifying them of their turn to be seen by a provider. Often, for reasons of confidentiality, providers just use a patient's first name when others are within earshot. Files and filing systems have been modified; electronic systems are omnipresent; and the handling of paper records has changed. The list of accommodations by the health care community to comply with regulations adopted in the wake of HIPAA is remarkable for its length and breadth.

HIPAA is the basis for providers' adoption of strict policies related to discussing a patient's health care with other professionals, the amount and type of information to be disclosed and to whom. HIPAA, and similar state statutes, require written contracts with business associates (e.g., legal, actuarial, accounting, management, administration, accreditation, financial services) before protected information can be shared with them. Likewise, HIPAA training—for employees and those who do business with the provider—is a common occurrence in health care provider organizations.

In the United States, the confidentiality of medical information is not specifically included within constitutional rights of privacy. Before HIPAA, there was no federal law that specifically governed patient information and its unique needs. HIPAA has three self-declared major objectives:

> 66 99
>
> 1. To protect and enhance the rights of consumers by providing them access to their health information and controlling the inappropriate use of that information;
> 2. to improve the quality of health care in the U.S. by restoring trust in the health care system among consumers, healthcare professionals, and the multitude of organizations and individuals committed to the delivery of care; and,
> 3. to improve the efficiency and effectiveness of health care delivery by creating a national framework for health privacy protection that builds on efforts by states, health systems and individual organizations and individuals.
>
> *Public Law 104–191*

Before HIPAA's enactment, patient information confidentiality was subject to state law, which varied from state to state and was not comprehensive. States may still enact laws regarding patient information,

stringent strict requirements, precise, exact

but the laws must be at least as **stringent** as those in HIPAA. HIPAA provides national guidelines for patient confidentiality, as well as criminal sanctions for those who do not comply. Someone found guilty of wrongfully disclosing private health information could face up to 10 years in jail and a $250,000 fine.

A former UCLA Health System employee became the first person in the nation to be sentenced to federal prison for violating HIPAA.

Huping Zhou, 47, of Los Angeles, was sentenced to four months in prison on April 27 after pleading guilty in January to four misdemeanor counts of accessing and reading the confidential medical records of his supervisors and high-profile celebrities, according to the U.S. Attorney's Office for the Central District of California. Zhou was also fined $2,000…

According to court documents, Zhou accessed the UCLA record system 323 times during the three-week period. In the plea agreement, Zhou admitted he obtained and read patient health information on four specific occasions—with no legitimate reason, medical or otherwise—after he was terminated from his job.

Dimick, C. (2010, April 29). Californian sentenced to prison for HIPAA violation. *Journal of AHIMA*. Retrieved from http://journal.ahima.org/2010/04/29 /californian-sentenced-to-prison-for-hipaa-violation/

Notably, Mr. Zhou did not use the information for personal gain or release it to others, but still received jail time, which is a first for HIPAA violation cases.

The HIPAA's objectives underscore the need for patient confidentiality, as was clearly stated by the U.S. Department of Health and Human Services:

> In short, the entire health care system is built upon the willingness of individuals to share the most intimate details of their lives with their health care providers. The need for privacy of health information, in particular, has long been recognized as critical to the delivery of needed medical care. More than anything else, the relationship between a patient and a clinician is based on trust. The clinician must trust the patient to give full and truthful information about their health, symptoms, and medical history. The patient must trust the clinician to use that information to improve his or her health and to respect the need to keep such information private… Individuals cannot be expected to share the most intimate details of their lives unless they have confidence that such information will not be used or shared inappropriately.

Federal Register. (2000, December 28). 65(250), p. 82465. Retrieved from https://www .gpo.gov/fdsys/pkg/FR-2000-12-28/pdf/00-32678.pdf

There is tradition and a history set by common law for maintaining the confidentiality of medical records. The following article provides an example of the strength of this tradition:

A state panel suspended a therapist's license for speaking publicly about her counseling sessions with Nicole Brown Simpson. Susan J. Forward, who was among the first to reveal Nicole Simpson's history of abuse at the hands of O.J. Simpson after Nicole Simpson's death, is barred from seeing patients for three months and placed on three years' probation for violating Nicole Simpson's confidentiality.

Deputy Attorney General Anne Le Mendoza, who represents the state Board of Behavioral Science Examiners, stated: "Therapy is based on privacy and secrecy, and a breach of confidentiality…destroys the therapeutic relationship."

Susan Forward, who is the author of the best selling *Men Who Hate Women and the Women Who Love Them*, acknowledged that she spoke to ten reporters about Nicole Simpson.

Therapist punished for Simpson revelations. (1995, November 24). *The Boston Globe*, p. 19.

Confidentiality

The expectation of confidentiality between patient and physician was first documented in 1134 B.C., when Greek physicians recorded case histories on columns in their temples. These primitive recordings included patient names, medical histories, and treatments. Patient confidentiality was protected by restricting temple access to authorized persons. During the Middle Ages, medical information was public, and during the nineteenth century, medical information was secret.

A patient's expectation of privacy, known as confidentiality in the patient–physician relationship, and the doctrine of **patient–physician privilege** in the legal arena have evolved from Hippocrates' fundamental concept:

patient–physician privilege legal concept that protects communications between a patient and a physician from disclosure in court

> ❝❞
>
> Whatsoever in my practice or not in my practice, I shall see or hear amid the lives of men, which ought not be noised abroad, as to this I will keep silence holding such things unfit to be spoken.
>
> *Hippocrates*

Because of the many professionals involved in patient care, maintaining confidentiality is a high-priority concern for everyone who has contact with patient records. The confidentiality of the patient–physician relationship extends to all who have access to patient information. Medical office professionals, including medical assistants, must maintain the same standards of confidentiality as physicians.

In 1991, Kirk B. Johnson, the American Medical Association general counsel said, "Confidentiality used to be a sacred principle in medicine, but it just isn't as sacred as it used to be... It is one of the things that got lost in the race to review everything in medicine and get it all computerized." Since 1991, HIPAA has turned the tides on the patient confidentiality.

Patients and health care providers recognize the ever-increasing availability of patient information, which raises concerns about confidentiality. HIPAA has reshaped attitudes toward safeguarding the confidentiality of patient information. UCLA Medical Center fired more than a dozen employees and suspended at least six others for accessing confidential medical records of pop star Britney Spears without authorization.

Such prying is also considered a violation of state and federal laws governing medical privacy. The laws allow for fines of up to $250,000, although such penalties are uncommon. Under different laws, separate fines are allowed if patients are receiving treatment for mental illness or substance abuse...

When employees look at a patient's records electronically, they leave an electronic trail. "We advise all of our workforce that their password is their PIN for lack of a better analogy, and it is their signature," Klove said. When it is used, the systems track which screens they view and for how long. ... Klove said that all workers must sign statements pledging to adhere to confidentiality rules when they are hired. The hospital is now considering having them sign such statements annually.

Ornstein, C. (2008, March 15). Hospital to punish snooping on Spears. *LA Times*. Retrieved from http://articles.latimes.com/2008/mar/15/local/me-britney15

Privileged Communication

Confidentiality also exists with privileged communications, also referred to as a privilege. Information that has been shared between people who have a special legal relationship is protected from disclosure so that it may not be disclosed at trial. The special legal relationship can be between a husband and a wife; a physician and a patient; an attorney and a client; or a priest and penitent, among others. The privilege is intended to encourage open and honest discussions within those relationships and avoid any concern that others will be able to learn about the content of the discussions.

In a typical patient–physician privilege, a physician cannot reveal confidential patient information in court unless the patient **waives** his or her privilege against disclosure. The patient–physician privilege belongs to the patient, not the physician. So, a physician may not waive the privilege. When a patient files a medical malpractice lawsuit, for example, the nature of the case requires that medical records be available, and the patient–physician privilege is implicitly waived.

waives to surrender a claim, privilege, or right the utterance of a false charge that damages another's reputation

CONFIDENTIALITY AND TECHNOLOGY

Chapters 2 and 7 discuss HITECH and the integration of the electronic medical record into the everyday practice of medicine. With HITECH's requirements to use EHR meaningfully also comes the responsibility of protecting patient information from improper disclose. High standards of confidentiality required by HIPAA can be breached if, for example, a physician decides to place patient information on the Internet without appropriate safeguards to ensure the information remains confidential.

Use of the Internet as a storage point for EHR is becoming more commonplace. World-famous medical organizations such as the Cleveland Clinic, Geisinger Health System, and others now keep patient records on the Internet, which permits access to appropriate health care personnel, as well as the patient. As this practice becomes more prevalent, it will be important for medical assistants to understand this use and how to protect patient confidentiality in this environment. Internet-based systems that permit different EHR systems to share information create many opportunities for improper disclosure of confidential patient information. Regardless of where the confidential patient information comes from, a key point to remember is that HIPAA applies.

Use of technology in health care creates an increasing number of ways that patient confidentiality can be compromised. For example, there have been several incidents where a hacker introduces malware to a health care provider's computer system. The malware allows the hacker to hold the computer system hostage, including patient records, and to demand ransom.

Hollywood Presbyterian Medical Center paid a $17,000 ransom in bitcoin to a hacker who seized control of the hospital's computer systems and would give back access only when the money was paid, the hospital's chief executive said Wednesday.

(Continues)

(Continued)

The assault on Hollywood Presbyterian occurred Feb. 5, when hackers using malware infected the institution's computers, preventing hospital staff from being able to communicate from those devices, said Chief Executive Allen Stefanek…

Ransom attacks are still relatively rare. But cyberattacks on hospitals have become more common in recent years as hackers pursue personal information they can use for fraud schemes. Last July, hackers may have accessed as many 4.5 million patient records in UCLA Health System's computer network.

Winton, R. (2016, February 18). Hollywood hospital pays $17,000 in bitcoin to hackers; FBI investigating. *LA Times.* Retrieved from http://www.latimes.com/business /technology/la-me-ln-hollywood-hospital-bitcoin-20160217-story.html

The confidentiality of EHR is important enough and has raised enough concerns to warrant security companies that are dedicated to researching the safety of health care provider's computer systems:

A two-year research project into the security of 12 hospitals and a variety of medical technologies has concluded that patient health is "extremely vulnerable" to digital attacks…

Its research involved attacking medical organizations in controlled settings, including compromises of patient monitoring systems, check-in kiosks and drug dispensers, the latter taking place after infections via USB sticks left around hospital premises. Those attacks, if they had been carried out by malicious hackers, would have ended in patient injury or death, the study concluded…

Hackers could "easily" compromise patient health, whether through theft of their data or by compromising medical data, the report claimed…

The report adds to an ever-expanding pile of evidence indicating poor security at medical facilities. A vast number of medical devices have been deemed vulnerable in the last year. In July 2015, a range of cancer scanning technology was found to use weak, easily-crackable passwords. Earlier this month, Sergey Lozhkin, senior researcher at Kaspersky Lab, revealed how easily he was able to penetrate the defenses of a Moscow-based hospital, breaking in via the hospital Wi-Fi (again, in a controlled environment).

Fox-Brewster, T. (2016, February 23). White hat hackers hit 12 American hospitals to prove patient life "Extremely Vulnerable." *Forbes.* Retrieved from http://www.forbes .com/sites/thomasbrewster/2016/02/23/hackers-tear-hospitals-apart/#c3881c740d7f

As a part of any medical office staff, you can contribute to the computer system security by strictly complying with all computer security policies in your office, not allowing anyone but yourself to use your password and not opening documents where the sender is unfamiliar, among others.

THE MEDICAL OFFICE

The High-Profile Patient

The media is always interested in gathering confidential information about public figures largely because the public is interested in hearing about it. Health care providers are required to keep the information of all patients confidential, even if the patient is the most popular Hollywood actor, the latest Internet celebrity, the highest-paid athlete, or the most disgraced politician. The high-profile patient need not have national or international fame: your local county commissioners, police chiefs, business owners, or corporate executives, among others, also have a right to confidentiality. Breaches of patient confidentiality, including high-profile patients, are very serious matters.

January 2011: University Medical Center in Tucson, Ariz., fired three employees for snooping in records after the shooting that left then-U.S. Rep. Gabrielle Giffords in critical condition. A contract nurse also was terminated.

July 2011: UCLA Health System agreed to pay $865,000 to the federal government to resolve allegations that its employees violated federal patient privacy laws by snooping in the medical records of two celebrity patients. Separately, in January 2010, a former UCLA employee pleaded guilty to four counts of illegally reading medical records, mostly from celebrities and other high-profile patients, and was sentenced to four months in federal prison.

July 2013: Five workers and a student research assistant were fired for inappropriately accessing records at Cedars-Sinai Medical Center in Los Angeles. One of those was reportedly reality TV star Kim Kardashian, who gave birth to her daughter at the hospital the prior month.

September 2014: Nebraska Medical Center in Omaha fired two workers for looking in the records of Dr. Rick Sacra, who had been treated at the hospital for the Ebola virus he contracted while volunteering in Africa.

Ornstein, C. (2015, December 10). Celebrities' medical records tempt hospital workers to snoop. Retrieved from http://www.npr.org/sections/health-shots/2015/12/10/458939656 /celebrities-medical-records-tempt-hospital-workers-to-snoop

Snooping in a medical record is not the only way high-profile patients might find their confidential information improperly disclosed. A breach of patient confidentiality can also occur when a member of the health care provider's staff improperly discloses the simple fact that a high-profile client is a patient.

Medical Office Personnel

The medical office offers many opportunities for confidentiality to be intentionally or accidently breached. For example, the simple clerical matter of sending a "checkup reminder" can cause problems:

A month after the death of a woman in a hospital, the family physician's office sent a notice to her home for a periodic checkup. Her husband and children were upset by the notice and informed the office in writing of her death and their distress.

Her husband subsequently filed a malpractice action against the physician for wrongful death, apparently for failure to diagnose her illness. Two more "checkup" reminders were received by the family, the second being sent to the daughter.

In its decision, the Court held that sending the first notice would not have constituted an action for invasion of privacy since it would have been mailed by mistake, but sending two more after the commencement of a malpractice lawsuit was grounds for a cause of action for invasion of privacy.

McCormick v. Haley, 37 Ohio App.2d 73 (Ohio App. 10 Dist., 1973)

Harry T. Paxton, in an article titled "Today's Guidelines for Patient Confidentiality," writes:

The other day I was in an office where a secretary yelled across a room to another secretary "Mr. Jones needs a vasectomy scheduled with Dr. Smith." There were a number of people in that room and they all heard that Mr. Jones was going to have a vasectomy. Matters like that are very personal. There's a potential lawsuit when something like this happens.

Paxton, H. T. (1988, February 1). Today's guidelines for patient confidentiality. *Medical Economics,* 198.

The two preceding examples illustrate, first, that state law still has a place in the issue of medical record privacy. Specifically, the first case would still obtain the result, not *because* of HIPAA but *in spite* of it. Simply put, HIPAA does not allow an individual to enforce its provisions; only the government has the authority to enforce the federally imposed requirements. The second case represents a clear violation of HIPAA; the personnel involved should be counseled and educated to avoid this kind of mistake in the future. If such conduct were to continue, the office would be justified in taking harsher actions such as suspension or termination.

Reminders to employees, physicians, and other professionals that someone may be listening to their conversations are posted in most hospitals. Confidentiality of a patient's symptoms, diagnosis, and treatment is essential to preserve a patient's privacy and to prevent others from recalling bits and pieces of information that could lead to wrong conclusions. Breaching confidentiality not only is unethical but may cause legal problems.

A woman who was employed by a caterer had a condition, which raised false positives on Wasserman tests [a diagnostic test for syphilis]. Her physician knew she did not have syphilis. The office nurse attended a social affair catered by the employer of the patient. The nurse told the hostess that the patient was being treated by her employer for syphilis. The information affected the patient's employment and the employer's business. The Court held that there was a good cause for slander against the nurse.

Schessler v. Keck, 271 P.2d 588 (Cal. App. 2 Dist., 1954)

The above case took place before HIPAA was enacted. Today, the same actions would constitute **egregious** HIPAA violations that could have criminal sanctions. The following letter from a "Dear Abby" column reveals how deeply disclosure of confidential information can affect a patient:

egregious outrageous, shockingly bad, awful

When I was twenty I had an abortion. Seven years later, when I was pregnant with my first child, my doctor asked if this was my first pregnancy, so I told him about the abortion. At one of my early prenatal visits, his nurse walked into the examining room, looked me straight in the eye, and said, "So, you've decided to keep this one?"… Never again will I disclose this information on my medical history.

The Patriot Ledger, p. 26 (1988, March 30).

Medical Records

The earlier trend toward loosening the rules of confidentiality and privileged communication has been reversed through HIPAA. The patient owns the patient–physician privilege, and the physician may not decide, absent extraordinary circumstances, to release confidential patient information without patient authorization to do so.

The plaintiff, the biological mother of a child years before placed for adoption, brought an action against a physician who had assisted the daughter in her search for the mother.

The daughter, at twenty-one years of age, became interested in finding her biological mother. She was unable to gain access to the confidential court file of her adoption but did locate the mother's obstetrician, who agreed to help her find her biological mother. In order to gain access to the confidential records concerning the daughter's birth and adoption, the physician/defendant fabricated a letter stating that although he could not find his records, he remembered giving the mother diethylstilbestrol (DES).

Hospital personnel, relying on the physician's letter, allowed the daughter to make copies of her mother's medical records, therefore making it possible for the daughter to find her mother. The Supreme Court of Oregon determined that the mother had a valid cause of action against the physician for breach of a confidential relationship and further stated that the duty of confidentiality could not be disregarded solely to satisfy the curiosity of a person who sought her biological mother.

Humphers v. First Interstate Bank of Oregon, 696 P.2d 527 (Or., 1985)

In this case, the mother would not be permitted to maintain a lawsuit under HIPAA. She might well sue under state law, but only the government can discipline the hospital or its staff formally for HIPAA violations.

Beverly Woodward tells of a friend, a physician who gave birth at a hospital—and soon found that ten of her colleagues had looked up her medical record on the hospital's computer system, eager to check on the status of mother and baby. "She has an extensive medical record, and she was appalled to realize her colleagues had instant access to everything in it," said Woodward, a sociology researcher at Brandeis University who has studied the problem of patient privacy. "When a medical record is on paper, a lot fewer people have access to it."

Bass, A. (1995, February 22). Computerized medical data put privacy on the line. *The Boston Globe*, p. 5.

The problem outlined in the preceding case indicates the very reason HIPAA was enacted: Congress understood that developing electronic storage of medical records was essential to simplify administration of the health care system. As the health care system has moved toward electronic storage of medical information, the possibility of confidential information being misused has increased. In response to increasing concern that federal regulation of information was necessary to secure and control such information, HIPAA was enacted. The privacy provisions are aimed at addressing concerns that this information would be released to employers, insurers, universities, police, courts, state and federal agencies, health researchers, and others.

Prior to the HIPAA safeguards, medical information was not as closely guarded. An example of a bizarre incident that violated confidentiality in computerized medical records occurred in Florida when a teenage girl called former hospital patients and told them they had tested positive for AIDS:

The 13-year-old's mother, an employee at University Medical Center, took her daughter to work because she could not find anyone to watch her. Getting telephone numbers of former emergency room patients from a computer, the child called seven people and told them they had tested positive for H.I.V. One of the victims tried to commit suicide. A call to one patient was traced to the child's home because the patient had Caller ID.

Girl accused of making false AIDS calls. (1995, March 1). *The New York Times*, p. 1.

By the same token, however, the technology of electronic data storage can sometimes be foiled. One of the ongoing concerns is hackers getting into medical data. In Massachusetts, a convicted child rapist working at a hospital used a former employee's computer password to invade nearly 1,000 confidential patient files and then used the telephone numbers he obtained to make obscene calls to girls. He was charged under a statute that makes it a criminal offense to use another person's password to gain access to a computer system.

Dr. Denise Nagel, president of the Massachusetts chapter of the Coalition for Patient Rights, reacted by saying, "People are being assured privacy as their medical records are being computerized and this is a sad example that there is no privacy once records are computerized."

Brelis, M. (1995, April 11). Patients' files allegedly used for obscene calls. *The Boston Globe*, p. 1.

LIMITS OF CONFIDENTIALITY

Keeping medical information confidential can breed conflict. The following situation demonstrates ethical dimensions involving a diagnosis of herpes:

The K's are prominent members of the community. Mrs. K is pregnant and Dr. O'Brien, her obstetrician, has been following the pregnancy. Mrs. K had an appointment with Dr. O'Brien in her office and upon examination Dr. O'Brien found an open lesion in her genital area. Dr. O'Brien diagnosed it as a genital herpes lesion and Mrs. K requested that the information not be entered into her medical record. Dr. O'Brien explained that if Mrs. K has open lesions at the time of delivery, a C-section would have to be performed to prevent infection to the child. Mrs. K pleaded with Dr. O'Brien to keep this information confidential, appealing as a friend and a trusted physician.

Purtile, R., & Sorrell, J. (1986, August).
The ethical dilemmas of a rural physician. *The Hastings Report*, 25.

The incident took place in a community where "everyone knew everyone else." The receptionist was Mrs. K's sister-in-law. The county public health clerk to whom this sexually transmitted disease should have been reported was Mrs. K's cousin. Other relatives worked as nurse's aides in the hospital where she would deliver. In this case, the physician did not record the information about the lesion in the patient's medical record. She did record the information in a second set of records she kept in a locked place accessible only to her and her partner. Emergency departments are often the scene of similar conflicts in patient confidentiality:

A teenager who's just been raped rushes in to the ER, requesting a pelvic exam and a morning-after pill but insisting that no one call the police. What do you do? In every state, rape is a reportable offense, one of a number of instances in which public welfare takes precedence over a patient's right to privacy…

AIDS, more than any other diagnosis, confuses issues of privacy and confidentiality. That's because disclosure has meant the loss of jobs, medical insurance, and even housing for many patients… HIV infection presents an additional dilemma: what to do when you know your patient has not informed his sexual partner of his diagnosis. Here, as in a case of child abuse, the welfare of a third party takes precedence over the patient's desire not to have this information disclosed.

Greve, P. A. (1990, December). Keep quiet or speak up?
Issues in patient confidentiality. *RN*, 53.

A landmark case involving conflict between the disclosure of information to a third party and patient–physician confidentiality follows:

⚖️

Poddar was undergoing treatment as a voluntary outpatient. He had become obsessed with Tatiana Tarasoff, a student he had met at a dance. He had tape-recorded conversations with her and spent hours replaying the tapes in order to determine her feelings for him. A friend became concerned and suggested that he seek professional help.

Poddar was seen by a psychiatrist, who did not believe that Poddar required hospitalization, but did prescribe medication and arranged weekly outpatient psychotherapy with a staff psychologist. During therapy, Poddar revealed his fantasies of harming, and perhaps even killing, Tarasoff. The friend told the psychologist that Poddar planned to purchase a gun. Poddar stopped therapy. The physicians believed that Poddar should be evaluated for hospitalization and requested help from the campus police.

The campus police went to Poddar's apartment and questioned him about his plans but then left when he denied any intention of harming Tarasoff. Two months later Poddar stabbed Tarasoff to death. He was convicted of second-degree murder, the conviction was overturned on the basis of improper jury instruction, and Poddar returned home to India.

Later, in a civil suit, the Tarasoff family sued the university, including both therapists and the campus police, for negligence. The court held that the therapists had a duty to warn Tarasoff.

Tarasoff v. Regents of University of California, 118 Cal. Rptr. 129 (1974)

The Tarasotff case makes clear that, in some instances, there are interests that outweigh a patient's right to confidentiality.

CONFIDENTIALITY AS AN ETHICAL DILEMMA

Intentionally disclosing confidential patient information raises issues as to what is right or wrong given the circumstances. For example, is it right or wrong to keep a patient's AIDS diagnosis confidential? Both state and federal laws play an important part in deciding whether to reveal private information. Failure to adhere to these laws can result in significant consequences for the violator. For individuals who believe that it is ethical to follow the rules at any cost, laws about confidentiality solve the ethical dilemma. For individuals who are motivated by other values or ethical thought systems, laws only add conflict to the dilemma.

DEVELOPING AN ETHICAL DECISION-MAKING PROCESS

To develop an ethical decision-making process for dealing with problems of confidentiality and privacy, distinguish between what is clinical, what is legal, and what is ethical in a given circumstance. Having identified the ethical issues, the next question becomes this: Who owns the problem? If you own the problem, how do you respond?

You can respond to the dilemma by refusing to disclose anything at any time except to those to whom you are immediately responsible. You can choose to adhere strictly to existing law about a patient's confidentiality. If you choose to follow another line of reasoning, the consequences of your action must be accepted by your peers, your superiors, and society, or you risk losing your job and the possibility of being sued. You must then balance the risk against personal internal conflict.

☑ SUMMARY

- *Privacy*, *confidentiality*, and *privileged communication* are terms used to define the relationship between medical professionals and their patients and between legal professionals and their clients. The terms refer to the tradition and precedence requiring the maintenance of silence by medical and legal personnel. Maintaining confidences often involves ethical conflict.

- HIPAA rules the confidentiality requirement of health care facilities and personnel. All factors must be reviewed when making decisions about breaking patient confidentiality. What is right for one individual may be wrong for another.

- EHR provides more opportunities for improper disclosure of patient information. No matter what the form of the information (electronic, written, verbal), HIPAA governs.

- High-profile patients are entitled to the same confidentiality as any other patient.

- There are limits to a patient's right to confidentiality when there is a greater interest in disclosing the information, which creates ethical dilemmas.

SUGGESTED ACTIVITIES

1. Review the quotation at the beginning of this chapter. Based upon the material you have just read, how is the quotation related to patient confidentiality? What does the author mean by "wings"?

2. Research methods of maintaining the confidentiality of medical records at a local emergency room or hospital.

3. Find out and document the procedure and charges to obtain a copy of your own medical record from your primary care physician.

CASES FOR DISCUSSION

1. "Gregg Wiatt was stunned. On his 28th birthday—six months before the death of the man he had thought was his natural father—his mother told him the truth. She told him he was the offspring of a semen donor. Long before, though, Wiatt had felt somehow different. 'It was like there was always this secret I could never put my fingers on,' says the 37-year-old Denver sales and marketing executive. 'When I finally learned the truth, it felt like I was living between Disneyland and the Twilight Zone.' Bill Cordray, 47, also felt odd. 'It was something that kept edging into my consciousness,' says the Salt Lake City architect. He and his dad were 'so different. My interests were artistic—music, building, creative. So different from everyone else. I felt like a stranger in my family.' Wiatt and Cordray are among tens of thousands of people literally born out of the high-tech merger of egg and sperm. And, like most of the others, they're still in the dark—because records are confidential" ("When Dad's a Sperm Donor," 1993). Develop arguments on both sides of the question: Should sperm donor records be confidential?

2. The Wisconsin Coalition Against Sexual Assault purchased a state surplus computer for 20 dollars and found that it contained the medical records of more than 600 people. Upon discovering the records, the coalition's executive director began erasing them from the computer. Before erasing all the records, she decided to make a copy of those that had not been erased. She then provided about 500 names and data to a state representative and erased all the original records. Upon receipt of the records, the state representative was concerned because he did not want patients upset because their medical records were made public and because it was a potential liability for the state. Wisconsin has a statute that prohibits the "knowing and willful" release of medical records and requires a showing that there was a willing disregard. Was there a willing disregard?

3. "A Simmons College survey of about 150 people who went to the South Shore Mental Health Center's crisis unit has prompted questions about whether the center violated patient confidentiality. The center gave a college research team the names, addresses and telephone numbers of randomly selected people who sought emergency help in September. The decision to turn over names and other information, which was used to conduct a 'consumer satisfaction' survey, has drawn complaints from two patients who say the center

violated their right to privacy... Simmons did the survey as a student research project. Those who were asked to participate had two chances to decline. Patients could call a telephone number to say 'no' after they got the letter, or they could withdraw when a student called them to conduct the phone interview. If they didn't call 'it was presumed that they were giving their consent' to be interviewed. The two patients felt that they'd lost their privacy. 'If you went to a crisis unit, would you want your name passed around by a bunch of college students?' asked one of the women, who went to the center because she was feeling 'suicidal.' The second woman said she doubted she would ever be able to trust the confidentiality of any counseling agency. 'This ices my going to another counselor anywhere,' she said. 'I don't believe there is any privacy'" (Lambert, 1996, p. 1). Did giving names, addresses, and telephone numbers violate or not violate the privacy of the patients? Justify your answer.

4. "In a case that has raised questions about the limits of confidentiality in self-help groups, a Larchmont carpenter is on trial again on charges of breaking into his childhood home and murdering the couple who had bought the house from his parents. The first trial of the carpenter, Paul Cox, 27, ended in a mistrial, with jurors deadlocked 11 to 1 in favor of conviction. In that trial more than a half dozen members of Alcoholics Anonymous testified under subpoena that Mr. Cox confessed to them that he thought he had committed the killings during a drunken blackout. As in the first trial, Cox had pleaded not guilty and intends to use a defense of temporary insanity" ("Retrial Begins in Murder Case," 1994, p. B7). Should privileged communication be extended to self-help groups?

5. Abigail Hinchy was in a relationship with Davion Peterson. During this time, Ms. Hinchy filled her prescriptions at a Walgreen pharmacy. Ms. Hinchy became pregnant with Mr. Peterson's child and gave birth to a son. After he was no longer dating Ms. Hinchy and had started dating a Walgreen's pharmacist, Audra Withers, Mr. Peterson learned that he had contracted genital herpes at some point in the past. Ms. Withers was concerned about how the herpes was spread and used Walgreen's records to research Ms. Hinchy's prescription history. Mr. Peterson learned of the records and confronted Ms. Hinchy because the records showed she had not refilled her birth control. Ms. Hinchy learned that "(1) a HIPAA/privacy violation had occurred, (2) Withers had viewed Hinchy's prescription information without consent and for personal purposes, and (3) Walgreen could not confirm that Withers had revealed that information to a third party." Ms. Hinchy sued Ms. Withers and Walgreens for several causes of action, including negligent training, negligent supervision, negligent retention, and negligence/professional malpractice. Who is to blame? Ms. Withers? Mr. Peterson? Walgreens? All of them? And, what is an appropriate remedy to make Ms. Hinchy whole?

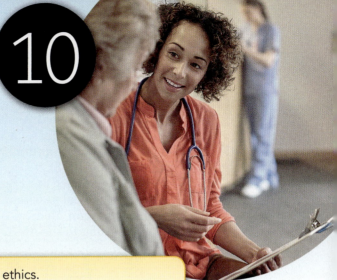

10

Professional Ethics and the Living

OBJECTIVES

After reading this chapter, you should be able to:

1. Paraphrase the creed of the American Association of Medical Assistants (AAMA), the Standards of Practice of the American Medical Technologists (AMT), the Preamble to the Code of Ethics of the American Medical Association (AMA), and provisions of the Uniform Anatomical Gift Act and of the Nuremberg Code.
2. Explain how the relationship between time, power, and ethics can influence a patient's medical office experience.
3. Identify some of the problems faced by medical professionals in allocating resources: transplant organs, money, and intensive care unit (ICU) beds.
4. Explain the ethics of medical research and experimentation.
5. Explain the need for and the propriety of drug testing in employment.
6. Recognize the importance of balancing autonomy and paternalism in patient care.

BUILDING YOUR LEGAL VOCABULARY

Autonomy
Calibration
Commitment

Creed
Paternalism
Personality traits

CREEDS

creed a statement of belief or principles

The **creed** of the AAMA is presented in Figure 10-1. Both the American Association of Medical Assistants (AAMA) and the Association of Medical Technologists (AMT) also have standards of conduct that address ethical and moral behavior for medical assistants (see Figures 10-2 and 10-3).

AMAA developed its creed to embody the highest ethical standards of the medical assistant. Its scope is narrower but closely aligned with the American Medical Association (AMA) Principles of Medical Ethics. According to the AMA, the Principles of Medical Ethics are nine

- I believe in the principles and purposes of the profession of medical assisting.
- I endeavor to be more effective.
- I aspire to render greater service.
- I protect the confidence entrusted to me.
- I am dedicated to the care and well-being of all people.
- I am loyal to my employer.
- I am true to the ethics of my profession.
- I am strengthened by compassion, courage and faith.

Figure 10-1 AAMA Medical Assistant Creed

The Medical Assisting Code of Ethics of the AAMA sets forth principles of ethical and moral conduct as they relate to the medical profession and the particular practice of medical assisting.

Members of AAMA dedicated to the conscientious pursuit of their profession, and thus desiring to merit the high regard of the entire medical profession and the respect of the general public, which they serve, do pledge themselves to strive always to:

A. Render service with full respect for the dignity of humanity.

B. Respect confidential information obtained through employment unless legally authorized or required by responsible performance of duty to divulge such information.

C. Uphold the honor and high principles of the profession and accept its disciplines.

D. Seek to continually improve the knowledge and skills of medical assistants for the benefit of patients and professional colleagues.

E. Participate in additional service activities aimed toward improving the health and well-being of the community.

Figure 10-2 AAMA Medical Assistant Code of Ethics

The American Medical Technologists is dedicated to encouraging, establishing and maintaining the highest standards, traditions, and principles of the disciplines which constitute the allied health professions of the certification agency and the Registry.

Members of the Registry and all individuals certified by AMT recognize their professional and ethical responsibilities, not only to their patients, but also to society, to other health care professionals, and to themselves. The AMT Board of Directors has adopted the following Standards of Practice which define the essence of competent, honorable and ethical behavior for an AMT-certified allied health care professional. Reported violations of these Standards will be referred to the Judiciary Committee and may result in revocation of the individual's certification or other disciplinary sanctions.

I.   While engaged in the Arts and Sciences that constitute the practice of their profession, AMT professionals shall be dedicated to the provision of competent and compassionate service and shall always meet or exceed the applicable standard of care.

II.   The AMT professional shall place the health and welfare of the patient above all else.

III.   When performing clinical duties and procedures, the AMT professional shall act within the lawful limits of any applicable scope of practice, and when so required shall act under and in accordance with appropriate supervision by an attending physician, dentist, or other licensed practitioner.

IV.   The AMT professional shall always respect the rights of patients and of fellow health care providers, shall comply with all applicable laws and regulations governing the privacy and confidentiality of protected healthcare information, and shall safeguard patient confidences unless legally authorized or compelled to divulge protected healthcare information to an authorized individual, law enforcement officer, or other legal or governmental entity.

V.   AMT professionals shall strive to increase their technical knowledge, shall continue to learn, and shall continue to apply and share scientific advances in their fields of professional specialization.

VI.   The AMT professional shall respect the law and pledges to avoid dishonest, unethical or illegal practices, breaches of fiduciary duty, or abuses of the position of trust into which the professional has been placed as a certified healthcare professional.

VII.   AMT professionals understand that they shall not make or offer a diagnosis or dispense medical advice unless they are duly licensed practitioners or unless specifically authorized to do so by an attending licensed practitioner acting in accordance with applicable law.

VIII.   The AMT professional shall observe and value the judgment of the attending physician, dentist, or other attending licensed practitioner, provided that so doing does not clearly constitute a violation of law or pose an immediate threat to the welfare of the patient.

IX.   AMT professionals recognize that they are responsible for any personal wrongdoing, and that they have an obligation to report to the proper authorities any knowledge of professional abuse or unlawful behavior by any party involved in the patient's diagnosis, care and treatment.

X.   The AMT professional pledges to uphold personal honor and integrity and to cooperate in protecting and advancing, by every lawful means, the interests of the American Medical Technologists and its Members.

Courtesy of the American Medical Technologists

Figure 10-3 AMT Standards of Practice

standards of conduct that define the essentials of physicians' honorable behavior. The Preamble to the Principles of Medical Ethics states, "The medical profession has long subscribed to a body of ethical statements developed primarily for the benefit of the patient. As a member of this profession, a physician must recognize responsibility to patients first and foremost, as well as to society, to other health professionals, and to self. The following Principles adopted by the American Medical Association are not laws, but standards of conduct which define the essentials of honorable behavior for the physician." (To read the full text of the Principles of Medical Ethics, go to the AMA website, www.ama-assn.org, and search for "Principles of Medical Ethics.")

Developing a code of ethics is difficult. Incorporating these ideals in everyday life is even more difficult. The role of health care professionals, such as medical assistants, does not usually involve making life-and-death ethical decisions. It does involve interpersonal interaction with patients and their families before and after difficult decisions have been made. It also involves support and understanding of the physicians involved in making these difficult decisions. It is important that each employee find his or her place in the office dynamics during intense, pressure-filled, decision-making moments. For example, someone who is not comfortable with abortion should seek employment in an office that is compatible with that moral perspective. A medical office, or any office, is an inappropriate place for moral debates or the airing of personal preferences. Working in an environment that is not morally comfortable puts intense stress on everyone and can potentially harm the patient. The internal discomfort of the incompatible employee will eventually result in burnout.

TIME

Health care professionals, like most people, prefer their weekends and evenings free. The economic environment in medicine has increased the pressure to be more cost conscious and profitable. As a result, health care professionals must find ways to use their facilities and equipment more efficiently. Weekends and evening hours have become additional opportunities to care for patients and increase revenue. Who must work on evenings and weekends? Is it the chief of staff, the resident, or the intern? Is it the head of a department, or the last one to join the organization? Who can change a weekend or evening assignment easily—the head of the department or the last one in? The answer to all these questions is usually the employee with the most power. Is it ethical to base these decisions on status within the organization?

The relationship between time, power, and ethics is also evident in the office or clinic waiting room. A constant sore spot in the physician–patient relationship is the amount of time patients spend waiting in reception and exam rooms. Wait time and increasing health care costs continue to raise serious questions for patients and providers. In many medical offices, physicians keep patients waiting. Is it ethical to keep all patients waiting the same amount of time, or do the most influential patients get in first? Are there different standards of care in attending to the needs of waiting patients? Does priority depend on the urgency of each case—for example, an emergency case? Do office ethics take into consideration the importance of time for everyone waiting? Is the physician's time more valuable than the patient's time? Time is a limited resource. There are ethical considerations with the allocation of time, as well as other resources.

ALLOCATION OF RESOURCES

Should everyone who needs expensive life-saving procedures, such as open-heart surgery and organ transplants, have an equal chance to get them regardless of ability to pay, social status, or other nonmedical factors? Is health care for everyone possible? Who will pay? If health care for everyone is not possible, who will receive life-saving services? Health care costs in the United States are high and rising; they currently account for more than 18 percent of the gross domestic product, with forecasts estimating it will be more than 20 percent by 2024. Americans spend much more than other countries, but are they getting what they pay for?

If you are dying in Miami, the last six months of your life might well look like this: You'll see doctors, mostly specialists, 46 times; spend more than six days in an intensive care unit and stand a 27% chance of dying in a hospital ICU. The tab for your doctor and hospital care will run just over $23,000. But spend those last six months in Portland, Ore., and you'll go to the doctor 18 times, half of those visits with your primary care doctor, spend one day in intensive care and stand a 13% chance of dying in an ICU. You'll likely die at home, with the support of a hospice program. Total tab: slightly more than $14,000...

While researchers are able to show differences in costs, the real question remains how much of those additional hospitalizations, tests and doctor visits resulted in better care or better quality of life? ...

(Continues)

> *(Continued)*
>
> Across the nation, some patients spend much of their final weeks seeing specialists, having tests, trying new drugs. Many die attached to machines, such as ventilators, in hospitals.
>
> For some patients, that's exactly the right care. Doing everything that can be done to save an 18-year-old motorcycle-crash victim makes sense. But what about an 85-year-old with heart failure, diabetes and cancer? Do you continue aggressive chemotherapy?
>
> Appleby, J. (2006, November 19). Debate surrounds end-of-life health care costs. *USA Today*. Retrieved from http://www.usatoday.com/money /industries/health/2006-10-18-end-of-life-costs_x.htm

Managed care is a response to the need to allocate limited resources for health care.

Managed Care

Chapter 1 discusses the business of health care and introduces many facets of managed care, and its various models. Today, more than 90 percent of the population with insurance is enrolled in some form of managed care, but in less restrictive models such as a preferred provider organization (PPO). This form of insurance is less effective than an HMO in controlling costs; however, it permits the patient greater latitude in choice of providers and is still less costly than the traditional fee-for-service (FFS) model. Ethical and legal conflicts abound for the individuals who operate the system: the physicians, nurse-practitioners, triage personnel, case managers, managed care organization administrators, risk managers, utilization reviewers, and corporate executives.

The former FFS system contributed to the rise of health care costs. To contain these costs, a total system change occurred. Because of the shift to managed care, the seriously ill patient needing more services became a burden. From the consumer's perspective, the single greatest threat posed by this shift is the potential for managed care systems to cut needed care to save health care dollars. Managed care often obscures the line separating insurers from providers. In addition, health care providers, paid on a capitation basis, who realize bonuses for fiscal restraint or who have portions of their salary withheld to control costs, make less money with a seriously ill patient. Inherent in the system is this major conflict:

Managed care is structured around a variety of incentives to encourage the practice of cost-effective medicine, and to minimize variation in clinical practice patterns. "Efficiency" here means providing a product, in this case health care, while minimizing resources used, most often dollars. Most often, efficiency is maximized by increasing productivity while fixing cost. Hence, managed care may create pressure to do more with less: less time per patient, less costly medicines, and fewer costly diagnostic tests and treatments.

Monetary incentives are often used to affect physician behavior, and may include rewarding physicians who practice medicine frugally by offering financial rewards, such as bonuses, for those who provide the most cost-efficient care. Those who perform too many procedures or are cost-inefficient in other ways may be penalized, often by withholding bonuses or portions of income. Nonmonetary inducements to limit care take the form of bringing peer pressure, or pressure from superiors, to bear on those who fail to take into account the financial well being of their employer. These monetary and nonmonetary incentives raise the ethical concern that physicians may compromise patient advocacy in order to achieve cost savings.

A related ethical concern pertains to the effect of managed care on physician–patient relationships. Many worry that managed care will undermine physician–patient relationships by eroding patients' trust in their physicians, reducing the amount of time physicians spend with patients, and restricting patients' access to physicians.

Jecker, N. S. (2008, April 11). *Ethics in medicine*. University of Washington School of Medicine. Retrieved from http://depts.washington.edu/bioethx/topics/manag.html

Negotiations between medical providers and insurers raise more ethical issues than service provided; they also can involve costs. A *Boston Globe* Spotlight Team series highlighted such a case in Massachusetts:

As his patient lies waiting in an adjacent exam room, Dr. James D. Alderman watches while an assistant reaches into a white envelope and pulls out a piece of paper that will determine where the man will be treated. Big money is on the line…

Usually he does the procedure…in Framingham. But he sometimes operates in Boston as part of a research program. One time of every four, by the luck of the draw, Alderman and his patient go to a big teaching hospital in the city.

(Continues)

(Continued)

If the white slip of paper directs him to do the procedure in Framingham, the insurance company will pay the hospital about $17,000, not counting the physician's fee. If Alderman is sent to…Boston, that hospital will get about $24,500—44 percent more—even though the patient's care will be the same in both places.

"It's the exact same doctor doing the procedure," said Andrei Soran, MetroWest's chief executive. "But the cost? It's unjustifiably higher."

Call it the best-kept secret in Massachusetts medicine: Health insurance companies pay a handful of hospitals far more for the same work even when there is no evidence that the higher-priced care produces healthier patients. In fact, sometimes the opposite is true: Massachusetts General Hospital, for example, earns 15 percent more than Beth Israel Deaconess Medical Center for treating heart-failure patients even though government figures show that Beth Israel has for years reported lower patient death rates.

Allen, S., Bombardieri, M., & Rezendes, M. (2008, November 16).
A healthcare system badly out of balance. *Boston Globe.* Retrieved from
https://www.bostonglobe.com/specials/2008/11/16/healthcare-system
-badly-out-balance/j2ushYtZTBiCSxxUtQegbN/story.html

In managed care, primary care physicians (PCPs) act as gatekeepers to control the cost-effectiveness of services offered to members and control access to specialists. In addition, many MCOs have adopted authorization requirements, where the MCO must approve certain procedures before the PCP orders them. These MCO payers are controlling access to health care by denying approval for certain procedures and allowing payment for others. They make decisions that reduce the number of hospital admissions, shorten the time until discharge, control the number of expensive diagnostic procedures, and, in the mental health field, substitute medication for therapeutic counseling treatment. Ethical questions arise when gatekeepers have a financial incentive to deny referrals to specialists, limit diagnostic treatments, and shorten hospital stays. And, when insurance companies make the decision to allow or deny diagnostic testing and hospital admissions, the well-being of the patient becomes an issue and ethical issues are front and center.

Transplants

The allocation of resources related to transplants gives rise to many ethical problems. Medical transplants are divided into three categories, depending on the tissue used. An *autograft* is the transplantation of a person's own tissue from one part of the body to another. This term also describes transplants between genetically identical children. A *homograft* is a transplant from one person to another, and the transplant of animal tissue into a human is a *heterograft*.

The current wave of transplant operations began in the late 1940s with corneal transplants from dead donors. Kidney transplants began in 1954 and are now commonplace. Liver and lung transplants followed, with the first recorded heart transplant to a human being attempted in 1964 with a chimpanzee's heart. In 2005, whole face transplants began in France, and in 2016, surgeons in Cleveland, Ohio, performed the first uterus transplant. The most common transplant, however, is a blood transfusion.

The rise in the number of transplants has increased competition for organs and blood. In an attempt to control the process, California was the first state to pass statutes allowing a citizen to dispose of his or her own body or to separate parts of it on death through a will or another written document. The Uniform Anatomical Gift Act was first drafted in 1968 and has been revised several times since then. The Act is intended to be adopted by states and used as a template to simplify the process of allowing individuals to specify their wishes. The main provisions of the Act are as follows:

1. Any individual of sound mind and 18 years of age or more may give all or any part of his body...the gift to take effect upon death.

2. In the absence of a gift by the deceased, and of any objection by the deceased, his or her relatives, in a stated order of priority (spouse, adult children, parents, adult brothers and sisters, etc.), have the power to give the body or any of its contents.

3. The recipients of a gift are restricted to hospitals, physicians, medical and dental schools, universities, tissue banks, and a specified individual in need of treatment. The purposes are restricted to transplantation, therapy, research, education, and the advancement of medical or dental science.

4. A gift may be made by will (to be effective immediately upon death without waiting for probate), or by a card or other document. If the donor is too sick or incapable of signing, it can be signed for him or her if two witnesses are present. A gift made by a relative can be made by document, or by telegraph or a recorded telephone message or other recorded message.

5. A gift may be revoked at any time.

6. A donee may accept or reject a gift.

All states use some form of the Act, and many allow individuals to indicate their choice to donate on their drivers' licenses. The use of organs from the dead and, later, from animals presented one set of ethical problems. The use of organs from the living presents even greater ethical dilemmas. Procedures that regulate living donor transplants have been developed through the courts.

Using live donors to obtain organs presents many problems. One is the discomfort of the provider. Many physicians will not take skin from a donor because of the pain inflicted. The removal of internal organs for transplant, in addition to the ethics involved with inflicting pain on one person for another's benefit, involves multiple dilemmas.

There is a high demand for donor organs. There are also strict protocols that govern organ harvesting, which do not always provide the needed protection for the prospective donor. For example:

On a winter night in 2006, a disabled and brain damaged man named Ruben Navarro was wheeled into an operating room at a hospital here. By most accounts, Mr. Navarro, 25, was near death, and doctors hoped that he might sustain other lives by donating his kidneys and liver.

But what happened to Mr. Navarro quickly went from the potentially life-saving to what law enforcement officials say was criminal. In what transplant experts believe is the first such case in the country, prosecutors have charged the surgeon, Dr. Hootan C. Roozrokh, with prescribing excessive and improper doses of drugs, apparently in an attempt to hasten Mr. Navarro's death to retrieve his organs sooner.

At the heart of the case is whether Dr. Roozrokh…was pursuing organs at any cost or had become entangled in a web of misunderstanding about a lesser-used harvesting technique known as "donation after cardiac death."

McKinley, J. (2008, February 27). Surgeon accused of speeding a death to get organs. *The New York Times*. Retrieved from http://www.nytimes.com/2008/02/27/us/27transplant.html

For centuries, human hair has been used by wig makers, and teeth have been implanted into the jaws of wealthy dental patients. As the number and kind of transplants increase, the demand for organs will also increase. Worldwide, there is consensus that dealing in human organs for profit is illegal, but consensus does not always make law. Illegal organ trafficking is no longer a myth but is rapidly becoming a growing problem.

The exchange of human organs for cash or any other "valuable consideration" (such as a car or a vacation) is illegal in every country except Iran. Nonetheless, international organ trafficking—mostly of kidneys, but also of half-livers, eyes, skin and blood—is flourishing; the World Health Organization estimates that one-fifth of the 70,000 kidneys transplanted worldwide every year come from the black market. Most of that trade can be explained by the simple laws of supply and demand. Increasing life spans, better diagnosis of kidney failure and improved surgeries that can be safely performed on even the riskiest of patients have spurred unprecedented demand for human organs. In America, the number of people in need of a transplant has nearly tripled during the past decade, topping 100,000 for the first time… But despite numerous media campaigns urging more people to mark the backs of their driver's licenses, the number of traditional (deceased) organ donors has barely budged, hovering between 5,000 and 8,000 per year for the last 15 years…

"Organ selling has become a global problem," says Frank Delmonico, a surgery professor at Harvard Medical School and adviser to the WHO. "And it's likely to get much worse unless we confront the challenges of policing it."

Interlandi, J. (2009, January 19). Not just urban legend. *Newsweek*. Retrieved from http://www.newsweek.com/id/178873

Funding

Financial resources for health care are limited. What is an adequate level of health care? Should everyone have the opportunity to get a transplant, if needed? Should everyone have the opportunity to get proper nutrition, exercise, and inoculations to prevent disease?

On the one hand, it is costly to fund transplant operations; on the other hand, it is costly to fund school lunch programs for indigent, undernourished children. Values and ethics become involved in this discussion. The artificial heart, for example, might bring four years of extended life to each of the 25,000 patients annually at a cost $100,000 per life extended. The school lunch program might ensure the improved physical development of hundreds of thousands of children, enabling each child to live healthier lives for 60 years or more and require less medical care. The appeal of the artificial heart is that it rescues people from certain death. The school lunch program does not provide that same level of excitement or emotional appeal. Would the money spent on the development of better artificial hearts be better spent to upgrade the standard of health for a larger segment of the population? All of these factors contribute to the health of the nation, but because society does not have unlimited funds for health care, ethical choices dictate the outcome.

Medical Tourism   Concerns about cost and allocation of resources have resulted in medical tourism, where patients travel—domestically or internationally—solely to seek medical care that is priced lower or otherwise not available locally.

In response to an article in The New York Times on Sunday about an American who went to Belgium to have his hip replaced because his insurer in the United States would not cover the procedure, hundreds of readers said they would be willing to follow that path.

Michael Shopenn's surgery in 2007 would have cost close to $100,000 in the United States. But it cost just $13,660—including all medicine, doctors' fees and round-trip airfare—at a private hospital in Torhout, Belgium. The Belgian government regulates medical fees, though most doctors' offices and hospitals are privately run.

"In the past few years, Americans are definitely more willing to go overseas and now appreciate that there is quality there, whereas seven years ago they didn't have that perception," said Jonathan Edelheit, the chief executive of the Medical Tourism Association, an industry group that supports and facilitates such travel.

The growing numbers of American medical tourists tend to be people who do not have insurance or whose insurance does not adequately cover the procedure they need. Their destination often depends on their cultural ties, Mr. Edelheit said. Spanish-speaking patients might favor Latin America, for example, he said.

While five years ago most American patients who went abroad for cheaper care went to countries like India and Thailand and over the border to Mexico, many are now going to Europe, where care at top hospitals frequently costs a fraction of what is charged in the United States. There are private facilitators who help make the arrangements, pairing patients with doctors and hospitals and arranging travel plans.

Rosenthal, E. (2013, August 6). The growing popularity of having surgery overseas. *The New York Times.* Retrieved from http://www.nytimes.com/2013/08/07/us/the-growing-popularity-of-having-surgery-overseas.html?_r=0

When Ben Schreiner, a 62-year-old retired Bank of America executive, found out last year he would need surgery for a double hernia, he started evaluating possible doctors and hospitals. But he didn't look into the medical center in his hometown, Camden, S.C., or the bigger hospitals in nearby Columbia. Instead, his search led him to consider surgery in such farflung places as Ireland, Thailand, and Turkey.

Ultimately he decided on San José, Costa Rica... Mr. Schreiner is what's known in the health care world as a "medical tourist." No longer covered under his former employer's insurance and too young to qualify for Medicare, Mr. Schreiner has a private health insurance policy with a steep $10,000 deductible...

"I didn't have to fork over my entire deductible," Mr. Schreiner said. "What's more, they bent over backwards there to take care of me—no waiting, a friendly staff, everyone spoke English."

At least 85,000 Americans choose to travel abroad for medical procedures each year, according to a recent report by the consulting firm McKinsey & Company... The cost of surgery performed overseas can be as little as 20 percent of the price of the same procedure in the United States, according to a recent report by the American Medical Association.

Konrad, W. (2009, March 21). Going abroad to find affordable health care. *The New York Times.* Retrieved from http://www.nytimes.com/2009/03/21/health/21patient.html?ref=health

Medical tourism does not always find the patient traveling outside the country. Sometimes, traveling to a different state, different region of your home state, or even to a different local hospital can make a difference in the cost or availability of a medical procedure.

I assumed that palm trees or streets teeming with foreign humanity were in my future as I began a quest to find a hip replacement at a price I could afford.

Because my severe osteoarthritis was deemed a preexisting condition, my insurance carrier would not pay for the surgery, so money was definitely an object.

Yet, after exploring so-called medical tourism options in Thailand, India, Hungary and Dubai, I settled on nothing so exotic. With rates that rival overseas alternatives, Oklahoma City beckoned me. It seems it has become a medical tourism hot spot.

Granted, I wasn't able to lounge on exotic beaches during my recuperation; instead, I toured a cowboy museum and the livestock market at Stockyards City. But the price was right.

Lytel, J. (2012, October 29). Medical tourism doesn't necessarily mean leaving the country to get treatment. *The Washington Post.* Retrieved from https://www.washingtonpost.com/national/health-science/medical-tourism-doesnt-necessarily-mean-leaving-the-country-to-get-treatment/2012/10/29/8d1bf5ce-d6710-11e1-b2d5-2419d227d8b0_story.html

Some employers have jumped on the medical tourism bandwagon by negotiating bulk rates for procedures in locations that require the patient to travel:

In 2008, Hannaford, an American supermarket chain, offered to pay the full cost of hip and knee replacements for its employees, including travel and patients' usual share—provided they would go to Singapore. None took up the offer...

And though American firms and insurers have mostly stopped scouring the globe for bargains, some have negotiated bulk rates with top-notch hospitals at home. Lowes, a home-improvement firm, offers workers all around the country in need of cardiac care the option of going to the Cleveland Clinic in Ohio. PepsiCo, a food giant, made a deal with Johns Hopkins in Maryland. Other firms are said to be working on similar schemes. The future of medical tourism may be domestic rather than long-haul.

Médecine avec frontiers: Why health care has failed to globalize. (2014, February 15). *The Economist*. Retrieved from http://www.economist.com/news /international/21596563-why-health-care-has-failed-globalise-m-decine-avec-fronti-res

Intensive Care Unit

Where there is a shortage of beds in the intensive care unit (ICU), the ethics of health care providers are put to the test. Who gets a bed—an elderly person or a young person? Someone whose prognosis is limited or one who will probably have many good years if properly treated? The patient who can pay or the one who cannot? The family man with five dependent children or the playboy with no responsibilities?

If there is a shortage of ICU beds, patients in the unit usually have a shorter stay than when there is a surplus. This may occur because the patients do not need additional care or because the bed is required for a more seriously ill patient. When hospitals keep patients in the ICU for a long time, it may be because the hospital did not wish to lower the ICU occupancy rate. Alternatively, some physicians might find their own workload reduced if a patient receives care in the ICU rather than on a regular medical ward.

Use of the ICU is just one example of the day-to-day ethical judgments that are made by medical professionals in the hospital setting. No two physicians will necessarily make the same decision for the same reason.

ETHICS IN MEDICAL RESEARCH

The mandates of the Tuskegee Experiment and the Nuremberg Code are the result of unethical behavior in medical research. All medical research in the United States, whether in an academic university or in a medical office, must abide by the rules created to ensure such research is ethical.

The Tuskegee Experiment

In 1972, a public health official objected to the "morality of an ongoing study being sponsored by the Public Health Service—a study compiling information about the course and effects of syphilis in human beings based upon medical examinations of poor black men in Macon County, Alabama. The men, or more accurately, those still living, had been coming in for annual examinations for forty years. They were not receiving standard therapy for syphilis… [This] has been called the longest running nontherapeutic experiment on human beings in medical history and the most notorious case of prolonged and knowing violation of subjects' rights—the Tuskegee study" (Caplan, November–December 1992, p. 29). Public anger over the immorality of the experiment spurred Congress to create a panel to review both the Tuskegee experiment and the adequacy of existing protections for subjects in all federally sponsored research.

The Centers for Disease Control and Prevention indicate that:

The study initially involved 600 black men—399 with syphilis, 201 who did not have the disease. The study was conducted without the benefit of patients' informed consent. Researchers told the men they were being treated for 'bad blood,' a local term used to describe several ailments, including syphilis, anemia, and fatigue. In truth, they did not receive the proper treatment needed to cure their illness. In exchange for taking part in the study, the men received free medical exams, free meals, and burial insurance. Although originally projected to last 6 months, the study actually went on for 40 years.

In July 1972, an Associated Press story about the Tuskegee Study caused a public outcry that led the Assistant Secretary for Health and Scientific Affairs to appoint an Ad Hoc Advisory Panel to review the study. The panel had nine members from the fields of medicine, law, religion, labor, education, health administration, and public affairs.

(Continues)

(Continued)

The panel found that the men had agreed freely to be examined and treated. However, there was no evidence that researchers had informed them of the study or its real purpose. In fact, the men had been misled and had not been given all the facts required to provide informed consent.

The men were never given adequate treatment for their disease. Even when penicillin became the drug of choice for syphilis in 1947, researchers did not offer it to the subjects. The advisory panel found nothing to show that subjects were ever given the choice of quitting the study, even when this new, highly effective treatment became widely used.

The advisory panel concluded that the Tuskegee Study was 'ethically unjustified'—the knowledge gained was sparse when compared with the risks the study posed for its subjects. In October 1972, the panel advised stopping the study at once. A month later, the Assistant Secretary for Health and Scientific Affairs announced the end of the Tuskegee Study.

In the summer of 1973, a class-action lawsuit was filed on behalf of the study participants and their families. In 1974, a $10 million out-of-court settlement was reached. As part of the settlement, the U.S. government promised to give lifetime medical benefits and burial services to all living participants. The Tuskegee Health Benefit Program (THBP) was established to provide these services. In 1975, wives, widows and offspring were added to the program. In 1995, the program was expanded to include health as well as medical benefits. The Centers for Disease Control and Prevention was given responsibility for the program, where it remains today in the National Center for HIV/AIDS, Viral Hepatitis, STD, and TB Prevention. The last study participant died in January 2004. The last widow receiving THBP benefits died in January 2009. There are 12 offspring currently receiving medical and health benefits.

Centers for Disease Control and Prevention. (n.d.). *The Tuskegee Timeline*. Retrieved from http://www.cdc.gov/tuskegee/timeline.htm

In 1974, Congress created the National Commission for the Protection of Human Subjects of Biomedical and Behavior Research, which was replaced in 1978 by the President's Commission for the Study of Ethical Problems in Medicine and Biomedical and Behavioral Research. Since then, there have been several commissions that have "differed in their composition, methods, and areas of focus, but they have shared a common commitment to the careful examination and analysis of ethical considerations that underlie our nation's activities in science, medicine, and technology," according to the current Presidential Commission for the Study of Bioethical Issues.

Nuremberg Code

Because no two patients are medically identical, some argue that therapeutic medicine is inescapably experimental. Society has developed guidelines, however, to deal with experimental medical research. The Nuremberg Code is the result of criminal trials related to medical atrocities conducted on prisoners by Nazi physicians during World War II.

On August 19, 1947, the judges of the American military tribunal in the case of the USA vs. Karl Brandt et. al. delivered their verdict. Before announcing the guilt or innocence of each defendant, they confronted the difficult question of medical experimentation on human beings. Several German doctors had argued in their own defense that their experiments differed little from previous American or German ones. Furthermore, they showed that no international law or informal statement differentiated between legal and illegal human experimentation. This argument worried Drs. Andrew Ivy and Leo Alexander, American doctors who had worked with the prosecution during the trial. On April 17, 1947, Dr. Alexander submitted a memorandum to the United States Counsel for War Crimes which outlined six points defining legitimate research. The verdict of August 19 reiterated almost all of these points in a section entitled "Permissible Medical Experiments" and revised the original six points into ten. Subsequently, the ten points became known as the "Nuremberg Code." Although the code addressed the defense arguments in general, remarkably none of the specific findings against Brandt and his codefendants mentioned the code. Thus the legal force of the document was not well established. The uncertain use of the code continued in the half century following the trial when it informed numerous international ethics statements but failed to find a place in either the American or German national law codes. Nevertheless, it remains a landmark document on medical ethics and one of the most lasting products of the "Doctors Trial."

United States Holocaust Memorial. (n.d.). *United States Holocaust Memorial Museum Note: Nuremberg Code*. Retrieved from https://www.ushmm.org/information /exhibitions/online-exhibitions/special-focus/doctors-trial/nuremberg-code

Today, research in the United States that includes human subjects must adhere to the terms of the Nuremberg Code, which are largely reflected in the Code of Federal Regulations. Even college students researching the opinions of classmates asking for confidential information (or the instructors who assign the project) are required to obtain clearance from an institutional review board to proceed. Given the potential for harm, research on human subjects is very carefully reviewed and regulated.

Clinical Trials

Articles cited earlier in this chapter indicate that an increasing number of American patients are traveling outside the United States to seek medical treatment. They are not alone. The *New England Journal of Medicine* reports that drug companies are also increasingly globalizing their clinical trials, raising several medical and ethical issues along the way.

Pharmaceutical and device companies have embraced globalization as a core component of their business models, especially in the realm of clinical trials. This phenomenon raises important questions about the economics and ethics of clinical research and the translation of trial results to clinical practice: Who benefits from the globalization of clinical trials? What is the potential for exploitation of research subjects? Are trial results accurate and valid, and can they be extrapolated to other settings?…

Clinical trials increasingly occur on a global scale as industry and government sponsors in wealthy countries move trials to less wealthy countries. Since 2002, the number of active Food and Drug Administration (FDA)—regulated investigators based outside the United States has grown by 15% annually, whereas the number of U.S.-based investigators has declined by 5.5%.

Glickman, S. W., McHutchison, J. G., Peterson, E. D., Cairns, C. B., Harrington, R. A., Califf, R. M., & Schulman, K. A. (2009, February 19). Ethical and scientific implications of the globalization of clinical research. *New England Journal of Medicine*. Retrieved from http://www.nejm.org/doi/full/10.1056/NEJMsb0803929#t=article

Clinical trials are sometimes halted because the mid-research results prove so conclusive that all patients should be given the option of going on the drug rather than potentially receiving a placebo. The following is one example of such success:

Drug maker Pfizer Inc. said Thursday that a late-stage clinical trial of its cancer drug Sutent has been stopped early, because it showed significant benefit for patients with a rare form of pancreatic cancer…

The trial results prompted an independent Data Monitoring Committee to recommended halting the test after concluding that Sutent…showed greater "progression-free survival" than a placebo.

Pancreatic drug trial halted on promising results. (2009, March 12). *U.S. News and World Report.* Retrieved from http://health.usnews.com/articles/health/healthday/2009/03/12/pancreatic-drug-trial-halted-on-promising-results.html

Private Office Medical Research

Many physician offices are now engaged in clinical trials with pharmaceutical companies, as this has become a new revenue source. Offices engaged in this kind of research must take special care in documenting administration of the medicine and the results. The trend of moving clinical trial research away from academic medical centers began in the early 1990s. The costs of conducting "community-based" research are lower than those for the same trials in an academic medical center. In addition, the research organizations conducting the trials for the pharmaceutical companies can produce results more quickly than an academic medical center. Although this trend raises ethical questions about the objectivity of the research and the treatment of people who serve as "guinea pigs," the practice continues to flourish.

Ethical questions arise regarding the motives of privately practicing physicians. Some of them bring to light positive reasons for adding an experimental medicine component to their practice. The office physicians follow clinical plans designed by the pharmaceutical company. The physician experiences conflict of interest when balancing the best interest of the patient against satisfying the pharmaceutical company's demands and the need to be paid for the experiments.

There is conflict of interest for a physician when participating in an experimental protocol with a drug company. On one side is the best interest of the patient; and on the other are the pharmaceutical demands for protocol fulfillment. In addition, there are benefits to the arrangement: (1) adding a level of continuity and personal contact to the process; (2) providing an enormous pool of potential research subjects; and (3) allowing patients and their physicians access to current and scientifically advanced therapies.

DRUG TESTING IN THE WORKPLACE

The following news report gives some idea of the range of issues involved and the damage done by disputed drug tests:

A Hailey man claims that a testing laboratory in Tennessee messed up his drug test and that the mistake cost him his job, his reputation, and put his family almost $6,000 in debt.

Jim Parker, 41, couldn't even collect unemployment until new tests on his original urine sample indicated that he was right. The laboratory, Advanced Toxicology Network in Memphis, has acknowledged that it got significantly

(Continues)

> *(Continued)*
>
> different results on a second test of the sample, but won't acknowledge that a mistake was made...
>
> Parker said he has no criminal record, not even a speeding ticket, but was shocked when a drug test result came back suggesting he was a morphine or heroin user.
>
> Smith, T. (2009, March 18). Fired worker wants justice. *Idaho Mountain Express.*
> Retrieved from http://www.mtexpress.com/index2.php?ID=2005125263

Screening the public for medical reasons is a part of our society. Within the medical community, certain testing procedures are recommended for mass screening: hypertension, cervical cancer, diabetes, and so on. The armed services instituted mass screening for anti-bodies to the human immunodeficiency virus (HIV). Such test results may contribute to medical research of the variables inherent in the disease process or may indicate latent disease in an unsuspecting individual. These results, used for the good of society, may justify the testing's infringement upon a patient's privacy.

There are other uses of medical testing that invade privacy but contribute less to the public good. One example is the Breathalyzer test administered to alleged drunk drivers. There are many inherent problems with the use of these machines: improper **calibration**, untrained personnel, the time span between ingestion and testing, broken machines, and false-positive tests.

Can you justify tests that invade rights of privacy in the following situations?

calibration the systematic standardization of quantitative measuring instruments

1. Psychological testing for employment:
   a. To assess **personality traits**
   b. To determine who will perform a given job well
   c. To generally screen all employees
   d. To assess for promotion

personality traits distinctive individual qualities of a person

2. Random lie detector tests on the job to discover employee theft

3. Drug tests for employees:
   a. After they have been warned about their behavior
   b. Prior to employment
   c. Prior to promotion
   d. Who drive vehicles or operate machinery

4. Drug tests to all high school athletes:
   a. Prior to championship games
   b. Randomly throughout the school year
   c. On a regular schedule throughout the season

5. Genetic testing to screen high-risk employees for disease:
   a. Cystic fibrosis
   b. Alzheimer's disease
   c. Sickle-cell trait

AUTONOMY VERSUS PATERNALISM

Being a patient often means being dependent on your physician. Both the physician and the patient have the same goal but perhaps different perspectives on how to reach that goal. One of the major issues that generates conflict between persons with different perspectives or different roles is the tension between **autonomy** and **paternalism**.

American culture highly values the autonomy of individuals, which includes their independence and self-reliance. Paternalism can be interpreted as interference with an individual's independence to benefit that individual. The principal goal of obtaining health care is to benefit from the caretakers' offerings. On the one hand, it is argued that those administering health care are obligated to take actions that benefit patients, even if those actions interfere with or neglect the patient's autonomy. On the other hand, it is argued, according to John Stuart Mill, that "over himself, over his own body and mind, the individual is sovereign." These conflicting positions produce ethical dilemmas.

autonomy allowing individuals control over themselves

paternalism providing for people's needs but giving them no responsibility or control over their destiny

"Sarah" was a 36-year-old woman, married with five young children, when she was admitted to hospice with late stage metastatic breast cancer. Friends had contacted a philanthropic organization and had arranged for Sarah and her family to receive an all-expense-paid holiday before Sarah's death. Sarah and her family were elated and talked about the trip and when they could go.

The oncologist, however, was opposed to the idea of a family trip. He continued to insist on aggressive chemotherapy treatments for Sarah, and the trip would interrupt her therapy. The oncologist was adamant that without these treatments, Sarah would have "no chance" and her disease would produce unbearable symptoms. He did not offer the option of discontinuing chemotherapy and providing palliative care. The treatments left her too weak and sick to travel. Sarah had great admiration for her oncologist and trusted him. He had treated her mom when she was dying of breast cancer, and Sarah felt a debt of gratitude for the care he had provided. When the hospice team asked Sarah what she wanted to do, she would look at her husband and say she had to keep trying for him and the children. She would repeat the doctor's statement that the chemotherapy was the only thing keeping her alive.

(Continues)

(Continued)

Sarah insisted that the oncologist had her best interests at heart, but she really wished she could take the trip with her family.

As the disease progressed, the hospice staff struggled with what they were observing. Sarah's condition continued to worsen, and her chemotherapy treatments created intolerable side effects. Sarah spent much of her last few months going back to the hospital. She and her family were conflicted over the seeming lack of choice and their inability to leave town for a final trip. The staff wanted to support Sarah in her decision, but they were unsure if they would undermine her relationship with the oncologist. The oncologist insisted that the family would have time for the trip after the chemotherapy. The staff wanted to encourage the family to question the usefulness of the chemotherapy treatment. Sarah continued with the treatments until she died. The trip never happened.

Snapp, J., & Meyer, B. (2006, October 24). *Sarah: Autonomy and Medical Paternalism.* Retrieved from Hospice Foundation website http://www.hospicefoundation.org

Often the lines between experiment and treatment are blurred as modern technology surges forward and the professional's desire to save life conflicts with the individual's desire to be autonomous and make informed decisions.

To what degree is society responsible for its citizens? Much money has been put into research showing that cigarettes are harmful to health, yet people still smoke. The Campaign for Tobacco-Free Kids estimates that tobacco "costs the U.S. approximately $170 billion in health care expenditures and more than $150 billion in lost productivity each year." Use of seat belts is mandatory in many states, yet many citizens refuse to wear them. In a related issue, there is a lot of litigation related to laws that require motorcyclists to wear helmets; many states have repealed or amended its helmet laws to require only protection for riders' eyes.

The involvement of the state infringes on the right of privacy when it uses its power to regulate personal behavior. At what point does the balance of the public's health outweigh an individual's right of privacy? Many states now prohibit smoking in public places or require that businesses have designated smoking areas. The smoking advocate would argue that this infringes on his or her right to enjoy a cigarette. Public health advocates argue that secondhand smoke endangers the health of those who have chosen not to smoke, thereby not only invading their privacy but injuring them as well. Who is right? For each of these questions, people often reach conflicting conclusions. Many states have laws that make the bar serving liquor responsible for actions of a drunken patron. What impact has this had on diminishing the responsibility of an individual for his or her own behavior? Mental health law regulates the autonomy of the patient. **Commitment** to mental health facilities, the administration of psychotropic drugs, and release from treatment are matters that involve state regulations and court hearings. When an individual is adjudicated mentally ill, the ability to make many decisions is taken from his or her hands. Conservators or guardians for the elderly require court appointment and monitoring.

In each of these areas, the autonomy of the individual must be weighed against the danger of the individual to self or to others. In restraining a person's liberty, the need for such restraint must be acceptable to society. When freedom is denied to an individual, the freedom of every individual is endangered.

commitment the process by which a person is placed into a mental health facility or a penal institution

 SUMMARY

- Professional organizations have creeds and codes of ethics that proclaim standards the membership strives to maintain. Those outside the organization use those standards to define correct professional conduct. Developing a code of ethics is difficult, but incorporating those ideals in daily life is even more difficult.

- Although medical office personnel do not make the headline ethical decisions, the interplay of power and scheduling of time is ethical in nature and affects both patients and personnel.

- One of the most pressing issues in health care is the allocation of resources. Scarcity of organs for transplant, limitation of funds for health care delivery systems, and decisions regarding ICU beds all fall under the allocation of resources.

- The ethics of human and medical experimentation were of concern even before the development of the Nuremberg Code.

- A professional's desire to save life sometimes conflicts with an individual's desire to be autonomous and make informed decisions.

SUGGESTED ACTIVITIES

1. Use your favorite Internet browser to research whether there are other creeds that apply to your profession.

2. Visit a local nursing home (with permission, of course) and listen to what the residents and the staff think about matters involving the autonomy of decision making. Ask the residents what matters they find most difficult to allow someone else to decide. Then talk with the social worker to gain another perspective on issues of autonomy and paternalism with the elderly.

3. In addition to scheduling decisions, think of other instances in which ethics enters into the behavior of medical office personnel.

4. You are the office manager. Develop a schedule for three employees, each of whom works a five-day week, sometimes including a Saturday. Two employees must be working at all times. Take into consideration each employee's need to have weekend time free. Two employees have children, and one does not.

5. You feel that the physicians could better schedule patients if they would spend one additional half-hour a day in the office. Write a memorandum to the physicians with your suggestion.

STUDY QUESTIONS

1. One of your patients is providing a kidney for transplant to her son. All the tests have been performed, and it has been determined that her tissue is compatible. She confides to you that she is frightened about the operation and living the remainder of her days with only one kidney. How do you handle the situation?

2. You are a medical assistant in a pediatrician's office. One of the patients needs a liver transplant. The matter has been in the newspaper, and additional newspapers are seeking interviews with the physician, the staff, and the patient. The newspapers will help advertise the need for an organ, but the family is too upset to handle the publicity. The pediatrician has told you to handle the press. What do you do?

3. A person comes into the office and says that he is in a time of financial hardship and wants to sell one of his kidneys. He is not a patient, and you know nothing about him, but one of your patients is waiting for a kidney. Your patient is wealthy and can afford to purchase a kidney. What do you do?

4. A former secretary tells you that she would like to be a surrogate mother. She is a friend of yours and tells you this over coffee. You know of a couple who wants a baby, but the wife is unwilling to carry the child because of her own health. How do you handle this situation?

5. A patient has been taken out of the ICU because the physicians believe he is terminal and the bed is needed for someone who can be helped. The patient's wife comes into the hospital and appears encouraged because her husband is being removed from the ICU. How do you handle the situation?

6. The physician wants everyone in the office to be tested for drugs on a routine basis. Are you in agreement? How will you handle the matter?

CASES FOR DISCUSSION

1. The defendant, as part of his defense in a criminal trial, requested the court to appoint a qualified cytogeneticist to carry out chromosomal testing of his blood at the county's expense. The purpose of the tests would be to determine whether the defendant had the XYY chromosome pattern. If so, the results would be used as part of his insanity defense and would be offered into evidence. Should evidence of chromosome abnormality be admissible as part of the defense of insanity in a criminal trial?

2. The plaintiff was diagnosed as a manic depressive and had been hospitalized and under treatment for many years. The plaintiff's psychiatrist testified that while in the manic phase of his illness, the plaintiff felt euphoric and invincible, and his judgment and behavior were grossly affected. While in such a state, the plaintiff bought from the defendant the privilege of selling a mechanical device to the government under a license that required considerable sales work. The plaintiff's attorney testified that neither he nor the plaintiff's wife intended to let him go through with the deal, but they thought it would be good therapy if he went through with the negotiations. The defendant did not know about the plaintiff's condition. Does a mental disorder that affects a person's judgment, but not the ability to understand, qualify an individual as an incompetent unable to contract?

3. In a civil action, the plaintiff was involuntarily committed as a mental patient for 15 years. Throughout his confinement, the plaintiff repeatedly demanded his release, claiming that he was dangerous to no one, that he was not mentally ill, and that the hospital was not providing treatment for his illness. Following release, the plaintiff sued the hospital's superintendent and other members of the hospital staff for intentionally and maliciously depriving him of his constitutional right to liberty. Do patients who are involuntarily committed to a state hospital have a right to treatment?

4. A prisoner in Florida was sentenced to die. A young child in Denver needed a kidney, and the prisoner asked to be taken to Denver to be tested to determine whether he was a suitable donor. Should the court allow him to go to Denver?

5. A man arranged to donate his body to a medical school. His mother, carrying out his directive, employed a funeral home to transport the body by ambulance to the medical school. She wished to ride in the vehicle with the body. The funeral home made an error, and the body was shipped by train. The railroad lost the body, and it took three days to trace it. The mother sued the funeral home for damages for mental anguish. Should she recover?

6. A wife told her husband that she wanted a divorce. The following day, a psychiatrist whom she had never met before arrived at her home but did not tell her that he was there to examine her. A few days later, the psychiatrist and another physician signed commitment papers for her, and she was forcibly removed from her home and taken to the hospital. She refused food and medication for six days and was refused permission to mail letters, use the telephone, or call her attorney. She finally was able to contact her relatives by telephone. Should she be released?

11

Birth and the Beginning of Life

 The two most important days in your life are the day you are born and the day you find out why.

Mark Twain

OBJECTIVES

After reading this chapter, you should be able to:

1. Recognize the impact of expanding technology on ethical questions involving birth and the beginning of life.
2. Identify ethical questions surrounding genetic research and its impact on future generations.
3. Recognize problems associated with all forms of artificial insemination.
4. Explain the rights of a fetus.
5. Explain the rights of a newborn.
6. Explain the rights of a child.
7. Identify the conflicts associated with adolescent autonomy in medical decisions.
8. Discuss issues of allocation of resources for children.

BUILDING YOUR LEGAL VOCABULARY

AIDS	Cloning
Amniocentesis	DNA
Chemotherapy	Embryonic stem cell

(continues)

Embryos	Sanctity
Fetus	Scientific investigation
Genetic	Survival action
HIV	Technology
Pluralistic	Wrongful death

INTRODUCTION

Advancements in health care technology bring much needed improvements, as well as more ethical and legal issues. Should a moratorium be placed on further scientific investigation to allow society to catch up? Probably not, but regulations may be placed on certain procedures while the scales of justice weigh issues of public policy versus private interest. There are no definitive answers to the new ethical issues, only additional questions.

Birth, the beginning of life, and the associated ethical issues are matters dealt with by every religion, questioned by each individual when working through his or her own personal developmental issues, and politicized by various groups for a host of reasons. The United States is a **pluralistic** society that allows for multiple positions on ethical issues. Advances in technology and medical knowledge provide additional fodder for these difficult ethical issues. *The New York Times* featured an article on the preimplantation testing of **embryos**. A woman in her late 20s was told that she carries the gene for a fatal neurological disease. She wanted to have children but did not want to pass the gene for the fatal disease on to her children. She and her husband chose to have in vitro fertilization so the embryos could be tested for the gene before implantation. They are now the parents of three children who do not carry the gene for the fatal disease. What are the ethical issues associated with creating embryos that will be discarded if they carry the gene for a fatal disease?

pluralistic pertaining to the belief that there is no single explanation for all the extraordinary aspects of life, particularly in a society of numerous distinct cultures

embryos fertilized eggs in the early stages of development

Genetic testing of embryos has been around for more than a decade, but its use has soared in recent years as methods have improved and more disease-causing genes have been discovered. The in vitro fertilization and testing are expensive—typically about $20,000—but they make it possible for couples to ensure that their children will not inherit a faulty gene and to avoid the difficult choice of whether to abort a pregnancy if testing of a fetus detects a genetic problem.

But the procedure also raises unsettling ethical questions that trouble advocates for the disabled and have left some doctors struggling with what they should tell their patients. When are prospective parents justified in discarding embryos? Is it acceptable, for example, for diseases like GSS, that develop in adulthood? What if a gene only increases the risk of a disease? And should people be able to use it to pick whether they have a boy or girl? A recent international survey found that 2 percent of more than 27,000 uses of preimplantation diagnosis were made to choose a child's sex.

In the United States, there are no regulations that limit the method's use. The Society for Assisted Reproductive Technology, whose members provide preimplantation diagnosis, says it is "ethically justified" to prevent serious adult diseases for which "no safe, effective interventions are available." The method is "ethically allowed" for conditions "of lesser severity" or for which the gene increases risk but does not guarantee a disease...

Preimplantation diagnosis often goes unmentioned by doctors. In a recent national survey, Dr. Robert Klitzman, a professor of clinical psychiatry and bioethicist at Columbia University, found that most internists were unsure about whether they would suggest the method to couples with genes for diseases like cystic fibrosis or breast cancer. Only about 6 percent had ever mentioned it to patients and only 7 percent said they felt qualified to answer patients' questions about it...

Janet Malek, a bioethicist at the Brody School of Medicine at East Carolina University, said that people who carry a gene like GSS have a moral duty to use preimplantation diagnosis—if they can afford it—to spare the next generation.

Kolata, G. (2014, February 3). Ethics questions arise as genetic testing of embryos increases. *The New York Times.* Retrieved from http://www.nytimes.com/2014/02/04 /health/ethics-questions-arise-as-genetic-testing-of-embryos-increases.html?_r=0

What are the ethical issues associated with people who carry genes with disease but who cannot afford the cost of in vitro fertilization and preimplantation embryonic testing? Should insurance companies be made to cover the cost of this procedure? **Embryonic stem cell** research also raises ethical issues, which are highlighted by the following article on changes in the U.S. policy:

embryonic stem cells cells that are derived from human embryos or human fetal tissues that are self-replicating

The embryonic stem cell research debate is steeped with religious arguments, with some faith traditions convinced the research amounts to killing innocent life, others citing the moral imperative to alleviate suffering, and plenty of religious believers caught somewhere in between.

President Barack Obama's order March 9, 2009 opening the door for federal taxpayer dollars to fund expanded embryonic stem cell research again brings those often colliding interests to the fore.

(Continues)

(Continued)

Cardinal Justin Rigali, chairman of the U.S. Conference of Catholic Bishops' Committee on Pro-Life Activities, called Obama's move "a sad victory of politics over science and ethics."

"This action is morally wrong because it encourages the destruction of innocent human life, treating vulnerable human beings as mere products to be harvested," Rigali, the archbishop of Philadelphia, said in a statement.

On the other side is the Rev. Susan Brooks Thistlethwaite, a United Church of Christ minister and a professor at Chicago Theological Seminary.

"There is an ethical imperative to relieve suffering and promote healing," she said. "This is good policy for a religiously pluralistic society that cares about human suffering and the relief of human suffering…"

Under Jewish law, an embryo is genetic material that does not have the status of a person… Some groups and faiths are divided on the issue. Muslims disagree over—among other things—whether an embryo in the early stage of development has a soul.

Gorski, E. (2009, March 19). Stem cell decision exposes religious divides. *San Jose Mercury News*. Retrieved from http://www.mercurynews.com/religion/ci_11954582

scientific investigation an investigation using scientific rules and concepts to validate a hypothesis

technology methods and materials used to achieve commercial or industrial objectives; the application of scientific methods to achieve a certain objective

The preceding represents views of three major religious groups in the United States. Ethical issues involving conception arise from moral positions typically founded on religious beliefs. Before advances in **scientific investigation**, birth and the beginning of life were shrouded in mystery. There is still an element of the unknown, but the issues have changed as technology allows people to control their destiny in new ways. Science and **technology** can manipulate the very beginning of life, and ethical dilemmas surround society's willingness to accept intervention in the conception–birth process.

GENETICS

genetic resulting from genes or attributable to them

There are thousands of human **genetic** diseases. At least 500 of these genetic diseases are linked to a defect in a single gene, and many of the diseases are extremely rare. They include cystic fibrosis, a disease that afflicts one in 3,000 Caucasians with often fatal chronic lung problems; sickle cell anemia, a blood disorder found in one in 500 African-Americans; hemophilia, a failure of blood clotting that subjects one in 4,500 (Hemophilia A) and one in 20,000 (Hemophilia B) boys to abnormal bleeding and bruising; and Tay-Sachs disease, a genetically defective enzyme that causes retardation and early death in one of 3,500 persons of Ashkenazic (Eastern European) Jewish ancestry.

Investigating an individual's genetic makeup may have positive effects on society or may produce negative outcomes. Genetic information can be used to invade an individual's privacy, to change a person's self-image, or to damage an entire family's identity. It may tarnish our concept of equality by adversely affecting opportunities for education, employment, and insurance. However, genetic information may also lead to treatments for diseases before they cause harm. It may advance the engineering of genes to remove harmful influences in the development process.

Testing for genetic information is relatively simple and just requires a **DNA** sample from solid tissues, blood, saliva, or other nucleated cells. Genetic data banks are found in both the public and private sectors of society and are usually developed for clinical research and public health programs. A genetic data search may be able to explain causes of death. For example, genetic technologies were used to determine whether Abraham Lincoln had Marfan syndrome.

DNA an essential component of all living matter and the basic chromosomal material transmitting the hereditary pattern

Amniocentesis allows physicians to perform genetic tests for defects before birth. Some diseases that produce dysfunction in humans later in life, such as Alzheimer's disease, have been found to have a genetic basis. Will society mandate abortion when a **fetus** exhibits certain genetic traits? Will society use genetic information to determine who will be educated and to what degree, or who will be treated medically and to what extent?

amniocentesis a medical technique used to determine whether a fetus has any abnormalities

fetus an unborn offspring in the postembryonic stage of gestation

Science also is investigating how to produce "perfect" specimens by **cloning**. Technology has reached the point where a fertilized egg can be cloned and implanted in the wombs of several females for incubation until birth. Is society willing to allow this to happen? What could be the repercussions of these practices?

cloning identically duplicating an organism

While there are no federal regulations related to human reproductive cloning, several states have enacted laws that prohibit human reproductive cloning. A handful of states prohibit state funds from being used on reproductive cloning. The United Nations and several other countries have banned reproductive cloning. Using technology to create a "designer baby" is not limited to cloning. Other methods are rapidly becoming viable options, raising several ethical questions for the medical community and society as a whole.

A Los Angeles clinic says it will soon help couples select both gender and physical traits in a baby when they undergo a form of fertility treatment. The clinic, Fertility Institutes, says it has received "half a dozen" requests for the service, which is based on a procedure called preimplantation genetic diagnosis, or PGD.

(Continues)

(Continued)

While PGD has long been used for the medical purpose of averting life-threatening diseases in children, the science behind it has quietly progressed to the point that it could potentially be used to create designer babies. It isn't clear that Fertility Institutes can yet deliver on its claims of trait selection. But the growth of PGD, unfettered by any state or federal regulations in the U.S., has accelerated genetic knowledge swiftly enough that pre-selecting cosmetic traits in a baby is no longer the stuff of science fiction.

"It's technically feasible and it can be done," says Mark Hughes, a pioneer of the PGD process and director of Genesis Genetics Institute, a large fertility laboratory in Detroit. However, he adds that "no legitimate lab would get into it and, if they did, they'd be ostracized."

But Fertility Institutes disagrees. "This is cosmetic medicine," says Jeff Steinberg, director of the clinic that is advertising gender and physical trait selection on its Web site. "Others are frightened by the criticism but we have no problems with it."

"If we're going to produce children who are claimed to be superior because of their particular genes, we risk introducing new sources of discrimination" in society, says Marcy Darnovsky, associate executive director of the Center for Genetics and Society...

In a recent U.S. survey...a majority said they supported prenatal genetic tests for the elimination of certain serious diseases. The survey found that 56% supported using them to counter blindness and 75% for mental retardation.

More provocatively, about 10% of respondents said they would want genetic testing for athletic ability, while another 10% voted for improved height. Nearly 13% backed the approach to select for superior intelligence, according to the survey conducted by researchers at the New York University School of Medicine.

Naik, G. (2009, February 12). A baby, please. Blond, freckles—Hold the colic. *The Wall Street Journal*. Retrieved from http://online.wsj.com/article/SB123439771603075099.html

What ethical issues are raised if parents use preimplantation genetic diagnosis (PGD) to ensure their child has a certain characteristic, such as blindness or deafness? What if parents wanted to use PGD to ensure their child had the height needed to be a basketball player, the muscles to be a gymnast, or the left-handedness to be a major league pitcher? Consider the **sanctity** and quality of life as you read the following sections.

sanctity the condition of being sacred

ABORTION AND THE RIGHT TO BE LEFT ALONE

Privacy, from a legal perspective, conveys the right to be left alone to make certain personal choices, including whether to abort a pregnancy. In the Tarasoff case described in Chapter 9, the patient forfeited the right to be left alone because he demonstrated an intent to harm a third party. In *Griswold v. Connecticut*, 381.U.S. 479 (1965), *Katz v. United States*, 389 U.S. 347 (1967), and *Roe v. Wade*, 410 U.S. 113 (1973), the U.S. Supreme Court cited several constitutional amendments that imply the right to privacy.

The human right to privacy is grounded in the basic moral tenet that each individual has an incalculable worth. Reflected in the Fourth Amendment of the U.S. Constitution, this right is a core issue of the abortion conflict. One side holds that an individual's incalculable worth extends to the fetus; the other side holds that the woman's worth—and what she does with her body—is a high priority.

For example, the well-known abortion decision of the U.S. Supreme Court, *Roe v. Wade*, protects a woman's right to privacy in a first-trimester abortion. This right to privacy allows the woman to communicate solely with her physician concerning an abortion. This decision has been challenged by those believing that having an abortion is tantamount to killing a child. Although the decision still stands as law, subsequent decisions further define the interplay of the right to privacy and abortions.

RIGHTS OF PARENTHOOD

Those who protect and represent children who have been abused often question the right of some individuals to parent. They reason that a person must have a license to drive a car, display a sense of financial responsibility to own a home, display emotional stability and a certain mental status to hold a job. Why are people not required to demonstrate an ability to parent before conceiving a child? When the state plans adoptions, potential adoptive parents are placed under intense scrutiny. Should potential biological parents not be subject to similar inquiry? For generations, society has discouraged, criminalized, and even prohibited marriages between relatives to prevent the passing of undesirable traits. Now that scientists can identify disease predispositions through genetic testing, should society allow these marriages but require premarital gene mapping or embryonic testing?

On the other side of the issue, does a couple have the right to have a child? Should the financial expense of a child born with a serious genetic disease be shared through insurance premiums? Should there be any criteria for becoming a parent via in vitro fertilization? Assisted reproductive technology introduces further questions about parenthood and ethics. Consider the following:

In April, 46 years after Kaur and Gill married, Kaur gave birth to a son named Arman. Kaur is in her early 70s. Gill is 79.

Kaur overcame the protestations of the Haryana fertility doctors, who ultimately agreed she was sufficiently fit — as well as sufficiently stubborn — to give birth. Arman was conceived through in vitro fertilization.

"I used to feel empty. There was so much loneliness," Kaur told the Agence France-Presse. "I feel blessed to be able to hold my own baby. I had lost hope of becoming a mother ever." Kaur's health appears to be as good as her spirits, as Barcroft TV noted she is breastfeeding her son, assuaging some of the clinic doctors' concerns…

Bina Vasan, a former president of the Indian Society for Assisted Reproduction, noted that Kaur and Singh have a combined age of 150. "This sends the wrong message to society, that anyone can give birth to a child at any age," she said in an interview with the Times of India. "We condemn such a practice."

Others take the view that denying women IVF procedures would be interfering their right to have a child. A strict upper limit on age is difficult to establish, Johns Hopkins University bioethicist Jeffrey Kahn told Time magazine in 2015, "because it contradicts reproductive liberties," drawing a parallel to men who father children at advanced ages.

Guarino, B. (2016, May 12). After nearly five decades of marriage, a woman in India finally gave birth. But some ethicists say 70 is too old. *The Washington Post*. Retrieved from https://www.washingtonpost.com/news/morning-mix/wp/2016/05/12 /after-a-decades-long-wait-for-a-child-a-woman-in-india-finally-gave -birth-but-doctors-say-shes-too-old/?utm_term=.4d6ce175f2e4

In vitro fertilization can be cost prohibitive for those whose insurance does not provide coverage. Is it ethical to offer in vitro fertilization only to those who can afford it?

Infertility treatments can be exorbitantly expensive, and 70 percent of people pay for them completely out of pocket. In vitro fertilization can cost anywhere from $15,000 to $70,000 per attempt, and it can take several attempts...

Seventy percent of people pay completely out of pocket. Fifteen states have some sort of mandate for fertility coverage. But it varies. Some insurance companies will cover fertility testing, but won't cover treatment. Or some will cover medications but not the whole IVF cycle, or they'll have limitations based on age. Or they say you have to be married, or they won't cover gay and lesbian couples.

Even in the best-case scenarios, insurance will most likely have a limit of one or two treatment cycles, or a $10,000 cap.

Andrews, M. (2009, March 17). Budgeting for infertility authors sterling, best-boss offer help for couples. *U.S. News & World Report.* Retrieved from http://health.usnews.com/health-news/blogs/on-health-and-money/2009/03/17/budgeting-for-infertility-authors-sterling-best-boss-offer-help-for-couples

The path to parenthood can vary greatly. Consider the ethical issues raised by the following scenarios: Bob and Elise had been married for six years and wanted to enrich their lives by having a child. After several months of trying, they visited a fertility specialist, who made the diagnosis that Bob did not have enough active sperm to fertilize an egg. They were offered the following options:

1. Adoption.
2. Homologous artificial insemination. The spermatozoa are those of the woman's husband. This is called artificial insemination by the husband (AIH).
3. Heterologous artificial insemination. The spermatozoa are taken from a donor who is not the husband of the woman. This is called artificial insemination by donor (AID).
4. Heterologous artificial insemination. The spermatozoa are taken from a donor who is not the husband and mixed with the husband's.

Now change the facts. The husband is able to donate the sperm, but the wife is unable to conceive. She has healthy eggs. Which of the following is personally preferable?

1. Her sister volunteers to allow an embryo to be implanted and to carry the child to term for the couple.
2. A stranger, a female who will become pregnant with the couple's embryo (sperm and egg), will carry the child to term for a fee.

chemotherapy the
chemical treatment of
disease

Let us change the facts again. The husband, at the age of 22 years, discovers that he has prostate cancer. He has the option, prior to surgery and **chemotherapy**, to have his sperm frozen. His wife could then be artificially inseminated with the sperm at a later date. The control of the cancer is successful, and the couple plans a child. It is determined that the wife cannot conceive because of scarred fallopian tubes. Eggs are surgically removed from the wife's ovaries, and conception takes place in a laboratory petri dish. Some of the embryos are frozen for future implantation. The first attempts to impregnate the wife are unsuccessful. The husband dies. Which of the following seems reasonable?

1. Continue to artificially implant the wife with the remaining embryos.
2. Impregnate a surrogate mother.
3. Throw the embryos away.

RIGHTS OF THE FETUS

Randy and Augusta Roman spent two years of infertility treatments trying to become pregnant. Ms. Roman's doctor retrieved 13 eggs from her ovaries, and fertilized six with her husband's sperm. Hours before the embryos were going to be implanted, Mr. Roman said he couldn't go through with it. The couple divorced 16 months later. During the separation of marital property, they could not agree on the disposition of the three remaining embryos that had survived the freezing process.

Augusta wanted to take possession and have [the embryos] implanted, agreeing to release Randy from any financial or parental obligation. Randy wanted the embryos destroyed, or at least frozen indefinitely. He argued that even though he did not want to raise children with Augusta, he would never disavow his genetic offspring. As he would point out in court, the couple had initialed a cryopreservation consent form stipulating that should they divorce, any frozen embryos "shall be discarded."

Roman vs. Roman now rests with the Supreme Court of Texas, one of a number of divorce cases nationwide in which the custody dispute has revolved around microscopic clumps of cells that are considered—by most states, at least—to be property and not human life.

Advances in assisted reproduction have created a legal landscape that judges and lawmakers could hardly have envisioned before 1984, when an Australian baby became the first created from a frozen embryo (the first U.S. birth came two years later). Since then, in vitro fertilization, or IVF, has become an immensely popular solution to fertility problems worldwide.

Sack, K. (2007, May 30). Her embryos or his? *Los Angeles Times.*
Retrieved from articles.latimes.com/2007/may/30/nation/na-embryo30

The *Roman v. Roman*, 193 S.W.3d 40 (Tex. App., 2006), appellate court ultimately upheld the terms of the written IVF consent agreement that included a provision to discard the embryos should the parties divorce. The repercussions of the disposition of frozen embryos affect other areas of society. Social security refused to pay benefits to Arizona twins Juliet and Piers Netting, conceived from their father Robert Netting's frozen sperm 10 months after he died of cancer. An administrative law judge ruled that the children are not entitled to benefits because they were not dependent on the father at the time of his death. A district court upheld the decision. However, a U.S. District Court of Appeals ruled differently.

Because the twins were Netting's legitimate children, the court held they were conclusively deemed dependent on Netting for purposes of Social Security and were entitled to benefits based upon his earnings.

The Court noted, however, that not "every posthumously-conceived child in Arizona would be eligible for survivorship benefits... If the sperm donor had not been married to the mother, Arizona would not treat him as the child's natural parent, and he likely would have no obligation to support the child if he were alive." In this type of situation, "no eligibility for benefits would exist unless the Commissioner made a determination that the claimant was the dependent child of the deceased wage earner..."

Gillett-Netting ex rel. Netting v. Barnhart, 371 F.3d 593 (9th Cir. 2004)

The life of the fetus is an area that is steeped in tradition and folklore, including the stork that flew babies to their new homes. Today, fetal rights are being defended in court. Again technology has entered human lives, providing options for medical treatment unavailable in the past and thereby redefining ethics and practice. In this area, courts and legislatures have taken the lead.

NEWS

Within the last five years, pregnant women have been arrested under fetal-harm statutes after falling down the stairs and driving with blood-alcohol levels of just half the legal limit. Other women have been forced against their will to undergo caesarean sections, or spend months on bed rest. The laws can affect people well beyond the woman herself, as in the recent Texas case of Marlise Muñoz, kept on life support for two months for the

(Continues)

(Continued)

purpose of saving her fetus, despite her family's wishes that she be allowed to die. In Wisconsin last summer, a pregnant woman named Alicia Beltran was taken to court in handcuffs after refusing to take an anti-addiction drug for a painkiller habit she had already kicked on her own. The court initially ignored her requests for a lawyer, but appointed a legal guardian for her 14-week-old fetus.

Lawyer and activist Lynn Paltrow, who is helping represent Beltran in a suit against several officials, coauthored a recent paper cataloging such cases and says she has found more than 700 instances since 1973 of women arrested, detained, or subjected to forced medical interventions because of issues related to their pregnancies. She is part of a group of legal scholars who are starting to raise the alarm about the breadth and meaning of what they see as a largely unappreciated shift in American law.

"What it means is that all fertile women are responsible for knowing at every single moment whether they're pregnant," says Paltrow, founder and executive director of the National Advocates for Pregnant Women. "Because at that moment an entirely different legal system comes into play."

Michele Goodwin, a law professor at the University of Minnesota who wrote a forthcoming article on the topic for the California Law Review, calls the issue a "new constitutional battlefront," turning pregnant women into unequal citizens in the guise of protecting them.

Though many "feticide" laws were pushed by conservative activists who see them as part of the fight against legal abortion, other fetal-rights cases have emerged in court rulings on laws intended to protect children from drugs, or protect pregnant victims of domestic violence. Whatever the motives, the laws have an effect with no real parallel elsewhere in the law: Essentially, two entities have begun to compete for rights in one body.

Underlying the phenomenon, the scholars are realizing, is an unsolved moral and philosophical question: how to establish protections for pregnant women without creating a second set of rights that can trump their own.

Graham, R. (2014, February 16). For pregnant women, two sets of rights in one body. *The Boston Globe.* Retrieved from https://www.bostonglobe.com /ideas/2014/02/16/for-pregnant-women-two-sets-rights-one-body /5Pd6zntIViRBZ9QxhiQgFJ/story.html

wrongful death death caused by negligence

survival action a lawsuit related to a death and brought by the decedent's survivors

The Unborn Victims of Violence Act became federal law in 2004 and made it a crime to harm a fetus while assaulting a pregnant woman during the commission of a federal crime. Adding to this, 38 states have fetus protection laws and case law in many others hold that a stillborn child's estate may seek recovery through a **wrongful death** and **survival action** for injuries sustained while in the womb.

Illinois judge Jeffrey Lawrence refused to dismiss a wrongful death suit against a fertility clinic in Chicago. The plaintiffs are a couple, Alison Miller and Todd Parrish. They allege that the defendant, the Center for Human Reproduction in Chicago, discarded their nine embryos and thereby ended the embryos' lives…

[T]he judge explained, a fetus qualifies as a deceased person for purposes of the Wrongful Death Act. Furthermore,…"a pre-embryo is a 'human being'… whether or not it is implanted in its mother's womb." For this conclusion, the judge cited another Illinois law that specifically finds that an "unborn child is a human being from the time of conception and is, therefore, a legal person."

Colb, S. (2005, February 23). Judge rules frozen embryos are people. *CNN.* Retrieved from http://www.cnn.com/2005/LAW/02/23/colb.embryos/index.html

Judge Lawrence's holding was reversed on appeal in 2008. The appellate court held that the Illinois wrongful death statute did not allow a cause of action or recovery for damages sustained by a preimplantation embryo created by in vitro fertilization.

With one in every 200 pregnancies ending in stillbirth in the United States—about 26,000 each year—there are numerous legal, ethical, and public policy questions surrounding the issue. This extends to questions about record keeping, with lawmakers debating whether stillborn children should be documented with birth certificates.

Last summer, three weeks before her due date, Sari Edber delivered a stillborn son, Jacob. "He was 5 pounds and 19 inches, absolutely beautiful, with my olive complexion, my husband's curly hair, long fingers and toes, chubby cheeks and a perfect button nose," she said…"The day before I was released from the hospital, the doctor came in with the paperwork for a fetal death certificate, and said, 'I'm sorry, but this is the only document you'll receive.' In my heart, it didn't make sense…we deserved more than a death certificate"… So Ms. Edber joined with others who had experienced stillbirth to push California legislators to pass a bill allowing parents to receive a certificate of birth resulting in stillbirth…19 states, including New Jersey, have enacted laws allowing parents who have had stillbirths to get such certificates. Similar legislation is under consideration in several more, among them New York…But politically, the birth-certificate laws, often referred to as "Missing Angels" bills, occupy uncertain territory, skirting the abortion debate while implicitly raising the question of fetal personhood.

Lewin, T. (2007, May 22). A move for birth certificates for stillborn babies. *The New York Times.* Retrieved from http://www.nytimes.com/2007/05/22/us/22stillbirth.html

Now that it has been determined that a fetus has rights, can a mother be charged for abuse to the fetus that results in a brain-damaged baby? If fetal neglect becomes a cause of action, would it mean that a pregnant woman is guilty of a crime if she does not eat properly, fails to drink enough milk, smokes, or drinks alcohol? Could this be extended to a cause of action against the state for not providing proper food and environment for indigent pregnant mothers?

In practice, the law has generally not been used to punish women for conduct during their pregnancy that might endanger the fetus. In recent years, that trend has seen some exceptions. Some raise questions of whether such prosecutions actually discourage pregnant women from seeking help for issues related to drugs, alcohol, or mental health. Consider the following case from Utah where a woman, originally charged with murder, was sentenced to 18 months' probation for child endangerment for allegedly delaying a cesarean section that may have saved one of her twins:

NEWS

Melissa Ann Rowland also was ordered into a drug treatment program… Prosecutors dropped their capital murder charge against Rowland earlier this month based on her mental health history. Rowland pleaded guilty to two counts of child endangerment and admitted using cocaine in the weeks before she underwent the C-section…that produced a stillborn boy.

District Judge Dennis Fuchs called it a travesty that the system "can't adequately deal with individuals like Miss Rowland." He described her as someone who has repeatedly fallen through the cracks.

Grace, F. (2004, April 29). Utah C-section mom gets probation. *CBS News*. Retrieved from http://www.cbsnews.com/stories/2004/03/12/national/main605537.shtml

There has been considerable scientific interest in using the fetus for transplants. Think about this issue using the following hypothetical situations:

Suppose an elderly patient is suffering from the degenerative progression of Parkinson's disease. There is hope that the ravages of the disease may be stopped or reversed by transplanting neural tissue from the human fetus. Experimentation done with monkeys has shown that symptoms similar to Parkinson's can be controlled by transplanting tissue into the brain of an afflicted adult animal.

1. A neurosurgeon at a large teaching facility wishes to transplant tissues from an aborted fetus into the brain of an elderly statesman.

2. The wife of the statesman wishes to become pregnant by having embryos the couple previously had frozen implanted in her uterus. Then she plans to abort the fetus to allow for the best tissue match.

3. The technique has never been performed in a human before.

Let us now change the facts. We find that the viable fetus is stillborn following a third-trimester miscarriage.

1. A cardiac surgeon wishes to transplant the heart of the stillborn child into an infant born prematurely who will not survive with her own deformed heart for more than two days.
2. The preemie has additional deformities of internal organs but no apparent physical deformities.
3. The stillborn child has both internal and physical deformities.
4. Because of the stillborn's physical anomalies, the pathologist wishes to preserve the child's body in formaldehyde to use as a teaching specimen.

RIGHTS OF A NEWBORN

A days-old infant sustained severe neurological injury after being asphyxiated during birth, but the dying baby's condition did not meet the criteria for brain death—long the only circumstance under which vital organs were procured…Family members also agreed to let surgeons there attempt to transplant the baby's heart into an infant born with complex congenital heart disease.

But to accomplish this, the potential donor heart had to stop working. The question: How long after cardiac functioning ceased should the retrieval team wait to ensure the baby's heart would not restart without intervention? The complicating factors: Odds of successful transplantation decrease as the wait after cessation of cardiocirculatory function increases. But acting too soon can make retrieval seem like death by organ donation.

The Denver team waited 75 seconds.

The infant who received that heart lived…

The clinical debate over whether 75 seconds without cardiac function after withdrawing life support is sufficient time to confidently declare death is unsettled, but the questions these cases raise go even deeper. Some bioethicists and physicians say the cases are merely the latest in the organ transplantation era to stretch the definition of death in ways that could potentially undermine Americans' trust in physicians and in the organ donation process.

O'Reilly, K. B. (2009, January 19). Redefining death: A new ethical dilemma. *American Medical News.* Retrieved from http://www.amednews.com/article /20090119/profession/301199972/4/

In the spring of 1982, an infant, identified only as Baby Doe, was born in Bloomington, Indiana. The diagnosis at birth was Down syndrome and an obstruction of the digestive tract that precluded normal feeding but was apparently surgically correctable. The parents refused to give consent to surgery, and the hospital took the matter to the court. The superior court concluded that when, as in this case, the parents were "confronted with two competent medical opinions, one suggesting that corrective surgery may be appropriate and the other suggesting that corrective surgery and extraordinary measures would only be futile acts, it was the parents' responsibility to choose the appropriate action without interference by the government." The child soon died.

The case was heavily covered by the press and appeared on television. The media portrayed the child as one who had been denied routine surgical treatment and allowed to starve to death for no reason other than a mild, unrelated handicap. On April 30, 1982, President Reagan sent a memorandum to officials in the government instructing them to take steps to prevent repetition of such an abuse. On May 18, 1982, a notice was sent to most of the nation's hospitals by the Department of Health and Human Services (HHS), explaining that the "discriminatory failure of a federally assisted health-care provider to feed a handicapped infant, or to provide medical treatment essential to correct a life-threatening condition," could be found to violate a federal rehabilitation act. The development of final so-called Baby Doe regulations took several more years and demonstrated the difficulty of legislating medical issues and the complexity of regulating ethical issues.

On April 15, 1985, the Department of HHS provided a final draft of the Baby Doe regulations for the treatment of handicapped children. Public policy behind these regulations prevents withholding of medical care from an infant with one or more noncongenital anomalies by defining the withholding of medical care as neglect. According to the rules, if there is treatment for the condition, it must be provided. There are three exceptions to the policy:

1. When the infant is chronically and irreversibly comatose.
2. When treatment would merely prolong dying.
3. When the treatment would be futile either because the child would not survive or the treatment would be inhumane.

This federal legislation requires the states to establish programs and/or procedures within their child-protective service system. It requires response to needs for treatment by disabled infants with life-threatening conditions.

RIGHTS OF A CHILD

Does a child have the rights of an adult? Is there equal access to health care for all children? What impact does race or socioeconomic conditions have on health care provided? A study conducted in Colorado provides some insights:

There has been a gradual decrease in the proportion of children covered by private health insurance in Colorado and the United States with a commensurate increase in those with public insurance or having no insurance which may impact access to care and outcomes.

Compared with those with private insurance, children in Colorado and the United States with public or no insurance have significantly higher rates of total hospital admission, as well as admission for chronic illness, asthma, diabetes, vaccine-preventable disease, psychiatric disease, and ruptured appendix. These children have higher mortality rates, higher severity of illness, are more likely to be admitted through the emergency department and have significantly higher hospital charges per insured child. Higher hospitalization rates occur in children who are nonwhite and/or Hispanic and those who are younger. If children with public or no health insurance in the United States in 2000 had the same hospitalization outcomes as children with private insurance, $5.3 billion in hospital charges could have been saved.

Todd, J., Armon, C., Griggs, A., Poole, S., & Berman, S. (2006, August 1). Increased rates of morbidity, mortality, and charges for hospitalized children with public or no health insurance as compared with children with private insurance in Colorado and the United States. *Pediatrics, 118*(2). Retrieved from http://pediatrics.aappublications.org/cgi/content/full/118/2/577

Improved technology offers many advances that can improve quality of life but also presents ethical dilemmas that cannot be anticipated. One promising technology is that of harvesting, freezing, and storing a baby's umbilical cord in case the child ever gets sick and needs it. But, the cost to store the cord is high. Can we do this for everyone, or is it just for the rich?

Cord blood is a hot commodity. Taken from a newborn's umbilical cord shortly after birth, it's a rich source of stem cells that can be used to treat dozens of disorders, including several forms of leukemia, lymphoma and anemia. Parents have the option to discard it, donate it or store it with a private cord blood bank.

(Continues)

(Continued)

Private cord blood banks store the blood for a fee, in the event that the family might need it in the future. The banks also let families donate the blood for free, where it can be matched with patients in need or used for medical research…

"It's a precious resource," said Dr. William Shearer, a professor of pediatrics and immunology at Baylor College of Medicine in Houston. But much of that resource is wasted. "Ninety percent of cord blood is discarded still today, and this is a life-saving treatment for a lot of people," said Jen Bruursema, senior director of global healthcare communications at Cord Blood Registry, a private bank in San Bruno, California…

The chance of baby later benefiting from his or her own banked cord blood is currently less than 0.04 percent, according to the ASBMT. Not only is that because the diseases currently treatable with cord blood are fairly rare, but with many, the child's cord blood would be unusable because those stem cells contain the same genetic defects, said Shearer, who co-authored the AAP policy statement.

Grant, K. (2015, July 29). Is cord blood banking worth the cost?
Here's what the experts say. *The NBC News*. Retrieved from
http://www.nbcnews.com/business/consumer/cord-blood-banking-n400561

Children may be conceived by parents for their assistance in the treatment of a serious illness of another family member. The following is an excerpt from an article in the *Chicago Tribune*:

Genetic testing of embryos outside the womb has led to the births of five babies selected to produce umbilical cord blood or bone marrow to save the lives of seriously ill siblings, Chicago doctors reported…

The controversial procedure, which employs cutting edge genetic tests during in vitro fertilization, expands the possibilities of the creation of so-called "savior babies" to provide stem cells for older children who lack compatible donors for bone marrow transplants…

Chicago scientists were able to create babies for five of nine couples whose other children already suffered from bone marrow failure…

Umbilical cord blood from one of the babies already has saved a sibling, another transplant is pending, and three of the affected children were in remission and may need the transplants later.

Gorner, P. (2004, May 5). 5 Babies born to save ill siblings, doctors say. *Chicago Tribune*.
Retrieved from http://articles.chicagotribune.com/2004-05-05/news/0405050257
_1_bone-marrow-transplants-reproductive-genetics-institute-cord-blood

HIV TESTING FOR PREGNANT WOMEN

The U.S. Centers for Disease Control and Prevention (CDC) reports that in 2014, there were approximately 45,000 new **HIV** cases in the United States, which is a 19 percent decrease compared to 2005. The Elizabeth Glaser Pediatric **AIDS** Foundation notes that drug therapies for preventing mother-to-child transmission of HIV has reduced the number of infected babies born in the United States to fewer than 200 per year. To continue decreasing that number, the foundation endorses voluntary, routine, and universal HIV testing of pregnant women as recommended by the CDC.

   Most of the HIV-infected babies born in the United States each year have mothers who are unaware of their own infections. Women may refuse to undergo testing for HIV because of the stigma associated with intravenous drug use or interaction with multiple sexual partners. Children infected with the HIV virus at birth may live for years without symptoms and without anyone knowing that they are infected. Physicians may fail to recognize that HIV is the source of children's illnesses. Has this become an ethical dilemma placing a baby's rights to medical care against a mother's rights to privacy?

HIV human immuno-deficiency virus, which causes AIDS

AIDS acquired immune deficiency syndrome

TEENAGE TREATMENT DECISIONS

Billy Best, 16 years of age, was a patient at Dana-Farber Cancer Institute in Boston when he was informed that he needed four more months of treatments to wipe out the remaining cancer around his windpipe. He was given an ultimatum by his physicians: continue chemotherapy treatments for Hodgkin's disease or face a painful death. His parents agreed with the physicians and required Billy to continue the treatments at the Dana-Farber Cancer Institute. At 16 years, he was considered a minor without the capacity to make this decision for himself.

   Billy determined he was no longer going to accept chemotherapy and ran away from home, crossing the United States from Boston to Texas. He claimed that the painful treatments were killing him and chose instead homeopathic drug treatment. His parents, after studying the alternative treatments, agreed with his decision, and Billy returned home. A year later tests revealed that the cancer had disappeared. Legally, Billy was unable to make the treatment decision in Massachusetts. Ethically, is it right that he should be forced to undergo treatment against his will?

TREATING CHILDREN'S BEHAVIOR ISSUES

There are many ethical dilemmas in current practices involving the psychopharmacological treatment of children. One controversy is the use of drugs versus the use of more traditional counseling and support therapy for children with suspected mental illnesses. In a review of the book *No Child Left Different*, Utrecht University researcher Kathy Davis highlights the extent of the problem:

Prescriptions for psychotropic drugs for children have skyrocketed in the past fifteen years. Currently one in ten white, middle-class, school age boys takes the stimulant Ritalin for attention deficit disorders (ADHD), and antidepressants (Prozac, Paxil, Zoloft, and others) are being prescribed to 2.4 percent of all U.S. children, making them more frequently prescribed than any other pediatric medication, including antibiotics. These statistics are alarming.

Davis, K. (2007, May–June). Rethinking normal. *Hastings Center Report*, 44.

Because the health care industry is determined to cut costs, managed care organizations emphasize drug treatment over counseling. Is it ethical that this policy dictates the care that today's children receive?

California regulators said…that insurers must provide speech, occupational and physical therapies to their autistic members but rejected pleas to require insurers to cover the cost of behavior therapy that aims to help patients live in society.

At issue is so-called applied behavior analysis, a therapy that teaches patients skills such as self-feeding and stopping injurious behaviors such as head banging. The therapy can cost as much as $70,000 a year per patient.

Parents of children with autism have argued in lawsuits and in complaints to regulators that insurers, by refusing to pay for an array of autism care, are ignoring the Mental Health Parity Act. The 2000 state law requires insurers to treat mental conditions the same as medical conditions.

Autism is the fastest-growing serious developmental disability in the U.S., more prevalent than childhood cancer, juvenile diabetes and pediatric AIDS combined. There are an estimated 185,000 Californians with autism…

The state's major insurers and HMOs routinely refuse to pay for applied behavior analysis, arguing, most recently, that it is an educational service, not medicine. The insurers also say that covering applied behavioral analysis will drive up premiums for everyone, although studies from other states have found such increases to be minimal.

Girion, L. (2009, March 10). Autism patients in California are dealt insurance setback. *Los Angeles Times*. Retrieved from http://articles.latimes.com/2009/mar/10/business/fi-autism10

It is important to consider the consequences of medicating children with drugs whose psychological effect may harm the body. It may be years before the medical community knows the effect of certain medications given to children during different stages of development.

☑ SUMMARY

- Ethical considerations involving the rights of embryos, fetuses, birth issues, the neonatal period, and the growing child are gaining prominence.

- Technology makes it possible to exercise more control over birth and the beginning of life by detecting genetic and chromosomal abnormalities.

- New techniques for artificial insemination raise questions of surrogate motherhood and paternal responsibility.

- Questions about fetal rights and maternal legal obligations during pregnancy take on new importance as technology's ability to intervene during pregnancy advances.

- Because of the value of fetal tissue in transplants, society has taken a new look at the need to protect the fetus.

- Because of conflicting ethical positions on sanctity versus quality of life, society takes steps to control procedures used to care for handicapped newborn infants.

- With the advent of newer methods for prolonging the lives of children with AIDS, pregnant women are under increasing pressure to submit to testing for the HIV virus.

- There are many questions but few answers at this point in time.

SUGGESTED ACTIVITIES

1. Contact a local agency involved in the care of children who have been neglected or abused and request a copy of their guidelines for responding to the medical needs of children in their care. Ask for particulars for children with failure-to-thrive syndrome, fetal-alcohol syndrome, HIV-positive status, and congenital abnormalities requiring surgery. Discuss the process required by the agency and compare it with what you would do if you were responsible for one of these children. During the discussion, consider the availability of the child for adoption.

2. Three major religions in the United States have commented on artificial insemination of women. Conduct research to determine if other religious organizations have moral positions on the matter.

STUDY QUESTIONS

1. If you were pregnant and had a family history of a genetic disease, would you have amniocentesis to determine if the fetus was defective? What factors would you consider when determining whether to abort the fetus?

2. Define *sanctity of life* and give an example of an ethical decision based on this philosophy.

3. Define *quality of life* and give an example of an ethical decision based on this philosophy.

4. What restrictions, if any, would you place on pregnant mothers?

5. Do you believe aborted fetal tissue should be used for transplant purposes? Why or why not? Do you believe the government should control this area of medicine? How?

6. Anencephalics will not live for an appreciable period of time. The organs in their bodies are often not large enough to be transplanted. What are your thoughts about keeping the body alive long enough to allow the major organs to reach a size at which they can be transplanted to other infants?

7. Children born with certain handicaps are born to a life of suffering and pain. If extraordinary means are used to keep these children alive, they may live for a few weeks but not without continual medical intervention. If allowed to die at birth without intervention, they will live a few hours at most. Try to develop philosophies for both sides of this issue.

8. Defend and differ with this statement: Parents should be required to cover the cost of medical care for every child born to them.

9. Defend and differ with this statement: The state should be required to cover the cost of medical care for every handicapped child.

CASES FOR DISCUSSION

1. The plaintiff became pregnant and bore a child after undergoing a sterilization operation. She sued the physician who performed the surgery for negligence, for the pregnancy, and for birth and the costs of rearing a normal, healthy child. Should she win?

2. The plaintiff gave birth to a daughter with Tay-Sachs disease. Children born with this incurable degenerative nerve disease do not live long. The plaintiffs claimed that the defendant physician was negligent in that he failed to take a proper genealogical history or to properly evaluate their genetic histories. The plaintiffs were Eastern European Jews, a fact that should have put the defendant on notice that there was a high risk the child would suffer from the disease. They also stated that if they had known of the risk involved, they would have taken tests and, if the results were positive, aborted the pregnancy. Both parents claimed that they underwent considerable anguish observing their child suffer prior to her death. Was there a cause of action against the defendant-physician?

3. A woman who was eight-and-a-half-months pregnant was in an automobile accident. During emergency surgery, the fetus was found dead. The mother died shortly afterward. Will a cause of action for wrongful death be allowed because the fetus, although stillborn, was viable at the time of injury?

4. The plaintiff contracted rubella in the first trimester of pregnancy and gave birth to a child with multiple birth defects. The plaintiff was hospitalized at the time of her illness and had asked the physician if her illness was rubella. The physician assured her that it was not. The plaintiff brought a cause of action against the physician for failure to advise her of the risk. What cause of action does the plaintiff have against the physician?

5. After seven years of marriage, it was medically determined that the defendant was sterile. His wife desired a child, by either artificial insemination or adoption. At first, the defendant refused his consent. Approximately 15 years into the marriage, the defendant agreed to artificial insemination of his wife. His wife became pregnant and gave birth to a baby boy. The couple separated four years after the child was born. The wife then became ill and applied for public assistance under the Aid to Needy Children program. The defendant refused to pay child support. The municipal court ordered him to pay support through the district attorney's office. The defendant appealed. Should the defendant have to pay support?

6. During a first marriage, a woman bore a child after consensual artificial insemination. Her husband was listed as the father on the birth certificate. The couple later separated and then divorced. Both the separation agreement and the divorce decree declared the child to be the offspring of the couple. The wife was granted support and the husband visitation rights. The woman remarried, and her second husband petitioned to adopt the child. The first husband refused his consent. The second husband then suggested that the first husband's consent was not required because he was not the parent of the child. Should the first husband's consent be necessary?

7. C.C. had a child who was conceived with sperm donated by C.M. C.C. wanted to have a child and wanted C.M. to be the father but did not want to have intercourse with him before their marriage. He therefore agreed to provide the sperm. After several attempts, C.C. did conceive a child. The relationship between the two parties broke off, and C.M. wanted visitation rights to the baby. C.C. does not wish to allow visitation rights. Should visitation rights be allowed?

8. The plaintiff, at 37 years of age, conceived a child. After conception, the plaintiff and her husband engaged the services of the defendants, specialists in obstetrics and gynecology. The baby was born with Down syndrome. The plaintiff contended that they were never advised by the defendants of the increased risk of Down syndrome in children born to women older than 35 years of age nor were they advised of the availability of an amniocentesis test. Do the plaintiffs have an action in wrongful life for their child and in their own right for the various sums of money they will spend for the long-term institutional care of their mentally challenged child? Should they sue as well for the emotional and physical injury suffered by the mother as a result of the birth of her child and the medical expenses stemming from her treatment?

Death and Dying

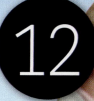

12

> Those who have the strength and the love to sit with a dying patient in the silence that goes beyond words will know that this moment is neither frightening nor painful, but a peaceful cessation of the functioning of the body.
>
> *Elisabeth Kübler-Ross, On Death and Dying (1969)*

OBJECTIVES

After reading this chapter, you should be able to:

1. Identify cultural perspectives on death.
2. Recognize the role individuals, families, hospitals, the medical community, courts, legislatures, and others play in dealing with the ethical, legal, medical, social, and political questions that arise from our ability to maintain life.
3. Articulate the need for a do-not-resuscitate (DNR) order from the patient's perspective.
4. Weigh both sides of the question in cases removing life support.
5. Identify provisions of the Patient Self-Determination Act (PSDA).

BUILDING YOUR LEGAL VOCABULARY

Advance directive
Assisted suicide
Cardiopulmonary arrest
Clear and convincing
Durable power of attorney
Euthanasia
Health care proxy

Hospice
Life-sustaining
Living will
Purist
Substitute judgment
Terminally ill

ATTITUDES TOWARD DEATH AND DYING

The questions asked in this chapter are very difficult, and your answers today will be challenged by your experience tomorrow. Death and dying issues question both the sanctity and the quality of life. Nurses, emergency medical technicians, and physicians are confronted with the reality of life-and-death situations, carrying out do-not-resuscitate (DNR) orders and removing life-support systems. All health care employees are affected by their nearness to and interaction with patients.

A variety of influences shape our thoughts and feelings about death and dying, including family, religion or spirituality, the media, society, and life experiences. How we each process death and dying depends on how those influences come together to define our own philosophies about the sanctity and quality of life.

Physicians, whose first obligation to a patient is to heal, cure, or postpone death for as long as possible, routinely face questions about death and dying. When a cure is not possible, the physician's obligation is to care for and comfort the dying patient. Dr. C. Everett Koop explains his resolution of the conflict:

There is this unique tumor of childhood called neuroblastoma in which I have been interested for more than thirty years. Because of this I have developed a broad clinical experience with the behavior of this tumor as it affects the lives of my patients... In a given situation I might have as a patient a five-year-old child whose tumor was diagnosed a year ago and who, in spite of all known treatment, has progressed to a place where although her primary tumor has been removed she now has recurrence... I know her days of life are limited and that the longer she lives the more likely she is to have considerable pain. She might also become both blind and deaf.

If this five-year-old youngster is quite anemic, her ability to understand what is happening to her might be clouded... I can let her exist with a deficient hemoglobin level knowing that it may shorten her life but also knowing that it will be beneficial in the sense that she will not be alert enough to understand all that is happening around her. On the other hand I could be a medical **purist** and give her blood transfusions until her hemoglobin level was up to acceptable standards... [S]he would be more conscious of the things happening around her, she would feel her pain more deeply, and she might live longer... [A]nd then there are the anticancer drugs which I know without any shadow of a doubt will not cure this child... Would it be better to let this little girl slip into death quietly...or should we prolong her life... I opt to withhold supportive measures.

Koop, C. E. (1976). *The right to live: The right to die*, pp. 98–99. Wheaton, IL: Tyndale House Publishers.

purist one who believes in and follows all traditional rules

Situations Where the Determination of Death Is Crucial
Executing wills and distributing estates A deceased person's will or intestate distribution cannot be made without a determination of death.
Life insurance Life insurance policies require a determination of death before they pay out on the policy.
Tort lawsuits Civil lawsuits that seek to recover damages for someone's death requires a determination of death.
Organ donation A determination of death is required to allow for the harvesting and use of a deceased person's organs.
Criminal matters involving death A determination of death is required to prosecute homicides.

Figure 12-1 Why a determination of death is important

Determination of Death

Ethical, legal, and medical issues arise that require a thorough analysis of the question, "When is a person is dead?" The Uniform Determination of Death Act (UDDA) was a response to that question. See Figure 12-1 for some of the reasons why a determination of death is important. The UDDA is a model act, which is intended to be a starting point for state legislations that want to adopt it. The UDDA defines the medical determination of biological death, and it has been adopted by all states with very few modifications.

The UDDA provides the following definition of death: "[a]n individual who has sustained either (1) irreversible cessation of circulatory and respiratory functions or (2) irreversible cessation of all functions of the entire brain, including the brain stem, is dead. A determination of death must be made in accordance with accepted medical standards."

ADVANCE DIRECTIVES

An **advance directive** asserts an individual's right to accept or refuse treatment and gives direction to relatives, friends, and medical professionals. The directive is necessary, according to former Senator John C. Danforth, R-MO, an Episcopal clergyman, because "[m]edical technology has outstripped ethics. For too many thousands of people, the end of life is a nightmare... [It is] turned over to technocrats whose job it is to eke out every last moment. This constitutes playing God by medicine." Supporting this position, and at the same time giving insight into the physician's behavior, James H. Sammons, former executive vice president of the American Medical Association (AMA), adds, "From the day [physicians]

advance directive a document signed and witnessed according to state statute authorizing one to make a decision for another, allowing treatment or refusal of treatment when the person for whom the document is made becomes incompetent

enter medical school they are taught to cherish and preserve life... While physicians should never directly cause death, they must always act in the best interest of the patients, and that sometimes includes allowing them to die." Advance directives can resolve many of the controversies that arise in situations where ethics, law, and medicine collide.

Consider the following: Terri Schiavo, a 41-year-old brain-damaged woman, was the subject of a national right-to-die legal battle. Ms. Schiavo collapsed in her home due to heart failure that led to severe oxygen-deprivation brain damage. Ms. Schiavo's parents, the Schindler's, fought to keep her feeding tube in while Ms. Schiavo's legal guardian, her husband, fought to respect her verbal wish not to be put on life support. The legal dispute between Ms. Schiavo's husband and her parents was exceptionally bitter. The legal battle included legislation passed by Congress that placed the dispute in the federal court system, as well as several appeals to the U.S. Supreme Court, who declined to hear the case.

The Schindlers "can know they have done everything possible under the law in letting government know that they wanted to fight for the life of their daughter," Gibbs said.

In his Supreme Court filing, Gibbs and other lawyers for the parents wrote that removing the tube represented "an unconstitutional deprivation of Terri Schiavo's constitutional right to life."

The Supreme Court's rejection came hours after the 11th U.S. Circuit Court of Appeals in Atlanta, Georgia, rejected the parents' petition 9-2. That court denied three similar requests from the parents last week.

In a concurring opinion of the Atlanta court's latest ruling, Judge Stanley Birch said Congress "chose to overstep constitutional boundaries" by passing a law to force the Schiavo case into federal courts...

[T]hree days after Schiavo's feeding tube was removed, Congress passed a bill transferring jurisdiction of the case from Florida state court to a U.S. District Court, for a federal judge to review. President Bush signed it into law the next day. But federal courts refused to overturn the state courts' decision...

Florida's 2nd District Court of Appeal heard a week of testimony from five doctors who examined her, including two picked by Michael Schiavo, two by her parents and one picked by the court.

Three doctors, including one appointed by the court, testified that Terri Schiavo was in a persistent vegetative state with no hope of recovery. The two doctors selected by the Schindlers testified they thought she could recover.

The appellate court concurred with a lower court decision that Schiavo had no hope of recovery and that her feeding tube could be removed.

Sosa, N., Franken, B., Phillips, R., & Candiotti, S. (2005, March 31). Terri Schiavo has died. *CNN.* Retrieved from http://www.cnn.com/2005/LAW/03/31/schiavo/index.html?iref=newssearch

Once doctors removed the feeding tube that had kept her alive for more than a decade, it was fewer than two weeks before Ms. Schiavo passed.

In the Terri Schiavo case, the court reaffirmed the **substitute judgment** requirement and found that it was based on **clear and convincing** evidence. In doing so, it allowed the removal of the feeding tube based on permitting her husband to become the decision maker and deciding that he was taking into account her value system and personal belief, as well as her earlier statements about medical treatments. The question was not whether the state had the right to prevent the removal of the tube but that it could not do so without clear and compelling evidence that she would make that same decision if so able. Advance directives are a result of the need for evidence. There are three major forms of advance directives: living will, durable power of attorney, and health care proxy.

substitute judgment one who makes a decision for another

clear and convincing that measure of proof that will produce in the mind of the trier of facts a firm belief or conviction as to allegations sought to be established

Patient Self-Determination Act (PSDA)

The Patient Self-Determination Act, enacted in 1990, requires health care facilities to provide written information to each adult admission regarding patient rights under state law to make decisions involving the acceptance or refusal of medical or surgical treatment. It also requires documentation of the patient's receipt of this information in the medical record as well as whether a patient has executed an advance directive. Institutions cannot condition care on the provision that the patient execute an advance directive or agree to accept treatment. Medical office professionals should know and be able to explain to patients the advance directives options available to them.

The PSDA governs all hospitals, nursing homes, rehabilitation facilities, home health agencies, and health maintenance organizations and **hospices** that receive Medicare/Medicaid payments. Each entity is required to maintain written policies and procedures regarding advance directives and provide information to patients at the time of admission or enrollment.

hospice a home or facility where the terminally ill are cared for

Under the PSDA, the regulated facilities must:

- provide written information to patients on admission informing them of their rights under state law to executive advance directives;
- provide written information about to carry out these rights;
- document whether an advance directive exists for each patient; and
- educate their staff and community on advance directives.

Living Wills

Most states recognize **living wills**, although state statutes vary in content for the requirement of a valid "living will." Over the past 30 years, living wills have been accepted by the courts, physicians, the President's

living will a will made by a person in which he or she requests to be allowed to die naturally rather than being kept alive by artificial means in the event there is no probable recovery from mental or physical disability

Commission for the Study of Ethical Problems in Medicine and Biomedical and Behavioral Research, and lawyers, but only a third of the population has a living will. Living will forms are easy to obtain: contact your state bar association or state department of elder affairs for information appropriate to your state.

Efforts to define policies on withholding or withdrawing life-sustaining procedures from hopelessly ill patients are a relatively recent development. All states have living will statutes that vary slightly. These statutes have differing requirements for the contents and authentication of living wills. A living will is a contract, and it must be executed by a competent person. Its intent is to extend the right to refuse artificial life-sustaining procedures into a possible future time of incompetency.

Durable Power of Attorney

durable power of attorney a document allowing the principal (the person writing the durable power of attorney) to delegate to another person the legal authority to act on the principal's behalf

The AMA suggests a medical directive as a substitute for the living will and suggests further that these be made available in physicians' offices and hospitals and included as part of the medical record. Assessing the relative merits of the living will and the **durable power of attorney** for health care, the AMA finds that the durable power of attorney can cover a broader range of illnesses than the living will, which is often linked to situations of terminal illness when death is imminent. In some states, the durable power of attorney may have a different name, such as medical power of attorney.

All 50 states recognize some version of the durable power of attorney, having adopted the Uniform Durable Power of Attorney Act or the Uniform Probate Code, or some variation of them. In a durable power of attorney, an individual designates, in writing, another as his or her attorney in fact. The document contains the words "this power of attorney shall not be affected by subsequent disability or incapacity of the principal," "[T]his power of attorney shall become effective upon the disability or incapacity of the principal," or similar words indicating the principal's intent that the authority conferred continues despite disability or incapacity. The authority differs from a regular power of attorney, which terminates upon disability or death.

In most cases, the durable power of attorney is accepted for the clauses of instruction contained within the document. If there is no direction to the agent regarding right-to-die issues, the document is interpreted to mean that the agent has no authority on these issues. Occasionally, the agent may be looked to by a hospital or physician to assist in a decision, but as a general rule, without instruction for medical treatment, the document cannot be used for that purpose.

Health care durable powers of attorney direct the person appointed to serve as a surrogate in health care decisions under certain circumstances. Some legal practitioners suggest that everyone who has a living will should also execute a durable power of attorney. Again, each state is different in its requirements, and state bar associations have the pertinent information.

Health Care Proxy

All states have enacted legislation empowering the patient to use a **health care proxy**. Sometimes known by other terms such as a *directive to physicians and family* or *surrogates* or some other title, in every case, the legislation provides that the document shall do the following:

1. Identify the principal and the health care agent;
2. Express the intention of the principal that the health care agent has authority to make health care decisions on behalf of the principal;
3. Describe any limitations on the authority of the health care agent;
4. Indicate that the authority of the health care agent to make health care decisions becomes effective upon a determination of incapacity; and
5. Be revoked by notifying the agent or health care provider orally, in writing, or by any other act evidencing specific intent to revoke; by execution of a subsequent health care proxy; or by divorce or legal separation of the principal and spouse when the spouse is the agent.

Most incompetent patients in need of **life-sustaining** treatment have not executed an advance directive. In this situation, it has become standard medical practice to seek consent from family members of incompetent patients. The President's Commission suggests the following:

health care proxy document appointing one person to act as a surrogate to make health care decisions for another under certain circumstances

life-sustaining maintaining or prolonging life in someone not able to do so naturally

> 66 99
>
> 1. The family is generally most concerned about the good of the patient.
> 2. The family will also usually be most knowledgeable about the patient's goals, preferences, and values.
> 3. The family deserves recognition as an important social unit that ought to be treated, within limits, as a responsible decision maker in matters that intimately affect its members.
> 4. Especially in a society in which many other traditional forms of community have eroded, participation in a family is often an important dimension of personal fulfillment.
> 5. Since a protected sphere of privacy and autonomy is required for the flourishing of this interpersonal union, institutions and the state should be reluctant to intrude, particularly regarding matters that are personal and on which there is a wide range of opinion in society.
>
> President's Commission. (1983). *Deciding to forego life-sustaining treatment*, p. 127. Washington, DC: Government Printing Office.

THE TERMINALLY ILL PATIENT

terminally ill fatally ill with a condition for which there is no cure

While advance directives can guide health care for patients unable to make decisions, caring for a **terminally ill** patient presents ethical issues in addition to those raised by advance directives. What is the purpose of providing care to a patient who has no prospect of recovery? In most cases, the objective is to alleviate suffering and ensure the patient is as comfortable as possible. Often in the last months of life, terminally ill patients will receive hospice care that provides palliative care and supportive services. Palliative care, which is coordinated medical care intended to provide relief from a seriously ill patient's physical or mental discomfort, is the keystone of medical care for terminally ill patients. Hospice care can take place in hospice-dedicated facilities or in patients' homes.

The National Public Radio program, *This American Life*, featured an episode dedicated to death and taxes. The segment on death focused on hospice care, as seen through the eyes of Nancy Updike, who experienced the natural death of a loved one who was in hospice. An excerpted transcript of the radio program follows.

Nancy Updike

… I had never seen the kind of expertise these nurses had. They knew death. They seemed to understand it, whereas I, even though I had just watched someone fade away and die right in front of me, all I could think was, what just happened?

…

Nancy Updike

… But there's a huge difference between dying and the very last part of dying, what Pattie and the other nurses call actively dying, a process that can take hours or even days. But it's different from what comes before. And being familiar with one doesn't mean you'll recognize the other.

…

Pattie Burnham

It's a weird thing, because when I came to work at the Kaplan house—and I was a registered nurse and had worked as a nurse for a while—I followed another nurse, Jeanette, for a month. And I was floored by the whole dying process, because it was nothing that I had learned. And I saw Jeanette say to a family—she woke them up and said, he's dying. He's dying right now.

And the man had been there, the patient had been there for a week. And I didn't know what was different. I didn't know what she saw that was different.

And when I asked her to explain it to me and to teach it to me, she said, you'll know. You just need about a month here and you'll know.

Nancy Updike

I talked to a palliative care doctor who told me that the most important thing she got better at with experience was looking for openings that allow you to be helpful, little windows, little moments. With hospice, part of that is trying to help people take in, bit by bit, the realness of what's happening. Some dying people—no surprise—are not at all OK with the fact that they're dying. And they don't often get a chance to just say so.

…

Dying is a constant series of judgment calls and decisions based on options that are very far from what anyone would want. And one thing the nurses are experienced at is trying to make the best of those narrow options.

…

But all the stories seemed to be trying to tackle the same huge question. How did we get here?

Pattie Burnham

Grief is one thing. But watching somebody die is a whole other thing.

…

Nancy Updike

I asked Pattie if anyone, at the end of that list, says, well, I'm just afraid of dying. I fear death. She said yes. And she listens if they want to talk about it, offers to bring in the chaplain or the social worker.

What else is there? That might be the biggest thing that she and the other nurses know that we don't. They know the limits of what they can do.

Updike, N. (2014, March 25). Death and taxes. *This American Life*. Retrieved from http://www.thisamericanlife.org/radio-archives/episode/523/transcript

Palliative care, including pain management, end of life issues, and emotional support, among others, squarely addresses issues of impending death. In some instances, terminally ill patients are in hospice because they have chosen to forego medical treatment that might extend their lives. In other instances, patients are in hospice because there are no other options. In both cases, most hospice patients find that palliative care allows them to focus on their families, themselves, and other practical issues related to death. What specific ethical issues arise from the care of a terminally ill patient?

THE RIGHT TO DIE

If refusing treatment may be an appropriate choice, just as choosing treatment may be an appropriate choice, then do physicians, with the intent of providing a "death with dignity," have the obligation to inform patients of the various ways of dying that are available to them or to assist them with dying? It appears that some physicians do and that they may have followers ready to assist them in helping patients to die. As recently as 2007, Michigan physician Jack Kevorkian completed eight years of a 10- to 25-year prison sentence for second-degree murder after he administered a lethal injection into a terminal patient. He was released on parole due to good behavior and, perhaps, changes in societal perceptions of a patient's right to die.

Given changes in societal attitudes toward medical intervention in death and dying, the spate of discussion regarding the right to choose medical procedures in the face of death is not surprising. In October 2015, California was the fourth state (in addition to Washington, Oregon, and New Hampshire) to enact a right to die statute, and a handful of other states are considering right to choose statutes.

The right to die debate continues, as do efforts to legalize such action. A contract to murder is an illegal contract and unenforceable under contract law. Each state has at least one statute that makes killing another person a felony. In some states, it is a crime to attempt to commit suicide, and in others, it is a crime to aid in a suicide.

Members of the families who have killed another family member with the intent of relieving suffering have been confronted by the criminal justice system. In Florida, a man shot his wife who was in advanced stages of Alzheimer's disease, and he was sentenced to life imprisonment. In Massachusetts, under similar circumstances, a husband suffocated his wife by placing her head in a plastic bag and sealing it with duct tape. He was not sentenced to prison but placed on probation.

The question is this: When does it appear that a disease has "mastered the patient"? There is a possibility that family or others can influence the decision. Further, how will competence be shown? Competence to enter into a contract is a legal issue that requires psychiatric evaluation.

The diagnosis of Alzheimer's disease is a verdict against the healthy spouse as well, sentencing him or her to a future life of poverty due to the length of the disease and the cost of treatment. State law requires couples to spend down to a certain level before either one of the parties is eligible for Medicaid. In some states, the family home will be lost to pay the expenses, whereas in others, a lien will be placed on the property to pay off whatever welfare spends during the time of crisis.

The durable power of attorney, living will, and health care proxies are legal instruments that ensure that personal preferences are known when competence is questioned. The moral implications of euthanasia are still questioned by society. The right to choose encompasses a spectrum of decisions related to the following questions: What medical efforts are permissible should a patient's experience cardiopulmonary arrest? When is it permissible to remove life support? And, is suicide or euthanasia an option?

Do-Not-Resuscitate Orders

As a result of the treatment of **cardiopulmonary arrest** with cardiopulmonary resuscitation (CPR), patients may be literally brought back to life after the traditional signs of a death have appeared. Whether CPR should be used on every patient is a question that haunts institutional professionals. This decision remains the province of the patient when they have executed an advance directive that includes an order to the physician not to resuscitate, a DNR order (in some states, referred to as a directive to physicians). It is estimated that approximately 80 percent of the two million people who die in the United States each year die in institutions. Each institution has professionals trained to respond to death with CPR. Is it practicing good medicine to require CPR for every patient, or should it be used like every treatment and prescribed on an individual basis? If CPR is not attempted, is the staff medically abandoning the patient? If an agreement is made between the staff and the patient that this particularly invasive procedure will not be utilized, is the patient psychologically abandoned? These are all ethical and legal questions that must be answered by the practicing professional.

Although awareness of the legal need to have DNR orders in effect, if that is what is desired, has increased, clear guidelines for making those wishes known have not been well established. This can lead to action that is not in accord with the patient's wishes.

cardiopulmonary arrest cessation of normal functioning of the heart and lungs

On Christmas Eve last year, the staff at Woodland Oaks Healthcare Center in Ashland failed to perform CPR on a dying resident, a state citation alleges, even though the resident had signed an order asking for resuscitation.

In February 2008, John Karem said, he arrived at Jefferson Manor Nursing Home in Louisville to find an emergency medical technician performing CPR

(Continues)

(Continued)

on his 95-year-old mother, Eva. This was done, her son says, even though the nursing home had do-not-resuscitate or DNR orders on file.

The two alleged incidents point to a gap in Kentucky law that can lead to errors at the bedside of the dying: There is no uniform regulation about how to denote a patient's wishes regarding resuscitation in a long-term care facility or a hospital, according to Sadiqa Reynolds, inspector general for the Cabinet for Health and Family Services...

Federal and state laws require that hospitals and nursing homes keep do-not-resuscitate orders in a patient's chart. But when it comes to how those orders are carried out at the bedside, it is up to the facility. Some use color-coded wrist bands, colored tape on residents' doors or stickers on their charts.

Spears, V. H. (2009, March 22). Gap in Ky. law leads to errors at bedside of dying patients. *Lexington Herald-Reader.* Retrieved from http://www.kentucky.com/living/health-and-medicine/article43994613.html

A DNR order only works if the health care provider knows that it exists. Whose responsibility is it to identify whether a patient has a DNR order? What are the ethical issues associated with a physician who refuses to acknowledge a patient's DNR order? What if the physician's refusal is based upon religious beliefs?

Removal of Life Support

Prolonging life today is often a treatment decision. The physician may make this decision, but it is the nurse who carries out the day-to-day patient care. The withholding of food and water is an indication that the medical community is no longer going to continue nurturing the patient. It is an intentional act. The case involving the removal of the feeding tube from a young woman mentioned earlier in this chapter, Terri Schiavo, became a rallying point for both those supporting the right to die and those supporting the right to life. Over the course of weeks, it led to numerous court actions, legislative action on the state and federal level, direct action by the President of the United States and the Governor of Florida, extensive media coverage, widespread protests, statements from religious leaders, and much more. It underscores the range of opinion and the deep emotional commitments surrounding such issues of life and death. The debate on the removal of feeding tubes shows that there are no easy answers, often just more questions.

As the following article shows, even the Catholic Church has had to struggle with the issues involved.

The ethical and moral dilemmas surrounding the end of life can be some of the most difficult and heartrending that most people ever face, and Ms. Schiavo's long coma and the struggle over who should decide what to do about it attracted huge attention and sent off political and social shock waves that still reverberate.

Even the Vatican, whose views on matters of life and death tend to be fairly absolute, had to deliberate for two years over how to answer a request for guidance on cases like Ms. Schiavo's that was posed by American bishops after she died in 2005…

Agence France Presse quotes the question posed by the bishops:

"When nutrition and hydration are being supplied by artificial means to a patient in a 'permanent vegetative state,' may they be discontinued when competent physicians judge with moral certainty that the patient will never recover consciousness?"

And the answer, from the Congregation for the Doctrine of the Faith, the Vatican office in charge of laying down the law:

"No. A patient in a 'permanent vegetative state' is a person with fundamental human dignity and must, therefore, receive ordinary and proportionate care which includes, in principle, the administration of water and food even by artificial means."

That word "must" makes the answer a pretty stark one: there would seem to be no room left even for a patient's own explicit wishes not to be kept alive in a coma past any hope of recovery, something that many people include in written "living wills" that are meant to spare their loved ones any doubts about such a potentially agonizing decision.

Lyons, P. J. (2007, September 14). Still more fallout from the Terri Schiavo case. *The New York Times*. Retrieved from http://thelede.blogs.nytimes.com/2007/09/14/still-more-fallout-from-the-terry-schiavo-case/?scp=2&sq=Terry%20Schiavo%20&st=cse

DNR orders are no longer hidden or camouflaged with purple dots. It has been legally recognized that individuals have the right to make decisions affecting their own death. Procedures are made available to document a dying person's wishes while the person is still considered legally competent. The ethical conflict in these cases is the tension between the obligation to prevent death and the obligation to prevent suffering.

Euthanasia

Euthanasia, Greek for "good death," usually refers to an act in which one person kills another, at the request of and for the benefit of the one who dies. Suicide is the taking of one's own life. There is a blurring of the terms **assisted suicide** and *euthanasia*. Euthanasia—mercy killing, or actively assisting someone to terminate their life at their request—is not a new subject. As far back as Hippocrates, "the physician is discouraged from invading the atrium of death" and instructed that, in certain circumstances, "attempts to cure must yield to attempts to comfort." Hippocrates' treatise *The Art* instructs physicians "(1) to do away with the sufferings of the sick, (2) to lessen the violence of their diseases, and (3) to refuse to treat those who are over mastered by their diseases realizing that in such cases medicine is powerless."

There are many arguments made against euthanasia:

1. There could be a mistake in diagnosis.

2. There may be difficulty in determining if euthanasia is voluntary—for example, where there is an undue influence exerted on the patient by a member of the family and/or beneficiary of a will for financial reasons.

3. It could lead to a slippery slope; for example, with the growth of managed care, there may be more financial pressure to hasten death for those who are elderly, uneducated, on welfare, or disabled.

4. Altering the role of physicians to include the practice of killing patients would bring about a psychological upheaval in the physician–patient relationship, and patients would become less trustful of their physician's role as healer.

In addition, some examples of euthanasia's slippery slope are from Holland, where there has been a right to die statute since 2002: A gay man in Holland who could not accept his sexuality sought to end his life; a sexual abuse victim who suffered from severe post-traumatic stress disorder sought to end her life, which prompted a second victim of sexual abuse to seek the same; and a woman who had a pathological fear of germs ended her life via the statute. Who decides what illnesses warrant permission to die in this manner here in the United States? What considerations are factored in to the decision?

Mercy killing differs from the Capute murder case discussed in Chapters 3 and 4 in that there is intent to kill. Mercy killing is known as **euthanasia**. According to *Black's Law Dictionary*, euthanasia is the act or practice of painlessly putting to death persons suffering from incurable and distressing disease as an act of mercy. It presents legal and ethical problems within the walls of a health care facility as well as without, as shown in the following article:

assisted suicide one person making it possible for another person to commit suicide

euthanasia ending someone's life to prevent pain or suffering

A county judge has ordered the early release of a 91-year-old man who was serving a four-year prison term for the "mercy killing" of his wife in 2008.

Robert Shaw, 91, was sentenced to prison by Lorain County Common Pleas Judge Mark Betleski in August and became eligible for early release after serving six months of his sentence.

Defense attorney Kenneth Lieux told Betleski during Tuesday's hearing that Shaw's family wanted him released and one of his daughters had driven to Pickaway Correctional Institution to pick up her father in the event he was ordered released…

Lieux said Shaw's family will help with caring for and housing his client when he is released. He said Shaw hasn't had any infractions since he was incarcerated and has even worked a job at the prison when he wasn't in the infirmary.

Shaw originally was charged with aggravated murder, murder and felonious assault for smothering his 84-year-old wife before calling Avon police Nov. 13, 2008. He claimed that he killed Virginia Shaw "to put her out of her misery" because of myriad health problems that had seen her in and out of the hospital in the months before her death.

Dicken, B. (2015, February 18). Judge grants early release to 91-year-old mercy killer. *The Chronicle-Telegram*. Retrieved from http://www.chroniclet.com/cops-and-courts/2015/02/18/Judge-grants-early-release-to-91-year-old-mercy-killer.html

The issue of euthanasia is a difficult one for society and the courts. For example, there have also been cases where courts ruled differently for a defendant in a similar case:

The Andersons, a couple who lived near Long Pond in Centerville, had been married for fifty-two years, but a stroke followed by two operations left the wife, Olive, an invalid. She was paralyzed on one side, could not talk and was incontinent after her second operation. Ten days after her return home from therapy following brain surgery, Anderson, a retired chef, placed a plastic bag over his wife's head and sealed it with duct tape. He then called his daughter, Shirley, who called police.

Anderson made no attempt to cover up his crime. When the Barnstable Police arrived, the tape and bag were still on his wife's face. Anderson pleaded guilty to first-degree manslaughter and was sentenced by the judge to one year on probation.

The Boston Globe (1985, October 31).

The issue of euthanasia also surfaced in the aftermath of Hurricane Katrina in the New Orleans Memorial Medical Center.

The New Orleans community has reacted with fury toward Foti's office and sympathy for head and neck surgeon Anna Pou, MD, and nurses Lori Budo and Cheri Landry, who were arrested in July upon Foti's announcement that his office had uncovered evidence the women intentionally euthanized four patients at Memorial Medical Center in the desperate days following Katrina. Physicians have responded with questions about the evidence Foti has gathered, and laypeople have reacted to what they view as the vilification of health care professionals who didn't have to stay with patients at all and were, many bloggers, editorial letter writers, and radio talk-show callers say, merely trying to ease the suffering of their patients…

Foti accuses Pou, an associate professor of otolaryngology at the Louisiana State University School of Medicine, and the two nurses of intentionally administering lethal doses of morphine and the anxiolytic midazolam (Versed) to four patients on Sept. 1, 2005—three days after Katrina hit New Orleans. The four were patients of Lifecare, a long-term acute-care unit located within Memorial Medical Center.

Flooding after the hurricane stranded the hospital, which had no electricity or safe water. Medical and food supplies were nearly gone, and the temperature inside was more than 100° F. Some patients had been evacuated, but most Lifecare patients were physically unable to get out on their own power, and the hospital staff were desperately trying to arrange evacuation.

Within days of the final evacuation of the hospital, rumors began spreading that an unnamed female physician had been seen entering patients' rooms carrying syringes, and that those patients later died. The four patients Foti listed in his complaint against Pou and the nurses included two men and two women, ranging in age from 61 to 90. At least one was paralyzed, two were described as extremely ill, and one was reportedly convalescing.

Foti stated in a press conference that toxicology reports showed lethal amounts of the drugs in the patients' bodies, and that Pou had allegedly told a Lifecare nurse executive that lethal doses were administered to patients too sick to be moved.

"This is a homicide. It is not euthanasia," Foti stated in announcing the case against the women.

ACH Media. (2006, September 1). *Arrest of Katrina Doctor, Nurses Stirs Up Strong Support for the Accused.* Retrieved from http://www.ahcmedia.com /articles/122579-arrest-of-katrina-doctor-nurses-stirs-up-strong-support-for-the-accused

The Grand Jury refused to indict Dr. Pou and the others for murder and the criminal charges were dropped.

Twenty-nine year-old Brittany Maynard suffered from terminal brain cancer. She moved to Oregon from California because of its right to die statute. Maynard ended her life on November 1, 2014, but she is partially credited with inspiring the passage of California's right to die statute.

Brittany Maynard, the terminally ill 29-year-old who spent her final days advocating for death-with-dignity laws, took lethal drugs prescribed by her physician on Saturday and died, a spokesman said, "as she intended—peacefully in her bedroom, in the arms of her loved ones."

Maynard, who was diagnosed earlier this year with a stage 4 malignant brain tumor, said last month she planned to die Nov. 1 in her home in Portland, Ore., with help from her doctor. And Saturday, she said farewell, having succeeded at reviving interest—and debate—in a charged subject that had been out of the news for some years…

Maynard's journey began on New Year's Day when she was diagnosed with brain cancer. By April, she was told she had six months to live. She looked at treatment options—and side effects. She considered hospice care.

Then she made her decision: doctor-assisted death.

"After months of research, my family and I reached a heartbreaking conclusion," she wrote in an op-ed for CNN. "There is no treatment that would save my life, and the recommended treatments would have destroyed the time I had left."

Bever, L. (2014, November 2). Brittany Maynard, as promised, ends her life at 29. *The Washington Post*. Retrieved from https://www.washingtonpost.com/news /morning-mix/wp/2014/11/02/brittany-maynard-as-promised-ends-her-life-at-29/

Suicide

What happens when rather than getting spouses or other loved ones involved in euthanasia, terminally ill patients decide to take their own lives? Suicide is a disaster for the family, who often experiences guilt and the feeling that "maybe if I had done just a little bit more it would not have happened." Following a suicide, there is nothing more that can be done to help the patient. The attention of professionals turns to the family to help them deal with their loss. There often is anger, speculation about momentary insanity, guilt, and sorrow. Many consider suicide a disgrace to the family, and in many religions suicide is prohibited. Compassion and understanding will do much to help them through a difficult time. In the words of Immanuel Kant, "Act so that you treat humanity, whether in your own person or that of another, always as an end and never as a means only."

☑ SUMMARY

- Each human being is faced with questions regarding death and dying. Working as a health care professional requires an ability to deal with these matters on a regular basis. The manner in which a professional handles these matters reflects personal philosophies.
- The durable power of attorney, living will, and health care proxy are legal instruments that ensure personal preferences are known when competence is questioned.
- The moral implications of euthanasia are still questioned by society.
- Technology has progressed to the point where it does not seem to be always in the patient's best interest to prolong life. Do-not-resuscitate orders are now recorded in nursing notes for patients; removal of life-support systems is allowed by the courts; and right to die statutes are being enacted.

SUGGESTED ACTIVITIES

1. Interview a physician and a religious professional. Document the standards each has about life-support systems and whether they should be used on a terminally ill patient. Note the development of their personal philosophies that has led to their current thinking. Ask what incidents might change their present beliefs.
2. Identify the options available to Dr. Koop for treating the five-year-old patient with neuroblastoma.
3. Research the criteria for death in your state.
4. Contact a local hospital to see if its ethics committee has a policy for DNR orders. If you can, get a copy.
5. Go to the Internet and find an example of a living will.
6. Look up the durable power of attorney or living will statute in your state. What types of legal protection does your state provide for people using these instruments?

STUDY QUESTIONS

1. Explain your philosophy regarding euthanasia.
2. Why would a patient want a DNR order?
3. What are the factors you consider when identifying your position on the right to die?

CASES FOR DISCUSSION

1. The patient was a man 34 years of age. He left a store and walked toward his car. The defendant, a young man of 18 years, tiptoed behind him and hit him on the head with a baseball bat. He then went into a building, changed his clothes, crossed the street, and entered the store where he worked. When asked why he had hit the man, he said, "For kicks." At the hospital, the victim was placed on an artificial respirator. Two days later, the victim's blood pressure, heartbeat, and pulse were not observable; he failed to breathe when taken off the respirator; and an electroencephalogram failed to reveal any cerebral electrical activity. In the opinion of the physician, the patient had reached the stage of irreversible brain death. Two days later, the patient was again taken off the respirator with the same outcome. After consultation with the patient's family, the respirator was removed and his heart stopped. The defendant was found guilty of first-degree murder with the requirement of death satisfied by the proof of brain death. The defendant appealed, stating that "death," as required by the law, never occurred. How should the court rule?

2. For reasons still unclear, the patient ceased breathing for at least two 15-minute periods. She received some ineffectual mouth-to-mouth resuscitation from friends. She was taken by ambulance to the hospital, where she had a temperature of 100°F and was unresponsive to deep pain. She lapsed into a coma. Medical evidence indicated that she suffered severe brain damage, leaving her in a "chronic and persistent vegetative state." The patient was kept alive through the use of respirators and other medical life support systems while her body underwent a continuing deteriorative process. There was no known treatment to improve her condition. Her father requested that life-support systems be withdrawn, but the attending physician refused because the patient did not meet the traditional medical standard for death. Her heart had not stopped nor was she brain dead. If the life-support systems are removed, should the physician be subject to civil or criminal liability?

3. The patient was 67 years old and had lived for 50 years in a mental institution. He became ill with acute myelogenous leukemia, a blood disease that leads to death within months if it is not treated. The disease process can be slowed by chemotherapy. This treatment has severe side effects and is effective in only 30–50 percent of the cases. Even when effective, the treatment prolongs life for little more than one year. Patients over 60 years of age have a particularly difficult time tolerating the treatment. At a hearing before the probate court, the patient's guardian ad litem recommended that he undergo the

treatment, since this is what most people elect. Should the court rule against the guardian ad litem and allow this incompetent person the right to refuse medical treatment?

4. The wife and son of a senile, 78-year-old man tried to stop the hemodialysis treatments that he had undergone for a year. The family and the physician believed that the request was what the patient would have wanted. The family went to probate court, where a guardian ad litem was appointed to represent the patient. An adversarial hearing was conducted, and the court issued an order to terminate the treatment. The guardian ad litem objected, insisting that there had to be some positive evidence of the patient's will, and not merely a "substituted judgment," before a court could order the termination of the treatment. This matter was continued through probate, appeals, and Supreme Court hearings. What should the court decide?

5. An 83-year-old monk entered the hospital for a routine hernia operation. During the course of the surgery, he suffered cardiopulmonary arrest. When resuscitated, it was found that he was in a chronic vegetative condition. The patient, following his religious convictions, agreed with the Catholic Church's teachings that heroic measures to prolong life were unnecessary. He had discussed those issues in conversations involving other cases and had clearly stated he did not want any extraordinary measures taken to prolong his own life. His guardian asked physicians to remove the respirator that was keeping him alive. They refused. The surgeon asserted that after such a medical procedure was started, it should not be withdrawn. A spokesman for the hospital stated that the hospital's mission was to do all that it could to maintain life. The guardian then went to court. What should the court decide?

6. At approximately midnight, a patient complained to his wife of a severe headache and lapsed into unconsciousness. Angiograms revealed he had an aneurysm at the apex of the basilar artery. The patient underwent a craniotomy following which a clip was inserted across the aneurysm. The patient never regained consciousness. The patient was put on a respirator. Nutrition was provided through a nasogastric feeding tube. He was later diagnosed as being in a semivegetative or vegetative state. Do-not-resuscitate orders were placed in the patient's chart, a gastrostomy tube was inserted, and the nasogastric tube removed. Although the patient's electroencephalogram was abnormal, it did indicate controlled electrical activity generated by millions of cortical nerves, which were normal. Apart from the brain injury, the patient was not terminally ill. The patient's wife, who was also his guardian, requested that the hospital staff remove the gastrostomy tube. They refused, and the matter went to court. Should the court allow removal of the tube?

7. The patient was an 84-year-old bedridden woman with serious and irreversible physical and mental impairment. She was confined to bed and unable to move out of the fetal position. In addition, she suffered from arteriosclerotic heart disease, hypertension, and diabetes, and her left leg was gangrenous to the knee. She had several decubitus necrotic ulcers on her feet, legs, and hips, and an eye problem that required irrigation. She was unable to speak, and her ability to swallow was limited. There was a urinary catheter in place, and she could not control her bowels. Experts determined that she was not brain dead, comatose, or in a vegetative state. Her nephew and guardian wanted to remove the nasogastric feeding tube. Should the court allow it?

Glossary

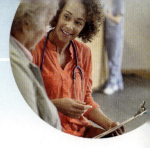

A

abandon to give up or cease doing.

acceptance an agreement to the terms of an offer.

adjudicate to hear and resolve a lawsuit by a judicial process.

advance directives written instructions about a person's future medical care.

adversary opponent.

affirmative duty responding to an incident in a predetermined manner.

age of majority the age, as determined by state law, at which a person becomes legally able to contract.

agent one who has authority to act on behalf of another.

AIDS acquired immune deficiency syndrome.

amniocentesis a medical technique used to determine whether a fetus has any abnormalities.

amoral without any consideration of morals.

arbitration a hearing held between two or more parties who disagree on an issue but agree in advance to abide by the decision of an impartial third person.

assault any deliberate attempt or threat to inflict bodily injury on another person and with apparent ability to do so.

assisted suicide one person making it possible for another person to commit suicide.

assumption of risk voluntary acceptance of a known danger.

autonomy allowing individuals control over themselves.

B

bargaining unit the labor union, or group of employees with similar interests, authorized to conduct negotiations on behalf of the employees who are members of the union or group.

battery illegal touching of another person.

beyond a reasonable doubt evidence so strong and credible that it leaves no more than a remote possibility that there is another explanation for what happened.

bioethics refers to life and death ethical issues and the implications of the application of biological research.

breach breaking a law, promise, or agreement.

burnout exhaustion from overwork.

bylaws regulations adopted by a corporation or association to govern its internal affairs.

C

calibration the systematic standardization of quantitative measuring instruments.

capitation payment in a lump sum to physicians, HMOs, and health care facilities to deliver health care to a segment of the population.

cardiopulmonary arrest cessation of normal functioning of the heart and lungs.

censure a formal statement of disapproval.

cert. denied when the U.S. Supreme Court refuses to hear a case on appeal.

certification a record of being qualified to perform certain acts after passing an examination given by an accredited professional organization.

chemotherapy the chemical treatment of disease.

civil the system of law concerned with lawsuits between individuals or between an individual and the state where the case does not relate to the violation of a criminal statute.

clear and convincing that measure of proof that will produce in the mind of the trier of facts a firm belief or conviction as to allegations sought to be established.

cloning identically duplicating an organism.

collective bargaining procedural attempt to achieve collective agreements between an employer and accredited representative of a group of employees, to improve the conditions of employment.

commitment the process by which a person is placed into a mental health facility or a penal institution.

common law law created by judge's decisions and by customs.

comparative negligence negligence measured by percentage, with the determined damages lessened according to the extent of injury or damage committed by the party proven guilty.

concurrent happening at the same time.

conglomerate a corporation diversifying operations by acquiring varied enterprises.

conservator a court-appointed person given authority to manage the financial affairs of an incompetent person.

consideration something promised that results in making an agreement a lawful, enforceable contract.

conspiracy an agreement among conspirators.

consumer one who buys products and services.

contingency something that may occur but is dependent on an uncertain future event.

contract a voluntary agreement, written or unwritten, between two parties that creates an obligation to do or not do something.

contributory negligence conduct by a plaintiff that is below the standard to which he or she is legally required to conform for his or her own protection.

creed a statement of belief or principles.

criminal the system of law concerned with crimes against the state or someone who has been proven guilty of such an offense.

cross-examination interrogation of a witness by a party other than the direct examiner.

D

data pieces of information.

defendant a person or party against whom a plaintiff's allegations are brought.

deposition a prior sworn statement by a witness to be used in court as testimony taken under oath and subject to cross-examination.

deterrence punishment used to discourage crime.

direct examination the first interrogation of a witness by the party for whom the witness has been called on behalf of that party's claim.

directors those elected and terminated by stockholders to manage a corporation.

disparate impact the force of impression of one thing on another.

disparate treatment a marked difference between two things.

district attorney the official prosecutor of a judicial district.

dividends distributed profits of a corporation.

DNA an essential component of all living matter and the basic chromosomal material transmitting the hereditary pattern.

durable power of attorney a document allowing the principal (the person writing the durable power of attorney) to delegate to another person the legal authority to act on the principal's behalf.

duress being influenced by threat to do something one would not ordinarily do.

E

egregious outrageous, shockingly bad, awful.

emancipated minor a person under the age of majority who is completely self-supporting and able to contract.

embryonic stem cells cells that are derived from human embryos or human fetal tissues that are self-replicating.

embryos fertilized eggs in the early stages of development.

enumerate to list a number of things.

ethical conforming to professionally proper behavior.

ethics the study of moral choices that conform to professional standards of conduct.

etiquette the prescribed code of courteous social behavior.

euthanasia an intentional action or lack of action causing the merciful death of someone suffering from a terminal illness or incurable condition.

expert witness a person whose education, profession, or specialized experience qualifies him or her with superior knowledge of a subject.

express contract a clear, definitive agreement between two or more parties.

F

facially neutral on the surface, the matter is impartial, or does not take an active part in either side.

fee-for-service basis of professional billing, either so much per hour or per identified procedure.

felony a crime more serious than a misdemeanor and punishable by imprisonment for more than one year or death.

fetus an unborn offspring in the postembryonic stage of gestation.

G

genetic resulting from genes or attributable to them.

grossly negligent failing intentionally to perform a necessary duty in extraordinary disregard of the consequences to the person neglected, particularly if it can be proven that there is more than a 50 percent chance the negligence caused an injury.

guardian a person entrusted to take care of the person, property, and rights of someone too young or otherwise incapable of managing his or her own affairs.

H

health care proxy document appointing one person to act as a surrogate to make health care decisions for another under certain circumstances.

HIV human immunodeficiency virus, which causes AIDS.

hospice a home or facility where the terminally ill are cared for.

I

immoral not moral.

implied contract an agreement not indicated by direct words but evident from the conduct of the parties.

incompetent persons those who lack the necessary qualifications to perform a duty.

inference a process of reasoning by which a fact is deduced as a logical consequence of other facts.

injunctive relief remedy preventing or requiring someone to perform or to refrain from performing a particular action.

insurance a contract binding a company to compensate someone for proven damages or injury caused by the party who has paid premiums in the contract.

interrogatory written questions about a case addressed to one party by another.

interstate commerce the movement of goods and services, or services that rely on the movement of goods, which cross state borders within the United States.

investment expenditure of resources (money, effort, etc.) to secure income or profit.

invitee a person who enters property for business as a result of express or implied invitation.

J

joint venture   a group of persons together performing some specific business undertaking that is limited in duration or scope.

judgment   a court's decision regarding the rights and obligations of the parties in a dispute.

L

larceny   stealing or removing someone's personal property to convert it illegally or deprive the owner of its possession; larceny is a felony.

legal capacity   legal ability to enter into contracts because no legal disabilities exist.

legal disability   lack of legal capacity for mutual agreement.

legal entity   an individual or organization that has legal capacity to contract, incur and pay debts, and sue and be sued.

licensee   a person who enters property with implied permission of the owner.

life-sustaining   maintaining or prolonging life in someone not able to do so naturally.

living will   a will made by a person in which he or she requests to be allowed to die naturally rather than being kept alive by artificial means in the event there is no probable recovery from mental or physical disability.

M

malice   an unjust intention to commit an illegal act to injure someone.

manslaughter   an unpremeditated taking of a human life.

mature minor   a person under the age of majority who has the mental capacity to make certain medical decisions without parental consent.

mediation   a neutral party meets with the plaintiff and defendant with the intent of persuading them to settle their dispute.

memorialize   to put something into writing.

mental incompetence   lack of reasoning faculties needed to enable someone to contract.

minors   persons who are under the age of majority as set forth by state law.

misdemeanor   an offense less serious than a felony and which may be punished by a fine or sentence to a local prison for less than one year.

mitigating   make less severe due to considerations of fairness and mercy.

motions   the application to a court or judge for a ruling in favor of the one applying.

murder   an act done with intent to kill the victim.

mutual agreement   common agreement of both parties.

N

negligence   failure to act with reasonable and prudent care given the circumstances.

negligent act   failure to take reasonable precautions to protect others from the risk of harm.

negligent per se   conduct that is against common knowledge that, by its act, without argument, can be declared negligence.

negotiated fee schedules   the process of the submission and consideration of offers until an offer is accepted. Fee schedule refers to the amount an insurance company or other third-party payer will reimburse for a medical procedure.

negotiation   exchange and consideration of offers until parties agree on a solution that is acceptable to both.

nonverbal communication   communicating with someone using body language.

notice   an announcement of pertinent information to those interested.

O

offer   a proposal to perform or refrain from a certain action.

officers   persons holding formal positions of trust in an organization, especially those involved in high levels of management.

P

paternalism   providing for people's needs but giving them no responsibility or control over their destiny.

patient–physician privilege legal concept that protects communications between a patient and a physician from disclosure in court.

peer review assessment of academic, professional, or scientific work by others who are experts in the same field.

per capita payment pay equally according to the number of individuals.

perjury a false statement under oath.

personality traits distinctive individual qualities of a person.

pharmacopoeia a book officially listing medical drugs along with information about their preparation and use; a stock of drugs in a pharmacy.

philosophy a basic viewpoint of an individual's or a society's value system.

plaintiff one who brings a court action against another.

pluralistic pertaining to the belief that there is no single explanation for all the extraordinary aspects of life, particularly in a society of numerous distinct cultures.

political administration of public affairs, particularly those of a government.

premises physical location, such as an office or building.

preponderance of the evidence the greater weight of the evidence that is more likely than not.

pretrial conference the first court conference of parties involved in a dispute.

principal the employer, or source of authority, of the agent or employee.

privileged communication a confidential communication (written or verbal) that is protected from disclosure in court.

probable cause (reasonable cause) having more evidence for than against.

product liability a tort making a manufacturer liable for compensation to anyone using its product if damages or injuries occur from defects in that product.

property right a right of ownership to a certain thing.

proximate cause an event from which an injury results as a direct consequence and without which the injury would not have happened.

purist one who believes in and follows all traditional rules.

Q

quality assurance responsibility to uphold the quality of care of patients receive.

qui tam lawsuit whistleblower brings suit and receives share of recovery as reward.

R

reasonable care the amount of care a rational person would use in similar circumstances.

reasonable person a prudent person whose behavior would be considered appropriate under the circumstances.

reformation the rehabilitation of a criminal; changed behavior.

registration fulfilling administrative qualifications for a licensed profession; may require special testing or training or other vetting.

remedies legal ways to make someone whole.

res ipsa loquitur ("the thing speaks for itself") evidence showing that negligence by the defendant may be reasonably inferred from the nature of the injury occurring to the plaintiff.

respectable minority a minority acceptable to its peer group.

respondeat superior legal theory that requires an employer be responsible (vicariously liable) for the behavior of an employee working within the scope of employment.

restraint restriction of liberty.

retribution something given or demanded in payment or as a punishment for criminal wrongdoing.

risk management the practice of considering the risk of actions taken and taking steps to minimize the risk associated with them.

robbery the forcible stealing of the personal property of another either from his or her person or in the immediate presence of the victim.

S

sanctioned   penalized for violating a law or accepted procedure.

sanctity   the condition of being sacred.

scientific investigation   an investigation using scientific rules and concepts to validate a hypothesis.

shares   units of stock giving the possessor part ownership in a corporation.

sociological   pertaining to human social behavior.

specific performance   the remedy of requiring someone to perform a contract as specified.

standard of proof   level of proof required, which is established by considering all evidence.

statute of limitations   the law setting a time limit within which one person can sue another.

statutory guidelines   legislative enactments defining legal rights and responsibilities.

stockholders   those who hold an interest (stock) in a corporation.

strict liability   responsibility of a seller or manufacturer for any defective product unduly threatening personal safety.

stringent   strict requirements, precise, exact.

subpoena   a written order to appear at a specified time and place to testify.

subpoena duces tecum   a written order to produce documents or things.

substitute judgment   one who makes a decision for another.

suit-prone   likely to sue someone or be sued.

survival action   a lawsuit related to a death and brought by the decedent's survivors.

T

technology   methods and materials used to achieve commercial or industrial objectives; the application of scientific methods to achieve a certain objective.

terminally ill   fatally ill with a condition for which there is no cure.

theft   stealing property without consent of the owner.

tort   a private wrong or injury, other than breach of contract, for which the court will provide a remedy.

trespasser   someone who enters a property illegally.

U

undue influence   any improper persuasion to make someone act differently from his or her own will.

utilization review   a process by which hospitals review patient progress to efficiently allocate scarce medical resources.

V

values   principles of thought and conduct that are considered desirable.

vicariously liable   legally obligated for the acts of others.

virtue   goodness conforming to the standard of moral excellence.

W

waives   to surrender a claim, privilege, or right the utterance of a false charge that damages another's reputation.

wanton   done with reckless disregard of another's rights or needs.

warranty   a promise that specifically named results will occur.

writ of certiorari   an order used by the U.S. Supreme Court to indicate the cases it wishes to hear.

wrongful death   death caused by negligence.

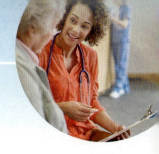

Bibliography

Cases

Adams v. State of Indiana, 229 N.E.2d 834 (Ind. 1973).

Alberts v. Devine, 395 Mass. 59 (1985).

Amadio v. Levin, 501 A.2d 1085 (Pa. 1985).

Anderson v. Somberg, 67 N.H. 291, 338 A.2d 1 cert. denied, 423 U.S. 929, S. Ct. 279 (1975).

Applebaum v. Board of Directors of Barton Memorial Hospital, 104 Cal. App. 3d 648, 163 Cal. Rptr. 831 (1980).

Arrest of Katrina doctor, nurses stirs up strong support for the accused. (2006, September 1). *Medical Ethics Advisor, 22*(9), 97–101.

Armstrong v. Svoboda, 49 Cal. Rptr. 701 (1966).

Ascher v. Gutierre, 175 U.S. App. D.C. 900, 533 F.2d 1235 (1976).

August v. Offices Unlimited, Inc., 981 F.2d 576 (1st Cir. 1992).

Avery v. Maryland, 292 A.2d 728 (Md. 1972).

Ayotte v. Planned Parenthood, 546 U.S. 320 (2006).

Backus v. Baptist Medical Center, 510 F. Supp. 1191 (1980).

Barnette v. Potenza, 79 Misc. 2d 51, 359 N.Y.S. 432 (1974).

Beadles v. Megayka, 311 P.2d 711 (Colo. 1957).

Becker v. Janiski, 15 N.Y.S. 675 (1891).

Becker v. Schwartz, 46 N.Y.2d 401, 413 N.Y.S. 895, 386 N.E.2d 807 (1978).

Bence v. Denbo, 183 N.E. 326 (Ind. Ct. App. 1932).

Berg v. New York Society for the Relief of the Ruptured & Crippled, 136 N.E.2d 513 (N.Y. 1956).

Bishop v. Byrne, 265 F. Supp. 460 (W. Va. 1967).

Bonner v. Moran, 75 U.S. App. D.C. 156, 126 F.2d 121 (1941).

Bouvia v. Superior Court of Los Angeles County, 179 Cal. App. 3d 1172, 225 Cal. Rptr. 297 (Ct. App. 1986).

Brophy v. New England Sinai Hospital, 398 Mass. 417 (1986).

Burton v. Leftwich, 123 So. 2d 766 (La. 1960).

Butler v. Louisiana State Board of Education, 331 So. 2d 192 (La. 1976).

Butterworth v. Swint, 186 S.E. 770 (Ga. 1936).

C.M. v. C.C., 152 N.J. Super. 160, 377 A.2d 821 (1977).

Caburnay v. Norwegian American Hosp., 2011 IL App (1st) 101740 (Ill. App., 2011).

Campbell v. Wainright, 416 F.2d 949 (1969).

Carr v. Shippolette, 82 F.2d 874 (D.C. Cir. 1936).

Carr v. St. Paul Fire & Marine Insurance Co., 384 F. Supp. 821 (Ark. 1974).

Carter v. Cangello, 164 Cal. Rptr. 361 (1980).

Christ v. Saliterman, 179 N.W.2d 288 (Minn. 1970).

Citizens for Health v. Levitt, 549 U.S. 941, 127 S.Ct. 43 (2006).

Cobbs v. Grant, 8 Cal. Rptr. 505, 502 P.2d 1 (1972).

Cochran v. Sears Roebuck, 34 S.E.2d 296 (Ga. 1945).

Commissioner of Correction v. Myers, SJC Mass. (1979).

Commonwealth v. Edelin, 3 Mass. Adv. 2795, 359 N.E.2d 4 (1976).

Commonwealth v. Golston, 366 N.E.2d 744 (1977).

Connell v. Medical & Surgical Clinic, 315 N.E.2d 278 (Ill. 1974).

Cook v. Rhode Island, 10 F.3d 17 (1st Cir. 1993).

Cooper v. Sisters of Charity, 272 N.E.2d 97 (Ohio 1971).

Corne & De Vane v. Bausch & Lomb, 390 F. Supp. 161 (1975).

Cox v. Stanton, 529 F.2d 247 (1975).

Crawford v. McDonald, 187 S.E.2d 542 (Ga. 1972).

Crow v. McBride, 153 P.2d 727 (Cal. 1944).

Crowe v. Provost, 374 S.W.2d 645 (Tenn. 1963).

Cruzan v. Director, Missouri Department of Health, 110 S. Ct. 2841 (Mo. 1990).

Delk v. Columbia Healthcare Corp., 523 S.E.2d 826 (Va. 2000).

DeMay v. Roberts, 9 N.W. 146 (Mich. 1881).

Doe v. Southeastern Pennsylvania Transportation, No. 93-5988 (U.S. Dist. Ct., E.D. Pa., December 5, 1994), 95 LWUSA 96, p. 8.

Donaldson v. O'Connor, 493 F.2d 507 (1974).

East Chicago Rehabilitation Center, Inc. v. NLRB, 710 F.2d 397 (1983).

Estate of Berthiaume v. Pratt, 365 A.2d 792 (Me. 1976).

Estate of Reiner, 383 N.Y.S. 2d 504 (1976).

Gashgai v. Maine Medical Association, 350 A.2d 511 (1976).

Geddes v. Daughters of Charity, 348 F.2d 144 (1965).

Gelder Medical Group v. Webber, 363 N.E.2d 573 (N.Y. 1977).

Gillanza v. Sands, 316 So. 2d 77 (Fla. 1975).

Gillette v. Tucker, 65 N.E. 865 (Ohio 1902).

Gillett-Netting ex rel. Netting v. Barnhart, 371 F.3d 595 (9th Cir. 2004).

Glanz v. Vernick, 756 F.Supp. 632 (D. Mass., 1991).

Goldman v. Kossove, 117 S.E.2d 35 (N.C. 1960).

Gotkin v. Miller, 379 F. Supp. 859 (E.D.N.Y. 1974), *aff'd* 514 F.2d 125 (2d Cir. 1975).

Gray v. Grunnagle, 23 A.2d 663 (Pa. 1966).

Greaves v. State, 528 P.2d 805 (1974).

Griece Mills v. Derwinski, 967 F.2d 794 (2d Cir. 1992).

Griffin v. Medical Society of New York, 11 N.Y.S.2d 109 (1939).

Griggs v. Duke Power, 401 U.S. 424 (1971).

Griswold v. Connecticut, 381 U.S. 479, 85 S. Ct. 1678 (1965).

Hand v. Tavera, 864 S.W.2d 601 (1971).

Hawker v. New York, 170 U.S. 189 (1898).

Hawkins v. McGee, 146 A. 611 (N.H. 1929).

Helling v. Carey, 83 Wash. 2d 514, 519 P.2d 981 (1974).

Helms v. St. Paul Fire & Marine Insurance Co., 289 So. 2d 288 (La. 1974).

Hiatt v. Grace, 523 P.2d 320 (Kan. 1974).

Hicks v. Arkansas State Medical Board, 260 Ark. 31, 537 S.W.2d 794 (Ark. 1976).

Holtzclaw v. Ochsner Clinic, 831 So. 2nd 495 (La. 5th Cir. 2002).

Hood v. Phillips, 554 S.W.2d 160 (Tex. 1977).

Horne v. Patton, 287 So. 2d 824 (1973).

Horton v. Niagara Falls Memorial Medical Center, 380 N.Y.S. 116 (1976).

Howard v. Lecher, 42 N.Y.2d 109, 397 N.Y.S.2d 363 (1977).

Humphers v. First Interstate Bank of Oregon, 696 P.2d 527 (Or., 1985).

Hurley v. Eddingfield, 156 Ind. 416, 59 N.E. 1058 (1901).

In re Adoption of Anonymous, 74 Misc. 2d 99, 345 N.Y.S.2d 430 (1973).

In re Conroy, 98 N.J. 321, 486 A.2d 1209 (1985).

In re Culbertson's Will, 292 N.Y.S.2d 806 (1968).

In re Osborne, 294 A.2d 372 (1972).

In re Quinlan, 70 N.J. 10, 355 A.2d 647 (1976).

In re Sampson, 317 N.Y.S.2d 241 (1970).

In re Smith, 295 A.2d 238 (Md. 1972).

In re Spring, 380 Mass. 629, 405 N.E.2d 115 (1978).

J. F. Kennedy Hospital v. Heston, 58 N.J. 576, 279 A.2d 670 (1971).

Jacobs v. Theimer, 519 S.W.2d 846 (Tex. 1975).

James v. Spear, 338 P.2d 22 (Cal. 1959).

Jefferson v. United States, 77 F. Supp. 706 (Md. 1948).

Jeswald v. Hutt, 239 N.E.2d 37 (Ohio 1968).

Johnson v. Woman's Hospital, 527 S.W.2d 133 (Tenn. 1975).

Johnston v. Black Co., 91 P.2d 921 (Cal. 1939).

Jones v. Fakehany, 67 Cal. Rptr. 810 (1968).

Katko v. Briney, 183 N.W.2d 657 (Iowa 1971).

Katz v. United States, 389 U.S. 347 (1967).

Kennedy v. Parrott, 243 N.C. 355, 90 S.E.2d 754 (1956).

Kirk v. Michael Reese Hospital, No. 81-2408 (Ill. App. Ct. August 28, 1995).

Leikvold v. Mahavier v. Beverly Enterprises, 540 S.W.2d 813 (Tex. 1976).

Lyons v. Walker Regional Medical Center, 868 So.2d 1071 (Ala. 2003).

Mazer v. Lipschutz, 327 F.2d 42 (1963).

McCormack v. Mt. Sinai Hospital, 44 N.Y.S.2d 702 (1981).

McCormick v. Haley, 307 N.E.2d 34 (Ohio 1973).

McCune v. Neitzel, No. 88-552 (Neb. Sup. Ct. Lawyer's Alert No. 215-23, July 13, 1990).

McGulpin v. Bessmer, 43 N.W.2d 121 (Iowa 1950).

McLaughlin v. Mine Safety Appliances Co., 11 N.Y.2d 62, 226 N.Y.S.2d 407, 181 N.E.2d 430 (1962).

McQuitty v. Spangler, 976 A.2d 1020 (Md. App. 2009).

Millsaps v. Bankers Life Co., 35 Ill. App. 3d 735, 342 N.E.2d 329 (1976).

Mone v. Greyhound Lines, 368 Mass. 358, 331 N.E.2d 916 (1976).

Mullins v. Duvall, 104 S.E. 513 (Ga. 1920).

National Federation of Independent Business v. Sebelius, 567 U.S. (2012).

National Treasure Employees Union v. Von Raab, 489 US 656 (1989).

Nolan v. Kechibrigian, 64 A.2d 866 (R.I. 1949).

Ochoa v. Vered, 186 P.3d 107 (Colo. App. 2008).

People v. Brown, 88 Cal. App. 3d 283, 151 Cal. Rptr. 749 (1979).

People v. Murray, unpublished decision (Cal App. 2014).

People v. Sorenson, 68 Cal. 2d 680, 66 Cal. Rptr. 7, 437 P.2d 495 (1968).

People v. Yukl, 83 Misc. 2d 364, 372 N.Y.S. 2d 313 (1975).

Price v. Sheppard, 239 N.W.2d 905 (Minn. 1976).

Rauhe v. Langeland Memorial Chapel, Inc., 205 N.W.2d 313 (1973).

Redder v. Hanson, 338 F.2d 244 (1964).

Reeder v. City of New York, 197 N.Y.S.2d 572 (1960).

Renslow v. Mennonite Hospital, 67 Ill. 348, 10 Ill. Dec. 484 (1977).

Reyes v. Wyeth Laboratories, 498 F.2d 1264, cert. denied, 419 U.S. 1096 (1974).

Reynolds v. McNichols, 488 F.2d 1378 (1973).

Riff v. Morgan Pharmacy, 508 A.2d 1247 (Pa. 1986).

Robins v. California, 370 U.S. 660, 82 S. Ct. 1417 (1962).

Rochester v. Katalan, 320 A.2d 704 (Del. 1974).

Rockhill v. Pollard, 259 Or. 54, 485 P.2d 28 (1971).

Roe v. Wade, 410 U.S. 113, 93 S. Ct. 705, 35 L. Ed. 2d 147 (1973).

Rogers v. Lawson, 170 F.2d 157 (D.C. Cir. 1948).

Roman v. Roman, 193 S.W.3d 40 (Tex. App., 2006).

Rudick v. Prineville Memorial Hospital, 319 F.2d 764 (1963).

Rule v. Cheeseman, 317 P.2d 472 (Kan. 1957).

Schachter v. Whalen, 581 F.2d 35 (1978).

Schessler v. Keck, 271 P.2d 588 (Cal. App. 2 Dist., 1954).

Sherlock v. Stillwater Clinic, 260 N.W.2d 269 (1977).

Shoemaker v. Friedberg, 183 P.2d 318 (Cal. 1947).

Simonsen v. Swenson, 177 N.W. 831 (Neb. 1920).

Skodje v. Hardy, 288 P.2d 471 (Wash. 1955).

Smalley v. Baker, 262 Cal. App. 2d 824, 69 Cal. Rptr. 521 (1968).

Smith v. Sibley, 431 P.2d 719 (Wash. 1967).

Snyder v. Holy Cross Hospital, 30 Md. App. 317 (1976).

St. John v. Pope, 901 S.W.2d 420, 38 Tex.Sup.Ct.J. 723 (Tex., 1995).

St. Joseph Hosp. v. Wolff, 94 S.W.3d 513 (Tex., 2002).

Stowers v. Wolodzko, 191 N.W.2d 355 (1971).

Strunk v. Strunk, 445 S.W.2d 145 (1969).

Sullivan v. O'Connor, 363 Mass. 579, 296 N.E.2d 183 (1973).

Superintendent Belchertown v. Saikwicz, 370 N.E.2d 417 (1977).

Tarasoff v. Regents of University of California, 118 Cal. Rptr. 129 (1974).

Tarasoff v. Regents of University of California, 17 Cal. 3d 342, 131 Cal. Rptr. 14 (1976).

Thomas v. St. Joseph Hospital, 618 S.W.2d 791 (Tex. Civ. App. 1981).

Traynom v. Cinemark USA, Inc., 940 F.Supp.2d 1339 (D. Colo. 2013).

United States v. Morvant, 843 F. Supp. 1092 (E.D. La. 1994).

Venner v. State, 30 Md. App. 599, 354 A.2d 483 (1976).

Vigil v. Rice, 397 P.2d 719 (N.M. 1964).

Wax v. Johnson, 42 S.W.3d 168 (Tex.App.-Hous. 1 Dist., 2001).

Whalen v. Roe, 429 U.S. 589, 97 S. Ct. 869 (1977).

Wickline v. State of California, No. B 10156 (Cal. Ct. 2d Dist., July 1, 1986).

Winters v. Miller, 446 F.2d 65, cert. denied, 404 U.S. 985 (1971).

Wong v. Chappell, 773 S.E.2d 496 (Ga. App. 2015).

Zeo v. Unemployment Comp. Bd. of Review (Pa. Commw. Ct., 2015).

Periodicals

ACH Media. (2006, September 1). Arrest of Katrina doctor, nurses stirs up strong support for the accused. Retrieved from http://www.ahcmedia.com/articles/122579-arrest-of-katrina-doctor-nurses-stirs-up-strong-support-for-the-accused

Allen, S., Bombardieri, M., & Rezendes, M. (2008, November 16). A healthcare system badly out of balance. *Boston Globe*. Retrieved from https://www.bostonglobe.com/specials/2008/11/16/healthcare-system-badly-out-balance/j2ushYtZTBiCSxxUtQegbN/story.html

AMA opposes taking organs from brain-malformed babies. (1996, January 7). *The New York Times*, p. 22.

Anderson, M. T. (1985, April). Reporting elder abuse: It's the law. *American Journal of Nursing*, 371.

Andrews, M. (2009, March 17). Budgeting for infertility authors sterling, best-boss offer help for couples. *U.S. News & World Report*. Retrieved from http://health.usnews.com/blogs/on-health-and-money/2009/3/17/budgeting-for-infertility-authors-sterling-best-boss-offer-help-for-couples.html

Annas, G. J. (1986, September). Made in the U.S.A.: Legal and ethical issues in artificial heart experimentation. *Law, Medicine and Health Care, 14,* 3–4.

Appleby, J. (2006, November 19). Debate surrounds end-of-life health care costs. *USA Today*. Retrieved from http://www.usatoday.com/money/industries/health/2006-10-18-end-of-life-costs_x.htm

Appleman, J. A. (1976, November/December). Malpractice insurance rates—What's the answer? *Journal of Legal Medicine*, 37.

Bailey, E. (2009, March 20). Umbilical cord blood banking: Smart move or not? *Salemnews*. Retrieved from http://www.salemnews.com/pulife/local_story_079005800.html?keyword=topstory

Barnicle, M. (1995, July 16). Father battles insane system. *The Boston Globe*.

Bass, A. (1995, February 22). Computerized medical data put privacy on the line. *The Boston Globe*, p. 5.

Bass, A. (1995, May 12). Children's mental health coverage often falling short. *The Boston Globe*, p. 1.

Beck, L. C. (1972, April 15). Patient information—when and when not to divulge. *Patient Care, 72,* 60.

Bergerson, S. R. (1984). Charting with a jury in mind. *Nursing, 2*(4), 5.

Besharov, D. J. (1988, Spring). Child abuse and neglect. *Family Law Quarterly, 22*(1), 8.

Bever, L. (2014, November 2). Brittany Maynard, as promised, ends her life at 29. *The Washington Post*. Retrieved from https://www.washingtonpost.com/news/morning-mix/wp/2014/11/02/brittany-maynard-as-promised-ends-her-life-at-29/

Bishop, J. E. (1981, December 16). Physical isn't needed yearly. *The Wall Street Journal*, p. 1.

Bowers, P. (2009, March 2). Final exit: Compassion or assisted suicide? *Time*. Retrieved from http://www.time.com/time/nation/article/0,8599,1882418,00.html

Brant, J. (1971/1972). Medical malpractice insurance: The disease and how to cure it. *Valparaiso University Law Review, 6,* 152, n. 41, 157, n. 31.

Brelis, M. (1995, April 11). Patients' files allegedly used for obscene calls. *The Boston Globe*, p. 1.

Brittain, R. S. (1978). Physician defines role of medical profession in claims prevention. *Lawyers Medical Journal, 7,* 203–205.

Brooke, J. W. (1970). *Willamette Law Review, 6,* 225, 232.

Brown, E. (2007, November). Diagnosis Medicare fraud. *AARP Bulletin Today*. Retrieved from http://bulletin.aarp.org/yourhealth/medicare/articles/outrage_diagnosis.html

California judge dismisses fetal abuse charges. (1987, February 28). Associated Press, San Diego, *The Boston Globe*.

Can I serve you now? (2009, January 29). *The Economist*. Retrieved from http://www.economist.com/science/displaystory.cfm?story_id=13014104

Capeci, J. (1985, March 8). Docs nabbed in abortion scheme. *The Boston Herald*.

Caplan, A. L. (1992, November–December). When evil intrudes. *Hastings Center Report, 29.*

Carroll, A. E. (2015, June 1). To be sued less, doctors should consider talking to patients more. *The New York Times*. Retrieved June 24, 2016, from http://www.nytimes.com/2015/06/02/upshot/to-be-sued-less-doctors-should-talk-to-patients-more.html?_r=1

Case conference: Fain would I change that note. (1978). *Journal of Medical Ethics*, 4, 207–209.

Cepelewicz, B. B. (1996, July). Telemedicine: A virtual reality, but many issues need resolving. *Medical Malpractice Law and Strategy*, 13(9), 2.

Chase, M. (1994, December 5). Can a doctor who's a gatekeeper give enough care? *The New York Times*, p. B1.

Chen, P. (2011, December 15). When the doctor faces a lawsuit. *The New York Times*. Retrieved from http://well.blogs.nytimes.com/2011/12/15/when-the-doctor-gets-sued-2/?_r=0

Colb, S. (2005, February 25). Judge rules frozen embryos are people. *CNN*. Retrieved from http://www.cnn.com/2005/LAW/02/23/colb.embryos/index.html

Cox, T. A risk management approach to computerizing a physician's office. *Forum of Health Law*, American Bar Association.

Crane, M. (2010, June 28). New study finds 91% of physicians practice defensive medicine. *Medscape Medical News*. Retrieved from http://www.medscape.com/viewarticle/724254

Davis, E. (2016). *HMO, PPO, EPO, POS—Which plan is best?* Retrieved from https://www.verywell.com/hmo-ppo-epo-pos-whats-the-difference-1738615

Davis, K. (2007, May–June). Rethinking normal. *Hastings Center Report*, p. 44.

Davis, M. (1996, August 1). An empty feeling. *The Patriot Ledger*, p. 15.

Davis, R. (1995, March 22). Online medical records raise privacy fears. *USA Today*, p. 1A.

Dennis, B. (2015, November 3). Nearly 60 percent of Americans—the highest ever—are taking prescription drugs. *The Washington Post*. Retrieved from https://www.washingtonpost.com/news/to-your-health/wp/2015/11/03/more-americans-than-ever-are-taking-prescription-drugs/

Dentzer, S. et al. (1986, May 5). Can you pass the job test? *Newsweek*, p. 46.

Dicken, B. (2015, February 18). Judge grants early release to 91-year-old mercy killer. *The Chronicle-Telegram*. Retrieved from http://www.chroniclet.com/cops-and-courts/2015/02/18/Judge-grants-early-release-to-91-year-old-mercy-killer.html

Dimick, C. (2010, April 29). Californian sentenced to prison for HIPAA violation. *Journal of AHIMA*. Retrieved from http://journal.ahima.org/2010/04/29/californian-sentenced-to-prison-for-hipaa-violation/

Dixon, J. (1995, July 29). Agency remains firm in refusal of benefits in frozen-sperm birth. *The Patriot Ledger*.

Doctor accused of trying to murder ex-boss. (1995, September 3). *The New York Times*, p. 28.

Doctor tries to sidestep child abuse reporting laws. (1990, January/February). *National District Attorneys Association Bulletin*, 9(1).

Doctors' union pres looking to enlist members. (1987, January 14). *The Patriot Ledger*.

Egan, M. (2016, August 9). A winning idea: How the cloud helps Olympic athletes avoid injury. *GE Reports*. Retrieved from http://www.gereports.com/a-winning-idea-how-the-cloud-helps-olympic-athletes-avoid-injury/

Estabrook, G. (1987, January 26). The revolution in medicine. *Newsweek*, p. 40.

Glasson, J., Plows, C. W., Clarke, O. W., Ruff, V., Fuller, D., & Kliger, C. H. Ethical issues in managed care. (1995, January 25). *Journal of the American Medical Association*, 273(4), 330–335.

Failure to report abuse charge leads to 5-year exclusion. (1991, May). *Civil Money Penalties Reporter, Medicare/Medicaid Fraud & Abuse*, 5(1), 1.

Family leave: A government survey. (1996, March 26). *The Wall Street Journal*, p. 1.

Florida man 75 gets life for mercy killing of ailing wife. (1985, May 10). *The Boston Globe*.

Four at a clinic are accused of Medicaid fraud. (1995, February 8). *The New York Times*, p. B2.

Fox-Brewster, T. (2016, February 23). White hat hackers hit 12 American hospitals to prove patient life "extremely vulnerable". *Forbes*. Retrieved from http://www.forbes.com/sites/thomasbrewster/2016/02/23/hackers-tear-hospitals-apart/#c3881c740d7f

Freudenheim, M. (1991, January 1). Guarding medical confidentiality. *The New York Times*.

Gage, S. M. (1981, Spring). Alteration, falsification and fabrication of medical records in medical malpractice actions. *Medical Trial Quarterly, 27*, 476.

Gaylin, W. (1980, August). XYY controversy: Researching violence and genetics. *The Hastings Center Special Supplement*.

Gaylin, W. (1994, June 12). Faulty diagnosis. *The New York Times*, sec. 4A, p. 1.

Gilbert, S. (1996, August 21). Life-saving medical history. *The New York Times*, p. 1.

Girion, L. (2009, March 10). Autism patients in California are dealt insurance setback. *Los Angeles Times*. Retrieved from http://articles.latimes.com/2009/mar/10/business/fi-autism10

Girl accused of making false AIDS calls. (1995, March 1). *The New York Times*, p. 1.

Glickman, S. W., McHutchison, J. G., Peterson, E. D., Cairns, C. B., Harrington, R. A., Califf, R. M., & Schulman, K. A. (2009, February 19). Ethical and scientific implications of the globalization of clinical research. *New England Journal of Medicine*. Retrieved from http://www.nejm.org/doi/full/10.1056/NEJMsb0803929#t=article

Goldberg, A. S. (2002, January). Healthcare technology and bio science, HIPAA and beyond. *The Health Lawyer, 14*(2). ABA Health Law Section, 1–5.

Gorner, P. (2004, May 5). 5 babies born to save ill siblings, doctors say. *Chicago Tribune*. Retrieved from http://articles.chicagotribune.com/2004-05-05/news/0405050257_1_bone-marrow-transplants-reproductive-genetics-institute-cord-blood

Gorski, E. (2009, March 19). Stem cell decision exposes religious divides. *San Jose Mercury News*. Retrieved from http://www.mercurynews.com/religion/ci_11954582 (accessed March 24, 2009)

Grace, F. (2004, April 29). Utah C-section mom gets probation. *CBS News*. Retrieved from http://www.cbsnews.com/stories/2004/03/12/national/main605537.shtml

Graham, R. (2014, February 16). For pregnant women, two sets of rights in one body. *The Boston Globe*. Retrieved from https://www.bostonglobe.com/ideas/2014/02/16/

for-pregnant-women-two-sets-rights-one-body/5Pd6zntIViRBZ9QxhiQgFJ/story.html

Grant, K. (2015, July 29). Is cord blood banking worth the cost? Here's what the experts say. *The NBC News*. Retrieved from http://www.nbcnews.com/business/consumer/cord-blood-banking-n400561

Greenhouse, L. (1996, June 14). [*Jaffee v. Redmond*, No. 95-266]. Justices uphold psychotherapy privacy rights. *The New York Times*, p. A1.

Greve, P. A. (1990, December). Keep quiet or speak up? Issues in patient confidentiality. *RN,* 53.

Groups spar over outcome of Kentucky medical record law. (1995, January 23/30). *American Medical News*, p. 29.

Groves, A. (2016, April 6). Temecula: Physician charged with additional felonies in amended complaint. *The Press Enterprise*. Retrieved from http://www.pe.com/articles/mcguire-786778-acts-sexual.html

Guarino, B. (2016, May 12). After nearly five decades of marriage, a woman in India finally gave birth. But some ethicists say 70 is too old. *The Washington Post*. Retrieved from https://www.washingtonpost.com/news/morning-mix/wp/2016/05/12/after-a-decades-long-wait-for-a-child-a-woman-in-india-finally-gave-birth-but-doctors-say-shes-too-old/?utm_term=.4d6ce175f2e4

Haralambie, A. M. (1988, Winter). Special problems in custody and abuse cases. *Family Advocate, 10*(3), 15.

Headlines. (1992, August). *American Journal of Nursing, 92*(8), 9.

Health care facility records: Confidentiality, computerization and security. (1995, July). *Forum on Health Law*, 13.

Hearn, W. (1996, October 21). When the president is the patient. *American Medical News*, p. 13.

Herbert, J. (1994, September 11). Profits before patients. *The New York Times*, p. E19.

Hirsch, H. L. (1978, Spring). Tampering with medical records. *Medical Trial Quarterly*, 450.

Holthaus, D. (1989, October). Employer's power to fight drug use. *Trustee*, 20.

Horsley, J. E. (1990, January). Legally speaking: Don't tolerate sexual harassment at work. *RN*, 69.

Hyer, M. (1987, March 12). *Petersburg Times*, p. 21A, col. 1.

Interlandi, J. (2009, January 19). Not just urban legend. *Newsweek*. Retrieved from http://www.newsweek.com/id/178873

Isler, C. (1979, February). Six mistakes that could land you in jail. *RN*, 66–67.

Jacobs, M. A. (1996, June 12). Women seek infertility benefits under disabilities law. *The Wall Street Journal*, p. B7.

Jecker, N. S. (2008, April 11). *Ethics in medicine*. University of Washington School of Medicine. Retrieved from http://depts.washington.edu/bioethx/topics/manag.html

Jones, L. (1995, March 13). HIV tests urged for pregnant women. *AMNEWS*, p. 5.

Jonsen, A. R. (1986, September). Bentham in a box: Technology, assessment and health-care allocation. *Law, Medicine and Health Care,14*(3–4), 174.

Judge rule favors mother. (1995, January 10). *The New York Times*, p. B5.

Kaiser Daily Health Policy Report. (2006, May 8). Retrieved from http://www.kaiserhealthnews.org/Daily-Report.aspx

Kearney, K. A. (1996). Legal liability and risk considerations for a medical call center. *The Health Lawyer, 9*(3), 20.

Kelasa, E. V. (1993, January). HIV vs. a nurse's right to work. *RN*, 63.

Kennedy, R. (1995, September 14). 20 arrested in drug dealing in Brooklyn VA hospital. *The New York Times*, p. B3.

Klein, C. F. (1995, Summer). Full faith and credit interstate enforcement of protection orders under the Violence Against Women Act of 1994. *Family Law Quarterly, 29*(2), 253–272.

Kolata, G. (2014, February 3). Ethics questions arise as genetic testing of embryos increases. *The New York Times*. Retrieved from http://www.nytimes.com/2014/02/04/health/ethics-questions-arise-as-genetic-testing-of-embryos-increases.html?_r=0

Konrad, W. (2009, March 21). Going abroad to find affordable health care. *The New York Times*. Retrieved from http://www.nytimes.com/2009/03/21/health/21patient.html?ref=health

Krupat, E. (1986, November). A delicate imbalance. *Psychology Today*, p. 22.

Kurkjian, S. (1996, May 2). Gloves are coming off. *The Boston Globe*, p. 1.

Kuvin, S. F. (2008, December 1). Our country is failing the AIDS test. *Washington Post*, p. A17.

Lachs, M. S., & Pillemer, K. A. (2015). Elder abuse. *New England Journal of Medicine, 373*, 1947–1956.

Ladd, J. (1982). The concepts of health and disease and their ethical implications. In B. Gruzalski & C. Nelson (Eds.), *Value conflicts in health-care delivery* (p. 23). Cambridge, MA: Ballinger Publishing Company.

Lambert, L. (1996, March 4). Mental health survey criticized. *The Patriot Ledger*, p. 1.

Landers, A. (1982, March 19). The inhumanity of some doctors. *The Boston Globe*, p. 33.

Landers, L. (1978, July). Why some people seek revenge against doctors. *Psychology Today*, p. 94.

Lane, M. B. (2013, April 11). Doctor to serve jail time for not reporting abuse of child. *The Columbus Dispatch*. Retrieved from http://www.dispatch.com/content/stories/local/2013/03/19/doctor-conviction-for-not-reporting-abuse.html

Lee, F. R. (1993, March 6). Difficult custody decisions being complicated by AIDS. *The New York Times*, p. 22.

Legal lines. (1986, August). *Professional Medical Assistant*, p. 16.

Legislator files an assisted-suicide bill. (2009, February 26). *Boston Globe*.

Letters to the editor. (1987, June 6). *The Baltimore Sun*.

Leung, S. (1996, August 10). Father of shooting victim sues owner of clinic site. *The Boston Globe*, p. B8.

Levine, J. (1986, September 29). A ray of hope in the fight against AIDS. *Time*, p. 60.

Levine, R. (1987, April). Waiting is a power game. *Psychology Today*, pp. 24–33.

Lewin, T. (1991, May 31). As elderly population grows, so does the need for doctors. *The New York Times*, pp. 1, A16.

Lewin, T. (1996, January 1). Blood banks starting to harvest umbilical cords. *The New York Times*, p. 12.

Lewin, T. (2007, May 22). A move for birth certificates for stillborn babies. *The New York Times*. Retrieved from http://www.nytimes.com/2007/05/22/us/22stillbirth.html

Loeb, N. (2015, April 29). Sofía Vergara's ex-fiancé: Our frozen embryos have a right to live. *New York Times*. Retrieved from http://www.nytimes.com/2015/04/30/opinion/sofiavergaras-ex-fiance-our-frozen-embryos-have-a-right-to-live.html?_r=0

Lyon, A. (2002, September/October). President's council on bioethics. *The Hastings Center Report, 32*(5).

Lyons, P. J. (2007, September 14). Still more fallout from the Terri Schiavo case. *The New York Times*. Retrieved from http://thelede.blogs.nytimes.com/2007/09/14/still-more-fallout-from-the-terry-schiavo-case/?scp=2&sq=Terry%20Schiavo%20&st=cse

Lytel, J. (2012, October 29). Medical tourism doesn't necessarily mean leaving the country to get treatment. *The Washington Post*. Retrieved from https://www.washingtonpost.com/national/health-science/medical-tourism-doesnt-necessarily-mean-leaving-the-country-to-get-treatment/2012/10/29/8d1bf5ce-d6710-11e1-b2d5-2419d227d8b0_story.html

Mahar, M. (2007, Fall). Making choice an option. *Dartmouth Medicine, 1*, 39.

Marshall, R. (1987, March 30). AIDS: The search for a vaccine. *Newsweek, 79*.

Marwick, C. (1996, January 10). Childhood aggression needs definition, therapy. *Journal of the American Medical Associatio , 275*(2), 90.

McConnell, M. (2014, April 21). Man suspected in armed robbery of Ferndale doctor's office arrested. *The Daily Tribune*. Retrieved from http://www.dailytribune.com/article/DT/20140421/NEWS/140429953

McGinley, L. (1992, April 21). Fitness exams help to measure worker acuity. *The Wall Street Journal*, pp. B1, B9.

McKinley, J. (2008, February 27). Surgeon accused of speeding a death to get organs. *The New York Times*. Retrieved from http://www.nytimes.com/2008/02/27/us/27transplant.html

Médecine avec frontiers: Why health care has failed to globalize. (2014, February 15). *The Economist*. Retrieved from http://www.economist.com/news/international/21596563-why-health-care-has-failed-globalise-m-decine-avec-frontires

Mittleman, M. (1980, February). What are the chances when malignancy leads to a malpractice suit? *Legal Aspects of Medical Practice, 42*.

Mooney, B. C. (1990, September 5). *The Boston Globe*, p. 23.

Mycek, S. (1991, May). Domestic violence goes public. *Trustee, 49*(5), 18.

Naik, G. (2009, February 12). A baby, please. Blond, freckles—Hold the colic. *The Wall Street Journal*. Retrieved from http://online.wsj.com/article/SB123439771603075099.html

Nossiter, A. (1995, March 16). A mistake, a rare prosecution, and a doctor is headed for jail. *The New York Times*, p. A1.

O'Reilly, K. B. (2009, January 19). Redefining death: A new ethical dilemma. *American Medical News*. Retrieved from http://www.amednews.com/article/20090119/profession/301199972/4/

O'Rourke, K. (1986, November 22). Tube feeding—A Catholic view. *America*.

Ornstein, C. (2008, March 15). Hospital to punish snooping on Spears. *The Los Angeles Times*. Retrieved from http://articles.latimes.com/2008/mar/15/local/me-britney15

Ornstein, C. (2015, December 10). Celebrities' medical records tempt hospital workers to snoop. Retrieved July 19, 2016, from NPR website, http://www.npr.org/sections/health-shots/2015/12/10/458939656/celebrities-medical-records-tempt-hospital-workers-to-snoop

Palinecsar, J., & Cobb, D. C. (1982). The physician's role in detecting and reporting elder abuse. *Journal of Legal Medicine, 3*, 413–441.

Pancreatic drug trial halted on promising results. (2009, March 12). *U.S. News and World Report*. Retrieved from http://health.usnews.com/articles/health/healthday/2009/03/12/pancreatic-drug-trial-halted-on-promising-results.html

Pappano, L. (1987, April 30). Tormented by fear of rejection. *The Patriot Ledger*.

Paris, J. H. (1980). Court intervention and the diminution of patients' rights: The case of brother Joseph Fox. *New England Journal of Medicine, 303*, 876.

Parker, B., & Hart, J. (1982, March 14). The wizard of Id. *The Boston Globe*.

Paxton, H. T. (1988, February 1). Today's guidelines for patient confidentiality. *Medical Economics*, 198.

Pear, R. (2016, January 16). New guidelines nudge doctors to give patients access to medical records. *New York Times*. Retrieved from http://www.nytimes.com/2016/01/17/us/new-guidelines-nudge-doctors-on-giving-patients-access-to-medical-records.html

Peratta, Ed. (1996, June 6). Wellesley doctor settles complaint stemming from patient's HIV test. *Wellesley Townsman*, p. 1.

Personal comments in medical records may cause trouble. (1976, January 12). *Medical World News*, p. 125.

Poulos, C. J. (1987, May/June). A case of fraud. *The Professional Medical Assistant, 14*.

Preiser, S. E. (1976, October 4). The high cost of tampering with medical records. *Medical Economics, 85*.

Purtile, R., & Sorrell, J. (1986, August). The ethical dilemmas of a rural physician. *The Hastings Report*, p. 25.

Rakowsky, J. (1995, August 3). Newton psychiatrist found guilty of fraud. *The Boston Globe*, p. 24.

Reese, M. (1985, May 6). A tragedy in Santa Monica. *Newsweek*, p. 10.

Report of the Ad Hoc committee of the harvard medical school to examine the definition of brain death. (1968, August). *Journal of the American Medical Association , 205*, 85.

Retrial begins in murder case tied to confession to an A.A. group. (1994, November 3). *The New York Times METRO*, p. B7.

Ristuben, K. R. (1996, June). Implications of managed care on patient care. *Health Law Section Newsletter*, Massachusetts Bar Association.

Robinson, D. (1989, May 28). Who should receive medical aid? *Parade Magazine*, p. 4.

Rosenthal, E. (1995, November 11). Public advocate says HMO's often mislead poor and elderly. *The New York Times*, p. B4.

Rosenthal, E. (2013, August 6). The growing popularity of having surgery overseas. *New York Times*. Retrieved from http://www.nytimes.com/2013/08/07/us/the-growing-popularity-of-having-surgery-overseas.html?_r=0

Roth, N. (1977). The medical malpractice insurance crisis. *Insurance Counsel Journal, 41*, 469–473.

Rovner, J. (1996). Analysis of the provisions of the health insurance portability and accountability act of 1996. *The Health Lawyer, 9*(3), 1.

Rubin, P. N., & Dunne, T. (1995, February). The ADA: Emergency response systems and TDD's, pp. 1–7. National Institute of Justice: Research in Action.

Ryan, J. Dispelling common myths about documentation: Advice from a defense attorney. *Forum of Health Law*, American Bar Association.

Sack, K. (2009, March 24). Her embryos or his? *Los Angeles Times*. Retrieved from http://articles.latimes.com/2007/may/30/nation/na-embryo30

Safeguarding the privacy of computer records. (1996, November 22). [*Knoxville News-Sentinel*]. *The Patriot Ledger*, p. 13.

Salcido, R. (1996, Mid-Winter). Application of the false claims act "knowledge" standard: What one must "know" to be held liable under the act. *The ABA Forum on Health Law, 8*(6), 1, 6.

Sanghavi, D. (2013, January 27). Medical malpractice: Why is it so hard for doctors to apologize? *The Boston Globe*. Retrieved from https://www.bostonglobe.com/magazine/2013/01/27/medical-malpractice-why-hard-for-doctors-apologize/c65KIUZraXekMZ8SHlMsQM/story.html

Santora, M. (2004, April 2). In Albany appeals court ruling, mother and fetus are one. *The New York Times*. Retrieved from http://www.nytimes.com/2004/04/02/nyregion/02baby.html?ei=5007&en=3f757abd39904d42&ex=1396328400&partner=USERLAND&pagewanted=print&position=

Schulz, E. E. (1995, June 29). Fudging medical claims can backfire. *The Wall Street Journal*, p. C1.

Smith, S. (2009, March 20). 'Young invincibles' OK with risk of no insurance. *CNN*. Retrieved fromhttp://www.cnn.com/2009/HEALTH/03/20/catastrophic.insurance.invincibles/

Smith, T. (2009, March 18). Fired worker wants justice. *Idaho Mountain Express*. Retrieved from http://www.mtexpress.com/index2.php?ID=2005125263

Snapp, J., & Meyer, B. (2006, October 24). Sarah: Autonomy and medical paternalism. Retrieved from Hospice Foundation Web site http://www.hospicefoundation.org

Snarey, J. (1987, June). A question of morality. *Psychology Today*, p. 6.

Sosa, N., Franken, B., Phillips, R., & Candiotti, S. (2005, March 31). Terri Schiavo has died. *CNN*. Retrieved from http://www.cnn.com/2005/LAW/03/31/schiavo/index.html?iref=newssearch

Spears, V. H. (2009, March 22). Gap in Ky. law leads to errors at bedside of dying patients. *Lexington Herald-Reader*. Retrieved from http://www.kentucky.com/181/story/734281.html

Stevens, W. K. (1982, March 28). High medical costs. *The New York Times*, pp. 1, 50.

Studdert, D. M., Mello, M. M., Sage W. M., DesRoches, C. M., & Peugh, J. (2005). Defensive medicine among high-risk specialist physicians in a volatile malpractice environment. *Journal of the American Medical Association, 293*, 2609–2617.

Sullivan, R. (1984, March 24). Queens hospital accused of denial of care. *The New York Times*, p. 17.

Tammelleo, A. D. (1990, October). Who's to blame for faulty equipment? *RN*, 67.

The Baltimore Sun. (1987, June 6).

The Boston Globe. (1985, October 31).

The Lakeberg Siamese twins: Were risks, costs of separation justified? (1992). *Medical Ethics Advisor, 9*(10), 121.

The Patriot Ledger, p. 26. (1988, March 30).

The Wall Street Journal, p. 1. (1982, July).

The Wall Street Journal, p. 1. (1990, February 13).

Therapist punished for Simpson revelations. (1995, November 24). *The Boston Globe*, p. 19.

Thobaben, M., & Anderson, L. (1985). Reporting elder abuse: It's the law. *American Journal of Nursing, 85*(4), 371–374.

Todd, J., Armon, C., Griggs, A., Poole, S., & Berman, S. (2006, August 1). Increased rates of morbidity, mortality, and charges for hospitalized children with public or no health insurance as compared with children with private insurance in Colorado and the United States. *Pediatrics, 118*(2). Retrieved from http://pediatrics.aappublications.org/cgi/content/full/118/2/577

U.S. Tort law's victims. (1985, April 2). *The Wall Street Journal*.

U.S. warns doctors, labs about kickbacks. (1994, October 14). *The Patriot Ledger*, p. 3.

Updike, N. (2014, March 25). Death and taxes. *This American Life*. Podcast retrieved from http://www.thisamericanlife.org/radio-archives/episode/523/transcript

Valente, R. L. (1985, Summer). Addressing domestic violence: The role of the family law practitioner. *Family Law Quarterly, 29*(1), 187–196.

When dad's a sperm donor. (1993, January 15–17). *USA Weekend*.

Wilson, P. T. (1975). Anesthesiology and malpractice lawsuits. *Medical Trial Technical Quarterly, 76*, 68–76, at 73.

Winslow, R. (1995, April 26). Drug-industry sales pitches to doctors are inaccurate 11% of the time, study says. *The Wall Street Journal*, p. B6.

Winton, R. (2016, February 18). Hollywood hospital pays $17,000 in bitcoin to hackers; FBI investigating. *LA Times*. Retrieved from http://www.latimes.com/business/technology/la-me-ln-hollywood-hospital-bitcoin-20160217-story.html

Wisenberg, B. (2006, October 24). PBM Medco Health Solutions agrees to settle Medicare fraud, kickback allegations for $155 million. *Dow Jones*. Retrieved from http://www.news-medical.net/?id=20754

Woman leaves hospital, finds out she died. (2016, June 11). Retrieved from http://www.nbcwashington.com/news/local/Woman-Leaves-Hospital-Finds-Out-She-Died-382568031.html

Books

American College of Legal Medicine. (1988). *Legal medicine: Legal dynamics of medical encounter*. St. Louis, MO: CV Mosby.

Belli, M. M. (1986). *Belli for your malpractice defense* (1st ed.). Oradell, NJ: Medical Economics Company.

Koop, C. E. (1976). *The right to live: The right to die*. Wheaton, IL: Tyndale House Publishers.

Ladd, J. (1982). *Value conflicts in health care delivery*. Cambridge, MA: Gruzalski Ballinger Publishing Co.

Landers, L. (1978). *Defective medicine*. New York: Farrar, Straus, and Giroux.

Nozick, R. (1974). *Anarchy, state and Utopia*. New York: Basic Books.

Pfeiffer, J. W. (1974). *Nonverbal communications: A collection of structured experiences for human relations training* (Vol. 2). La Jolla, CA: University Association.

Provost, G. (1985). *Fatal dosage*. New York: Bantam Books.

Scott, R. (1981). *The body as property*. New York: The Viking Press.

Hamilton, A. *The Papers of Alexander Hamilton*, Report on Public Credit, Edited by Harold C. Syrett et al. 26 vols. New York and London: Columbia University Press, 1961-79.

Miscellaneous

American Association of Medical Assistants. (n.d.). *Medical Assisting Code of Ethics*. Retrieved from http://www.aama-ntl.org/about/overview#.V5O4BriAOko

American Association of Medical Assistants. (n.d.). *Medical Assisting Creed*. Retrieved from http://www.aama-ntl.org/about/overview#.V5O4BriAOko

American Medical Association, Code of Ethics: Opinions on Patient-Physician Relationships, June 2016.

American Medical Association. (2016, June). *Opinions on privacy, confidentiality, and medical records, 3.3.1. Management of Medical Records*.

American Medical Association. (n.d.). *Frequently asked questions about HIPAA*. Retrieved from http://www.ama-assn.org/ama/pub/physician-resources/solutions-managing-your-practice/coding-billing-insurance/hipaahealth-insurance-portability-accountability-act/frequently-asked-questions.page

American Medical Technologists. (2013, October 1). *Standards of practice*. Retrieved from http://www.americanmedtech.org/Portals/0/PDF/Stay%20Cert/2013%20standards%20of%20practice.pdf

American Telemedicine Association. (n.d.). *Telemedicine frequently asked questions (FAQs)*. Retrieved from http://www.americantelemed.org/main/about/telehealth-faqs-

Bonnie, R. J., & Wallace, R. B. (Eds.) (2003). *Elder mistreatment: Abuse, neglect and exploitation in an aging America*. Washington, DC: National Research Council Panel to Review Risk and Prevalence of Elder Abuse and Neglect.

Bureau of Labor Statistics, U.S. Department of Labor. (2015). *Occupational outlook handbook, 2016–17 edition; Medical assistants*. Retrieved from http://www.bls.gov/ooh/healthcare/medical-assistants.htm

Centers for Disease Control and Prevention. (n.d.). *Meaningful uses*. Retrieved from http://www.cdc.gov/ehrmeaningfuluse/introduction.html

Centers for Disease Control and Prevention. (n.d.). *The Tuskegee timeline*. Retrieved from http://www.cdc.gov/tuskegee/timeline.htm

Child Abuse and Neglect Program, MCLE/NELI. (1984, October 25). Boston College, Massachusetts Continuing Legal Education, Inc.

Child Welfare Information Gateway. (2008, April). *General information packet*. Retrieved from http://www.childwelfare.gov/

Children's Bureau (Administration on Children, Youth and Families, Administration for Children and Families) of the U.S. Department of Health and Human Services. (2014). *Child Maltreatment 2014*.

Department of Health and Human Services. (n.d.). *Individuals' right under HIPAA to access their health information 45 CFR § 164.524*. U.S. Retrieved from http://www.hhs.gov/hipaa/for-professionals/privacy/guidance/access/index.html

Excerpt from the decision at 331 F.2d 100 (D.C. Cir.), cert. denied, 377 U.S. 978 (1964). Reprinted as it appears in J. Katz (Ed.). (1972). *Experimentation with human beings* (pp. 551–552). New York: Russell Sage Foundation.

Federal Register. (2000, December 28). *65*(250), p. 82465. Retrieved from https://www.gpo.gov/fdsys/pkg/FR-2000-12-28/pdf/00-32678.pdf

Gillespie, K. (1997). *Perspectives: Malpractice law evolves under managed care*. Princeton, NJ: The Robert Wood Johnson Foundation.

Gold, J. (2011, January 18). *Accountable care organizations, explained*. Retrieved from http://www.npr.org/2011/04/01/132937232/accountable-care-organizations-explained

Issue: Facsimile transmission of health information. (1994, May). American Health Information Management Association (AHIMA) Position Statement.

Marken, S. (2016). *U.S. uninsured rate at 11.0%, lowest in eight-year trend*. Retrieved from http://www.gallup.com/poll/190484/uninsured-rate-lowest-eight-year-trend.aspx

Medicare Part B Intermediary Letter No. 84-9: Payments to Respiratory Therapists by Durable Medical Equipment Suppliers and the Illegal Remuneration Provisions of the Social Security Act. (September 1984).

National Center for Child Abuse and Neglect Specialized Training.

National Coalition Against Domestic Violence. (2015). *Domestic violence national statistics fact sheet*. Retrieved from http://ncadv.org/files/National%20Statistics%20Domestic%20Violence%20NCADV.pdf

National Council on Aging. (n.d.). *Elder abuse facts*. Retrieved from https://www.ncoa.org/public-policy-action/elder-justice/elder-abuse-facts/

Office of the Attorney General, Eastern District of New York. (2015, November 4). *Riverhead physician assistant arrested for conspiracy to illegally prescribe oxycodone, United States Department of Justice*. Retrieved from https://www.justice.gov/usao-edny/pr/riverhead-physician-assistant-arrested-conspiracy-illegally-prescribe-oxycodone

President's Commission. (1983). *Deciding to forego life-sustaining treatment*, p. 127. Washington, DC: Government Printing Office.

Public Law 104–191, Health Insurance Portability and Accountability Act of 1996.

Sexual Harassment Survey, Massachusetts Department of Education, 1385 Hancock Street, Quincy, MA 02169.

The United States Department of Justice, Office of the Attorney General. (2015, June 18). Press Release.

The United States Department of Justice. (n.d.). *What is Domestic Violence?* Retrieved from https://www.justice.gov/ovw/domestic-violence

Trials of war criminals before the Nuremberg military tribunals under control council law (No. 10, Vol. 11). (October 1946–April 1949). Nuremberg.

United States Holocaust Memorial. (n.d.). *United States Holocaust Memorial Museum Note: Nuremberg Code*. Retrieved from https://www.ushmm.org/information/exhibitions/online-exhibitions/special-focus/doctors-trial/nuremberg-code

Index

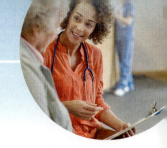